ANNUAL REVIEW OF NURSING RESEARCH

VOLUME 35, 2017

SERIES EDITOR

Christine E. Kasper, PhD, RN, FAAN, FACSM
Department of Veterans Affairs
Office of Nursing Services, Washington, DC
and
Professor, Daniel K. Inouye School of Nursing
Uniformed Services University of the Health Sciences,
Bethesda, MD

VOLUME EDITORS

Charles A. Vacchiano, PhD, CRNA, FAAN
Professor, School of Nursing
Duke University

Kenneth A. Wofford, PhD, CRNA, CDR, NC, USN
Assistant Professor
Daniel K. Inouye Graduate School of Nursing
Uniformed Services University of the Health Sciences

Annual Review of Nursing Research

Anesthesia and Pain Management

VOLUME 35, 2017

Series Editor

CHRISTINE E. KASPER, PhD, RN, FAAN, FACSM

Volume Editors

CHARLES A. VACCHIANO, PhD, CRNA, FAAN
KENNETH A. WOFFORD, PhD, CRNA, CDR, NC, USN

SPRINGER PUBLISHING COMPANY
NEW YORK

Springer Publishing Company, LLC
11 West 42nd Street
New York, NY 10036
www.springerpub.com

Acquisitions Editor: Joseph Morita
Composition: Exeter Premedia Services Private Ltd

ISBN: 978-0-8261-4284-9
e-book ISBN: 978-0-8261-4285-6
ISSN: 0739-6686
Online ISSN: 1944-4028

17 18 19 / 5 4 3 2 1

The author and the publisher of this Work have made every effort to use sources believed to be reliable to provide information that is accurate and compatible with the standards generally accepted at the time of publication. Because medical science is continually advancing, our knowledge base continues to expand. Therefore, as new information becomes available, changes in procedures become necessary. We recommend that the reader always consult current research and specific institutional policies before performing any clinical procedure. The author and publisher shall not be liable for any special, consequential, or exemplary damages resulting, in whole or in part, from the readers' use of, or reliance on, the information contained in this book. The publisher has no responsibility for the persistence or accuracy of URLs for external or third-party Internet websites referred to in this publication and does not guarantee that any content on such websites is, or will remain, accurate or appropriate.

Contents

Controversies in Clinical Care

Progress and Problems in Anesthesia Pharmacology

About the Volume Editors

Charles A. Vacchiano, PhD, CRNA, FAAN, earned a BSN at Wright State University in 1979, a Bachelor of Science in Anesthesia from George Washington University in 1984, and a PhD in Physiology from the Medical University of South Carolina in 1995. He spent 26 years in the U.S. Navy as a practicing nurse anesthetist, educator, and researcher. During this time, he provided anesthesia care at stateside and overseas hospitals and aboard naval combat vessels, taught and performed clinical research in the Navy Nurse Corps Anesthesia Program, and was the Director of the Biomedical Sciences Division at the Naval Aerospace Medical Research Laboratory.

Following his retirement from the U.S. Navy, Dr. Vacchiano became director of the Gooding Institute, Bay Medical Center Nurse Anesthesia Program. He has published in multiple journals (including *American Journal of Physiology*, *Cardiovascular Research*, *Shock*, and the *American Association of Nurse Anesthetists Journal*) and serves as a reviewer for several agencies and journals. Dr. Vacchiano is the author of a chapter on regional anesthesia in the only anesthesia textbook written by nurse anesthetists. He was named the American Association of Nurse Anesthetist Researcher of the Year in 2007. He served as the president of the board of directors for the National Board of Certification and Recertification for Nurse Anesthetists (NBCRNA) in 2012 and 2013. He was selected as a fellow of the American Academy of Nursing in 2014.

Dr. Vacchiano joined the faculty at the Duke University School of Nursing in 2008 where he teaches in the nurse anesthesia program and is involved in various research projects and related activities. Dr. Vacchiano's research has been funded by several government and private agencies. His research interests include extremes of oxygen exposure in cell, animal, and human models, and clinical studies in anesthesia and critical care.

Kenneth A. Wofford, PhD, CRNA, CDR, NC, USN, enlisted in the Navy in 1992 as a Hospital Corpsman and has since served in diverse locations including California, South Carolina, Guam, Okinawa, Korea, Florida, Iraq, and Maryland. He received his Bachelor of Science from Jacksonville University in 1997, his Master of Science from Georgetown University in 2004, and his Doctor of

Philosophy from Duke University in 2012. He is currently an Assistant Professor in the Daniel K. Inouye Graduate School of Nursing at the Uniformed Services University of the Health Sciences in Bethesda, Maryland, where he teaches evidence-based practice and statistics. In addition to teaching, CDR Wofford practices clinically at Walter Reed National Military Medical Center, peer-reviews for several national journals, and serves as chair of the Airway Management Recognition Panel of the NBCRNA Continuous Professional Certification Program.

CDR Wofford's first research study examined the effect of varying spinal needle orientation during injection on block characteristics. His dissertation work investigated the impact of surgery and anesthesia on the mental and physical well-being of Veterans with chronic posttraumatic disorder. His current research interests include the impact of surgery and anesthesia on mental health, training for low incidence/high mortality event management, and trauma resuscitation in the austere setting. He resides in Bethesda, Maryland with his wife and two children.

Contributors

Edwin N. Aroke, PhD, CRNA
Staff CRNA
University of Massachusetts Medical Center
Millbury, MA

Paul N. Austin, PhD, CRNA
Professor
Texas Wesleyan University
Graduate Programs of Nurse Anesthesia
Fort Worth, TX

Chuck Biddle, PhD, CRNA
Professor and Director of Research
Department of Nurse Anesthesia
Virginia Commonwealth University
Richmond, VA

Thomas Corey Davis, PhD, CRNA
Assistant Professor
Vice Chair of Clinical Affairs
Virginia Commonwealth University
School of Allied Health Professions
Department of Nurse Anesthesia
Richmond, VA

Matthew D'Angelo, DNP, CRNA
Associate Professor
Daniel K. Inouye Graduate School of Nursing
Uniformed Services University of the Health Sciences
Bethesda, MD

Jennifer Dungan, PhD, RN
Assistant Professor of Nursing
Duke University School of Nursing
Durham, NC

Ladan Eshkevari, PhD, CRNA, LAc
Associate Professor
Department of Nursing
Department of Pharmacology & Physiology
Georgetown University
Washington, DC

Amanda C. Faircloth, PhD, DNAP, CRNA
Staff CRNA
Department of Anesthesiology
Adjunct Faculty
Department of Nurse Anesthesia
Virginia Commonwealth University Medical Center
Richmond, VA

Vincent Ford, BSN, MEd
Student Registered Nurse Anesthetist
Department of Nurse Anesthesia
Virginia Commonwealth University
Richmond, VA

Jennifer Greenwood, PhD, CRNA
Associate Professor
Department of Nurse Anesthesia
Rosalind Franklin University of Medicine and Science
Northern Chicago, IL

R. Kyle Hodgen, DNP, CRNA, Maj., NC, USAF
Assistant Professor
Daniel K. Inouye Graduate School of Nursing
Uniformed Services University of the Health Sciences
Bethesda, MD

Rex A. Marley, MS, CRNA, RRT
Staff Nurse Anesthetist
Northern Colorado Anesthesia Professional Consultants
Fort Collins, CO

Brett Morgan, DNP, CRNA
Assistant Professor of Nursing
Assistant Director, Nurse Anesthesia Program
Duke University School of Nursing
Durham, NC

Lisa Osborne-Smith, PhD, CRNA, CAPT, NC, USN
Associate Professor
Daniel K. Inouye Graduate School of Nursing
Uniformed Services University of the Health Sciences
Bethesda, MD

Joseph E. Pellegrini, PhD, CRNA
Associate Professor
Director
Nurse Anesthetist Program
University of Maryland
Baltimore, MD

Kaycee Simon, MS, CRNA
Staff Nurse Anesthetist
Norther Colorado Anesthesia Professional Consultants
Fort Collins, Colorado

Kenneth A. Wofford, PhD, CRNA, CDR, NC, USN
Assistant Professor
Daniel K. Inouye Graduate School of Nursing
Uniformed Services University of the Health Sciences
Bethesda, MD

Steven R. Wooden, DNP, CRNA, NSPM-C
President
Wooden Anesthesia PC
East-Central, NE

Foreword

The historical dawn of nurse anesthesia emerged on the battlefields of the United States Civil War when early forms of anesthesia were delivered by nurses to the wounded. While not often recognized, nurses were the first professional group to administer anesthesia and emerged as the first clinical nursing specialty. Shortly thereafter in the period 1899–1906, the first anesthesia research papers were published by Alice Magaw of St. Mary's Hospital, now Mayo Clinic, on the safe delivery of anesthesia. It should be noted that the discipline of anesthesia was originally a nursing specialty, which was then taught by the nurse anesthetists to other allied health professions. It is unfortunate that this historical fact is often deliberately forgotten by other health-care disciplines.

It is upon this long history of nursing led research and innovative clinical practice that we feature the scientific descendants of the original nurse researchers in anesthesia. The research topics for the chapters were carefully chosen and compiled into this review of nursing research by Drs. Charles A. Vacchiano, PhD, CRNA, FAAN, professor of nursing at Duke University, and Kenneth A. Wofford, PhD, CRNA, CDR, NC, USN, assistant professor, Uniformed Services University of the Health Sciences. Daniel K. Inouye Graduate School of Nursing, who have served with distinction as the volume editors. They have both excelled as leaders in the study of anesthesia in human and animal models. As series editor, it is my hope that these topically based chapters will be used not only by those conducting research studies, but also by undergraduate and graduate students as texts and supplements to nursing curricula.

This volume is comprised of 13 chapters divided into five sections on: Airway and Ventilation, Information Exchange, Pain and Palliative Care, Controversies in Clinical Care, and Progress and Problems in Anesthesia Pharmacology. Beginning with the first section, Kenneth A. Wofford reviews anesthesia in patients who cannot be intubated in Chapter 1. In Chapter 2, Jennifer Greenwood reviews the research of anesthesia in obesity and obstructive sleep apnea. Rex A. Marley and Kaycee Simon discuss lung-protective ventilation in Chapter 3. In the second section, Lisa Osborne-Smith and R. Kyle Hodgen review the important studies of communication in operating room settings in Chapter 4. The issue continues with an in-depth review by Thomas Corey Davis on anesthesia information management systems in Chapter 5. The third section focuses on the important areas of pain and palliative care. In Chapter 6, Steven R. Wooden reviews the use of anesthesia in controlling chronic post-surgical pain. In Chapter 7, Ladan Eshkevari reviews research in the use of acupuncture and pain management. In Chapter 8, Amanda C. Faircloth reviews the anesthesia involvement in palliative care. The fourth section reviews the current controversies in clinical care. In Chapter 9, Joseph E. Pellegrini investigates research into the delivery of anesthesia in the causation of hypotension during cesarean section in obstetrics. Chapter 10 by Paul N. Austin reviews the use of forced-air warmers and surgical site infection. The final section addresses progress and problems in anesthesia pharmacology. Chapter 11 by Chuck Biddle and Vincent Ford discusses the neurotoxicity of anesthesia in the developing and aged brain. In Chapter 12, Matthew D'Angelo and R. Kyle Hodgen review fluid therapy in anesthesia. Finally, in Chapter 13, Brett Morgan, Edwin N. Aroke, and Jennifer Dungan review the literature on the pharmacogenomics of anesthetic agents.

The science involved in the care of patients and the alleviation of pain through anesthesia is one of the foundations of clinical patient care. We are fortunate that this field of nursing science is populated by a large number of highly trained certified registered nurse anesthetists who are also researchers. It is a field that truly accomplishes one of nursing's fundamental objectives, that of the alleviation of human suffering and the restoration of quality of life.

Christine E. Kasper, PhD, RN, FAAN, FACSM
Series Editor

Preface

So God empal'd our Grandsire's (Adam) lively look,
Through all his bones a deadly chilness strook,
Siel'd-up his sparkling eyes with iron bands,
Led down his feet (almost) to Lethe's Sands';
In briefe, so numm'd his Soule's and Bodie's Sense,
That (without pain) opening his side, from thence
He took a rib, which rarely He refined,
And thereof made the Mother of Mankind.
—Guillaume de Salluste Du Bartas, 16th century poet.

While the era of "modern" anesthesia practice is often associated with the introduction of the muscle relaxant curare into clinical practice in 1942, Du Bartas suggested that God was the first practitioner of anesthesia having painlessly removed a rib from Adam to create Eve. In 1983 Dr. Richard Knapp, an anesthesiologist, authored a short treatise on the history of modern anesthesia titled "The Gift of Surgery to Mankind" in which he noted his amazement at the speed of change within the specialty during his 20 years of practice. It is with equal wonder that the editors of the current volume have observed and experienced the advances in the science of anesthesia practice in the years since 1983. Few of the drugs considered mainstays of clinical practice in that year are in use today and the techniques and technology available to deliver and monitor anesthesia care have expanded and improved exponentially in the intervening years. These advances have been driven by a persistent search for best practices based on a foundation of evidence-based care. Best practice by definition bridges the gap between research and practice and affords a basis for translation of research into clinical care. It is this interest in translation of research to practice that spawned this edition of the *Annual Review of Nursing Research*, the first of this series to address anesthesia care. Our goal was to identify current topics in anesthesia care that generate discussion and disagreement with respect to the available research and evidence and therefore application of best practices. This was not a difficult task as most anesthesia providers who routinely provide direct patient care are aware of these topics and the controversies associated with them. What these providers often lack is access to the accumulated literature on these topics and/ or the time to digest the arguments and determine how the evidence informs their practice.

This edition of the *Annual Review of Nursing Research* bridges that gap for all those involved or interested in clinical anesthesia care including nurse anesthetists, physician anesthesiologists, anesthesia assistants, and postanesthesia care unit nurses. The volume is unique among publications in the field in that it contains a collection of contemporary anesthesia issues for which there is a body of literature that occasionally provides sound evidence for practice change, but more often generates more questions than answers and suggests the need for additional research before a practice change can be recommended. The need for additional research is no more apparent than in the chapters discussing the current body of work related to lung-protective ventilation, communication in the operating room environment, the use of acupuncture for chronic pain management, treatment for spinal anesthesia induced hypotension in the cesarean section patient, surgical site infections associated with the use of forced-air warmers, the potential neurotoxicity of general anesthetics, the administration of intraoperative intravenous fluids, and the role of pharmacogenomics in anesthesia. Other chapters, including preparation for managing a cannot intubate or ventilate situation, implications of obesity compounded by obstructive sleep apnea, the source and treatment of chronic postsurgical pain, the adoption of anesthesia information systems, and anesthesia involvement in palliative care, review the extant literature and offer more definitive recommendations for practice. Each author was specifically selected for their interest, expertise, and knowledge of the chapter topic but just as importantly for their direct exposure to the issue within their personal clinical experience. The material will provide the busy clinician with the most up-to-date information and recommendations on topics germane to everyday practice.

Charles A. Vacchiano, PhD, CRNA, FAAN
Volume Editor

CHAPTER 1

Preparing Anesthetists to Manage Cannot Intubate/Cannot Ventilate Situations

Kenneth A. Wofford

ABSTRACT

Cannot intubate/cannot ventilate (CICV) situations during anesthesia are rare, potentially catastrophic to the patient, and difficult to predict. Widely adopted practice guidelines advocate an algorithmic approach to CICV situations in which the anesthetist: (a) recognizes the CICV situation, (b) calls for help, (c) steadily progresses through a variety of methods to ventilate the patient and secure the airway, (d) restores ventilation via an infraglottic airway if the patient cannot be safely awakened prior to becoming moribund. Despite widespread consensus that rapid progression to placement of an infraglottic airway is critical to the survival of the patient in a CICV situation, the rarity of CICV is a substantial barrier for anesthetists attempting to gain and maintain skill at placing infraglottic airways.

Peer-reviewed literature reveals a number of themes relevant to training anesthetists in infraglottic airway placement. Specific training in infraglottic airway access consistently decreased the time required for anesthetists to decide to place an infraglottic airway. No one approach or method for placing an infraglottic airway was consistently faster or more successful. Model fidelity (i.e., the use of low-fidelity task trainers vs. high-fidelity simulated patients) during teaching

http://dx.doi.org/10.1891/0739-6686.35.1

did not affect the performance of anesthetists at placing infraglottic airways, and performance rapidly plateaued after five repetitions during teaching. Finally, skill at placing an infraglottic airway was sustained for 6 to 12 months after training.

These findings have implications for how nurse anesthetists should learn and sustain the skill of infraglottic airway placement. Nurse anesthetists should undergo initial training that requires the repetitive placement of infraglottic airways, and receive sustainment training every 6 to 12 months thereafter. Although rarely used, the skill of an anesthetist in infraglottic airway placement can mean the difference between life and death for the patient in a CICV situation.

INTRODUCTION

Unanticipated difficult intubation and mask ventilation are rare, potentially catastrophic to the patient, and difficult to predict. The incidence of co-occurring difficult intubation and mask ventilation in adult patients undergoing general endotracheal anesthesia has been reported as 2.3 per 10,000 (Norskov et al., 2015). The incidence of cannot intubate/cannot ventilate (CICV), defined as the absolute inability to intubate or ventilate by any means, has been reported as 0.3 per 10,000 (Tachibana, Niiyama, & Yamakage, 2015). Furthermore, a survey of members of the Canadian Anesthesiologists' Society indicated that only 56.8% of respondents had encountered a CICV situation during their careers (Wong, Lai, Chung, & Ho, 2005). Thus, an anesthetist may complete his or her entire career without encountering a CICV situation.

Although rare, CICV situations are overrepresented as causes of patient morbidity and mortality. Difficult intubation and/or inadequate ventilation constitutes 56% of respiratory events and 9% of all damaging events reported between 1990 and 2007 in the American Society of Anesthesiologists (ASA) Closed Claims Database (Metzner, Posner, Lam, & Domino, 2011). Taken together, claims for injury associated with difficult ventilation and/or intubation are three times more common than injuries associated with the two next most common sources, aspiration (3%) and central venous catheters (3%); see Metzner et al. (2011). When a difficult airway event is reported in the Closed Claims Database the results are likely to be catastrophic, as death or permanent brain damage is cited as the outcome of 58% of injuries associated with difficult airway management between 1985 and 1999 (Peterson et al., 2005). Findings from the United Kingdom (UK) indicate that 10.5% of major airway complications leading to death, brain damage, emergency surgical airway placement, unanticipated admission to the intensive care unit (ICU), or prolonged ICU stay are associated with CICV situations (Cook, Woodall, Frerk, & Fourth National Audit Project, 2011).

PREDICTION OF DIFFICULT VENTILATION, INTUBATION, AND CICV

In an effort to prevent patient harm due to CICV, expert panels have published consensus statements recommending a comprehensive airway examination. For example, the Task Force on Management of the Difficult Airway recommends assessment of the patient for 14 historical factors and 11 physical characteristics reported to be associated with difficult ventilation and/or intubation, while acknowledging that the list is not exhaustive (Apfelbaum et al., 2013). Although less specific, the UK-based Difficult Airway Society also recommends comprehensive airway assessment to identify factors associated with difficult ventilation and/or difficult ventilation (Frerk et al., 2015). The objective of this recommended targeted assessment is to identify patients at risk of difficult ventilation and/or difficult intubation so that they may be managed in such a way as to minimize the need for mask ventilation and/or placement of an endotracheal tube after the induction of anesthesia.

However, assessment of the patient's history and airway is an imperfect predictor of difficult ventilation and/or intubation. Given the rarity of unanticipated difficult intubation, difficult ventilation, or CICV situations, most clinical trials are insufficiently powered to detect the sensitivity and specificity of specific assessment techniques. Two recently published studies, one Danish and one Japanese, leverage national-level data collection to estimate the accuracy of current preanesthetic assessment practices in identifying patients at risk for experiencing unanticipated difficult intubation, difficult ventilation, or CICV (Norskov et al., 2015; Tachibana et al., 2015). In a sample of 182,050 patients in whom endotracheal tube placement was attempted, Norskov et al. (2015) reported a difficult intubation rate of 1.86%, 93% of whom were not predicted to be difficult to intubate prior to induction. In a sample of 129,962 patients in whom mask ventilation was attempted, Norskov et al. (2015) reported a difficult mask ventilation rate of 0.66%, 94% of whom were not predicted to be difficult to mask ventilate prior to induction. Of the 129,962 patients in whom mask ventilation was attempted 0.33% were also difficult to intubate, 89.4% of whom were predicted to be neither difficult to mask ventilate nor ventilate. Thus in Denmark between 2008 and 2011, between 89.4% and 94% of cases of difficult mask ventilation, difficult intubation, or combined difficult mask ventilation/intubation were not predicted to be difficult prior to induction of general anesthesia (Norskov et al., 2015). Particular strengths of this study are its large size, heterogeneous sample, and clear method of excluding patients managed with advanced airway techniques, such as fiber optic laryngoscopy or awake tracheotomy, designed to avoid provoking a CICV situation (Norskov et al., 2015).

In contrast, CICV (i.e., the complete inability to mask ventilate or secure the airway by nonsurgical means) appears to be more rare and more readily recognized during preoperative assessment: In a survey of 20 Japanese hospitals reporting 97,895 cases of airway management under general anesthesia, Tachibana et al. (2015) identified three cases of CICV between 2010 and 2012, only one of which was not predicted to be difficult to mask ventilate or intubate prior to the induction of anesthesia. Thus, even with conscientious assessment some proportion of patients who are difficult to mask ventilate and/or intubate will not be recognized as such until after induction.

MANAGEMENT OF UNANTICIPATED DIFFICULT VENTILATION, INTUBATION, AND CICV

In an effort to decrease the risk of patient injury or death due to unanticipated difficult ventilation or intubation, guidelines have been developed and promoted for application across the discipline of anesthesia for managing these situations. The ASA Practice Guideline for Management of the Difficult Airway (aka, the ASA Difficult Airway Algorithm [ASA-DAA]) was first published in 1993 and updated in 2003 and 2013 (American Society of Anesthesiologists Task Force on Management of the Difficult Airway, 1993, 2003; Apfelbaum et al., 2013), and the Difficult Airway Society (DAS) guidelines for management of unanticipated difficult intubation in adults were first published in 2004 (Henderson, Popat, Latto, Pearce, & Society, 2004) and updated in 2015 (Frerk et al., 2015). Differences exist in the scope of the two sets of guidelines, as the ASA guideline addresses both anticipated and unanticipated difficult ventilation and intubation (Enterlein, Byhahn, & American Society of Anesthesiologists Task Force, 2013), while the DAS guideline addresses only unanticipated difficult ventilation and intubation (Frerk et al., 2015).

However, practice guidelines from both groups advocate an algorithmic approach in which the anesthetist: (a) recognizes the situation as a potentially difficult ventilation or intubation, (b) calls for help, (c) steadily progresses through a variety of methods to ventilate the patient and secure the airway without repeating techniques previously demonstrated to be ineffective, (d) limits the number of laryngoscopy attempts in favor of restoring ventilation by mask, supraglottic airway (SGA) device placement, or awakening the patient, and (e) restores ventilation via an infraglottic technique (e.g., percutaneous cricothyrotomy, surgical cricothyrotomy, or tracheostomy) if the patient cannot be safely awakened prior to becoming moribund (Apfelbaum et al., 2013; Frerk et al., 2015). This recommendation for infraglottic airway access as the terminal and definitive method of restoring ventilation in the CICV airway has been constant across all versions of both guidelines (American Society of Anesthesiologists Task Force on Management of the Difficult Airway, 1993, 2003; Apfelbaum et al., 2013; Frerk et al., 2015; Henderson et al., 2004).

INFRAGLOTTIC AIRWAY ACCESS TECHNIQUES AND PRACTICE PATTERNS

Infraglottic Airway Access Techniques

There are four principal routes of infraglottic airway access: narrow-gauge percutaneous cricothyrotomy, wide-gauge percutaneous cricothyrotomy, surgical cricothyrotomy, and tracheostomy. In narrow-gauge percutaneous cricothyrotomy, the anesthetist introduces a 12–14-gauge over-the-needle catheter percutaneously through the cricothyroid membrane in a caudad direction (Stothert, Stout, Lewis, & Keltner, 1990). Once the catheter is threaded into the lumen of the trachea, a jet ventilator is connected and oxygen is intermittently injected via a manual jet ventilator at a pressure of 50 psi or less. Adequate time must be allowed for exhalation to occur passively through the nose and mouth. Stothert et al. (1990) recommend an inspiratory to expiratory (I/E) ratio of 1:9 as shorter ratios (e.g., 1:4) are associated with barotrauma, tension pneumothorax, cardiovascular collapse, and death in live animal models. Thus, oxygen is injected for 1 second and then the subject is allowed to exhale for 9 seconds. Given the increased resistance to exhalation, hypercarbia and respiratory acidosis are inevitable, and barotrauma, tension pneumothorax, and cardiovascular collapse due to increased intrathoracic pressure are possible (Cook, Bigwood, & Cranshaw, 2006; Stothert et al., 1990). Additional limitations of the technique include subcutaneous emphysema and/or pneumomediastinum due to catheter misplacement or dislodgement (Patel, 1999), interruption of ventilation due to catheter kinking (Ross-Anderson, Ferguson, & Patel, 2011), and inability to suction blood or secretions from the trachea due to the narrowness of the catheter. In addition, meta-analysis of studies of narrow-gauge percutaneous cricothyrotomy use in the prehospital setting estimates the success rate at only 65.8% (Hubble, Wilfong, Brown, Hertelendy, & Benner, 2010). Thus narrow-gauge percutaneous cricothyrotomy is best viewed as a short-term technique to stave off cardiovascular collapse until a definitive airway can be secured.

Preemptive placement of narrow-gauge percutaneous cricothyrotomy has been used with automated high-frequency jet ventilation to manage patients at high risk of CICV during airway surgery (Ross-Anderson et al., 2011). Ross-Anderson et al. (2011) report utilizing a 13-gauge catheter connected to a high-frequency jet ventilator in 44 patients with preoperative airway compromise. The narrow-gauge catheter was inserted before induction; after induction, initial high-frequency jet ventilator settings were: driving pressure 1 bar (14.5 psi), ventilation rate 100 per minute, I/E ratio 1:2.5; pause pressure 10 mbar (0.2 psi), and oxygen concentration 100%. Note that shorter I/E ratios may be used in automated high-frequency jet ventilation as the volume of each delivered breath is small (typically less than physiological dead space) and gas flow is bidirectional, ameliorating the air trapping that limits I/E ratio in manual jet ventilation. Driving pressure was increased to a maximum of 3 bar (43.5 psi) to obtain a pulse oxygen saturation greater than 95%, and ventilation rate and I/E ratio decreased if the pause pressure exceeded 10 mbar (0.2 psi). Anesthesia was maintained using a total intravenous technique. The authors did not report the subjects' arterial or end-tidal carbon dioxide partial pressures, but all patients survived their procedure without major complications (Ross-Anderson et al., 2011).

Wide-gauge percutaneous cricothyrotomy is performed using one of a variety of commercially available kits, which can be divided into two categories: kits that use wire-through-needle (Seldinger) technique and kits that use a direct puncture technique (Langvad, Hyldmo, Nakstad, Vist, & Sandberg, 2013). In the Seldinger technique, a small-gauge needle is used to locate and pass a wire through the cricothyroid membrane (Eisenburger et al., 2000). After removal of the small-gauge needle, a wire-guided dilator is utilized to enlarge the defect in the cricothyroid membrane and a wide-gauge cricothyrotomy tube is inserted. In the direct puncture technique, a rigid, sharp trochar that passes through a 4 to 6-mm internal diameter cricothyrotomy tube is used to puncture the skin and cricothyroid membrane (Assmann, Wong, & Morales, 2007). After the cricothyroid membrane is punctured, the cricothyrotomy tube is threaded off into the lumen of the trachea. Both types of device allow ventilation via standard 15-mm connectors and are large enough to allow suctioning of the trachea (Assmann et al., 2007; Eisenburger et al., 2000). In addition, cuffed versions assist in reaching desired tidal volumes and theoretically provide some measure of protection against aspiration.

In surgical cricothyrotomy, an incision is made in the skin of the neck, a tissue spreader is used to expose the laryngeal and cricoid cartilages, and the cricothyroid membrane is identified by visualization and palpation (Brantigan & Grow, 1976; Jackson, 1909). Once identified, the cricothyroid membrane is incised, the trachea elevated with a hook, and a cuffed tube inserted directly through the defect in the cricothyroid membrane. Alternatively, the tracheal hook can be omitted and a tissue dilator or gum elastic bougie can be inserted through the defect to guide the tube into the trachea with a small saving in time (Quick, MacIntyre, & Barnes, 2014). Meta-analysis of studies of surgical cricothyrotomy in the prehospital setting suggests that with regular training success rates are estimated to be 90.5% (Hubble et al., 2010).

In contrast, a tracheostomy is inserted percutaneously via the Seldinger technique between the first and second or second and third tracheal rings, or surgically by incising the skin and cutting a window through the second tracheal ring (Durbin, 2005). After dilation or incision of the tracheal defect, a tube is passed directly into the trachea. Of the methods, tracheostomy is the most complex, as it requires the operator to extend the patient's neck and identify and avoid, divide, or mobilize the isthmus of the thyroid gland (Durbin, 2005).

Given the complexity of tracheostomy, infraglottic techniques that access the trachea via the cricothyroid membrane (narrow-gauge percutaneous cricothyrotomy, wide-gauge percutaneous cricothyrotomy, and surgical cricothyrotomy) may be most appropriate for the anesthetist attempting to restore ventilation in a CICV situation. To address the proliferation of commercially available kits to facilitate the performance of narrow-gauge, wide-gauge, and surgical cricothyrotomy, Langvad et al. (2013) conducted a systematic review of the literature to determine if one approach or commercial product was superior to the others. A total of 24 studies were included in the review, representing nine comparisons: (a) among different wide-gauge Seldinger technique kits, (b) between wide-gauge Seldinger and non-Seldinger technique kits, (c) between wide-gauge Seldinger technique kits and surgical techniques, (d) between a wide-gauge Seldinger technique kit and a narrow-gauge technique, (e) between two wide-gauge non-Seldinger technique kits, (f) between a wide-gauge non-Seldinger technique kit and a surgical technique, (g) between a wide-gauge non-Seldinger technique kit and a narrow-gauge technique, (h) between two surgical techniques, and (i) between a surgical technique and a narrow-gauge technique. After examining the available evidence the authors concluded that no single approach or product demonstrated clear superiority, although the heterogeneous populations, small sample sizes, variable outcome measures, and divergent simulation models (e.g., human cadaveric, excised pig trachea) would make identifying a superior technique difficult if one existed (Langvad et al., 2013). Furthermore, the authors suggest that operator skill and familiarity with a particular technique or kit may be more important than the particular technique or product used (Langvad et al., 2013).

Infraglottic Airway Access Practice Patterns

Currently, all board-certified nurse and physician anesthetists are tested in basic knowledge of infraglottic airway access techniques during the process of certification (American Board of Anesthesiology, 2011; National Board of Certification and Recertification for Nurse Anesthetists, n.d.). However, the specific techniques taught and degree of emphasis likely vary between institutions, across geographical regions, and over time. In a 2003 survey of 452 American anesthesiologists, 74%, 14%, 30%, and 12% of respondents indicated that they were skilled in using narrow-gauge percutaneous cricothyrotomy, wide-gauge percutaneous cricothyrotomy, surgical cricothyrotomy, and tracheostomy in clinical practice, respectively (Ezri, Szmuk, Warters, Katz, & Hagberg, 2003). In a 2014 survey of 997 Canadian anesthesiologists, 44%, 52%, 28%, and 6% of respondents felt comfortable performing narrow-gauge percutaneous cricothyrotomy, wide-gauge percutaneous cricothyrotomy, surgical cricothyrotomy, and tracheostomy in clinical practice, respectively (Wong, Mehta, Tam, Yau, & Wong, 2014). Thus, practice patterns appear to have changed over time, with a smaller proportion of anesthesiologists endorsing narrow-gauge percutaneous cricothyrotomy and a greater proportion of anesthesiologists comfortable with wide-gauge percutaneous cricothyrotomy compared to 10 years ago. Unfortunately, similar data are not available for nurse anesthetists.

INFRAGLOTTIC AIRWAY USE IN CICV CASES

Data for how compliant anesthetists are in following the recommendations of the ASA and DAS algorithms to limit the number of laryngoscopies in favor of progression to the definitive step of infraglottic airway access are limited but suggestive. Specific case descriptions were available for two of the three CICV events reported by Tachibana et al. (2015): Both patients became difficult to mask ventilate only after multiple direct and video laryngoscopies, both experienced severe desaturation, both were salvaged with emergency tracheotomy performed by a surgeon, and both recovered without apparent neurological sequelae. The patient for whom limited information was presented suffered severe hypoxic brain injury and was pending litigation (Tachibana et al., 2015). Although anecdotal, these cases suggest that a willingness on the part of the anesthetist to progress to the terminal state of the ASA and DAS difficult airway algorithms was effective in salvaging patients even after effective ventilation was lost. In contrast, data from 75 ASA Closed Claims cases of CICV demonstrated similar precipitating events but poorer outcomes (Peterson et al., 2005). In these claims, multiple laryngoscopies were performed in 46% of CICV cases, the definitive end point of attempted surgical airway placement was reached in 76% of CICV cases, and death or brain damage was the result in 84% of CICV cases that received a surgical airway and 83% of CICV cases that did not (Peterson et al., 2005).

A possible factor accounting for the difference in incidence of brain injury and/or death attributable in CICV cases between the Japanese and American data (33% vs. 83%–84%) may be the expeditiousness with which a surgical airway was placed: The two case descriptions by Tachibana et al. (2015) suggest that a surgical airway was placed without delay once ventilation became inadequate, while Peterson et al. (2005) concluded that invasive airway access was attempted too late in two-thirds of CICV cases. Thus, more than 20 years after initial publication of the ASA guidelines (American Society of Anesthesiologists Task Force on Management of the Difficult Airway, 1993) and more than a decade after initial publication of the DAS guidelines (Henderson et al., 2004), there still appears to be resistance among anesthetists to the end state of infraglottic airway access when laryngoscopy fails and ventilation becomes difficult.

Overcoming Decisional Barriers

In order to successfully salvage a patient from a CICV situation, the anesthetist must rapidly overcome both decisional and technical barriers. First, the anesthetist must recognize that the situation warrants the placement of an infraglottic airway and take steps to initiate the procedure. Second, the anesthetist must be equipped with the technical skills to safely place a functioning infraglottic airway device under stressful conditions. In recent years, high-fidelity simulation has been used to assess the impact of various interventions on anesthetists' decisional and technical performance in CICV situations.

In order to salvage a patient from a CICV situation the anesthetist must recognize that ventilation cannot be restored by other means and make a decision to initiate placement of an infraglottic device. Studies testing interventions designed to help anesthetists overcome decisional barriers to appropriate infraglottic airway placement used high-fidelity simulation as a teaching and/or testing environment (Borges et al., 2010; Hubert, Duwat, Deransy, Mahjoub, & Dupont, 2014; Kuduvalli, Jervis, Tighe, & Robin, 2008; You-Ten, Bould, et al., 2015). Adherence to airway management guidelines was a consistent performance standard across studies, but individual studies also examined behavioral indicators of the decision to secure infraglottic access such as time to request, pick up, or start placement of the infraglottic airway, time to finish placement of the infraglottic airway, and/or time to initiate ventilation through the infraglottic airway (Borges et al., 2010; Hubert et al., 2014; Kuduvalli et al., 2008; You-Ten, Bould, et al., 2015).

Kuduvalli et al. (2008) assessed the performance of 21 anesthesiologists during a medium fidelity simulation of a CICV situation designed to end in infraglottic airway placement. After completion of a baseline CICV simulation, participants underwent a half-day of training in the DAS guidelines for difficult airway management, to include instruction and practice on task trainers in SGA-facilitated intubation, narrow-gauge percutaneous cricothyrotomy, and surgical cricothyrotomy. Nineteen participants were reassessed at 6 to 8 weeks and 15 participants were reassessed at 6 to 8 months by repeating the identical CICV scenario. Compared with baseline performance, adherence to the DAS guideline was significantly improved at both follow-up time points. Time to restore ventilation via narrow-gauge percutaneous cricothyrotomy placement was faster at 6 to 8 weeks, but no different from pre-training by 6 to 8 months.

Borges et al. (2010) assessed the performance of 36 anesthesiologists during a high-fidelity simulation of a CICV situation designed to end in infraglottic airway placement. After the first simulated CICV scenario, participants underwent an hour-long debrief during which their individual performance, the ASA-DAA, and wide-gauge percutaneous cricothyrotomy were reviewed. Immediately after the debriefing, participants repeated an identical simulated CICV scenario. Despite practice and debriefing, similar numbers of participants deviated from the ASA-DAA during the post-debrief simulation by failing to call for help, performing more than two laryngoscopies, and/or failing to place an SGA (Borges et al., 2010). Furthermore, significantly fewer participants asked for surgical assistance with infraglottic airway access during the second simulated CICV scenario (Borges et al., 2010). However, simulation and debriefing were effective in decreasing time to decide to place an infraglottic airway and time to restore ventilation, as participants started the wide-gauge percutaneous cricothyrotomy an average of 26 seconds sooner and restored ventilation an average of 88 seconds faster during the second simulation (Borges et al., 2010).

Hubert et al. (2014) conducted a similar but more extensive study in 27 third-year anesthesia residents. One month after baseline assessment during a simulated CICV scenario, all participants underwent 2 days of instruction. The first day was devoted to didactic instruction in difficult airway management, followed by training in difficult airway management including narrow-gauge percutaneous, wide-gauge percutaneous, and surgical cricothyrotomy. Task trainers were used to reinforce infraglottic airway placement skills. The second day was devoted to applying the learned skills in simulated difficult ventilation and/or intubation scenarios. The participants were randomized to repeat the initial CICV simulation at either 3, 6, or 12 months after training. At all three follow-up assessments, adherence to the French Anesthesiology and Critical Society difficult airway algorithm (Langeron, Bourgain, Laccoureye, Legras, & Orliaguet, 2008) was significantly improved and time to place an infraglottic airway significantly faster than baseline (Hubert et al., 2014).

A critical weakness of Kuduvalli et al. (2008), Borges et al. (2010) and Hubert et al. (2014) was the use of single-group, repeated measures designs. You-Ten, Bould, et al. (2015) attempted to address these limitations by examining the effect of cricothyrotomy training on ASA-DAA compliance in a randomized, after-only trial. Twenty-one anesthesia residents were given 60 to 90 minutes of didactic instruction on the difficult airway algorithm, including wide-gauge percutaneous infraglottic airway access. Ten residents were then randomized to receive additional instruction on wide-gauge percutaneous cricothyrotomy, to include practicing simulated cricothyrotomy five times on a low-fidelity task trainer, while 11 received no additional training. After 2 to 3 weeks, participant performance was assessed in a high-fidelity simulated CICV scenario. Compared to participants without hands-on training, participants who received hands-on training had greater compliance with the ASA-DAA and asked for the cricothyrotomy kit sooner, but waited longer to call for help and took a similar length of time to initiate the cricothyrotomy (You-Ten, Bould, et al., 2015).

These studies were heterogeneous in design and participants, but suggest implications for effective interventions to improve compliance with difficult airway management algorithms and encourage rapid progression to infraglottic airway placement. First, in simulated CICV scenarios any training in the difficult airway algorithms was associated with *decreased time* to decide to place an infraglottic airway (Borges et al., 2010; Hubert et al., 2014; Kuduvalli et al., 2008), but *adherence* to the difficult airway algorithm only improved in studies where task trainers were used to reinforce the skills of infraglottic airway placement, (Hubert et al., 2014; Kuduvalli et al., 2008; You-Ten, Bould, et al., 2015). Second, training in infraglottic access was associated with *delays* in calling for assistance in simulated CICV situations in some studies. Third, improvements in the cognitive aspect of adherence to difficult airway management guidelines appeared to be sustained for 6 to 12 months after training (Hubert et al., 2014; Kuduvalli et al., 2008), but the psychomotor skill of placing an infraglottic airway decayed within 6 to 8 months after a half-day training session (Kuduvalli et al., 2008), and was sustained for 12 months after a two-day training session incorporating multiple rounds of high-fidelity simulation (Hubert et al., 2014). Thus, training to reinforce difficult airway management skills should incorporate the use of task trainers in infraglottic access, should reinforce that individual competency or training in infraglottic access is no substitute for a team approach to the CICV situation, and should be repeated every 6 to 12 months, depending on the length of the training session.

Overcoming Technical Barriers

In the ideal CICV situation, the anesthetist would attempt to sustain or restore ventilation via mask or SGA while a proficient surgeon places the infraglottic airway device (Frerk et al., 2015). In the absence of a proficient surgeon the anesthetist will have to initiate infraglottic access to salvage the patient; thus several studies have investigated skill-related barriers to infraglottic airway placement. Studies investigating technical barriers to infraglottic airway access have sought to establish the number or repetitions necessary to establish initial technical skill at infraglottic airway access (Wong, Prabhu, Coloma, Imasogie, & Chung, 2003), establish the rate of decay of skill at infraglottic airway access (Boet et al., 2011), compared different teaching/training paradigms and different training models or environments (e.g., the use of task trainers or low- vs. high-fidelity simulation; Friedman, You-Ten, Bould, & Naik, 2008; You-Ten, Wong, et al., 2015).

Wong et al. (2003) investigated the number of repetitions necessary to attain proficiency in wide-gauge percutaneous cricothyrotomy in a sample of 81 anesthesiologists and 21 anesthesia residents. After an initial orientation to the wide-gauge percutaneous cricothyrotomy device, each participant performed cricothyrotomy 10 times on a moderate fidelity mannequin. Time from palpation to ventilation and success, defined as correct placement of the device, was recorded after each attempt. Both time to place the cricothyrotomy and success rate plateaued after five repetitions, with additional repetitions yielding little decrease in time or improvement in success rate. Shetty, Nayyar, Stachowski, and Byth (2013) conducted a similar study in 30 anesthesia residents. After viewing a demonstration video, participants attempted wide-gauge percutaneous cricothyrotomy five times on a mannequin. By the fifth attempt, all participants were successful, defined as successfully placing the device within 60 seconds of palpation. Taken together, Wong et al. (2003) and Shetty et al. (2013) provide some evidence that five repetitions are necessary and sufficient to establish initial familiarity in wide-gauge percutaneous infraglottic airway placement.

Boet (2011) investigated the rate of decay in skill at wide-gauge percutaneous cricothyrotomy placement in 38 anesthesiologists. Immediately after baseline assessment during a simulated CICV scenario designed to end in infraglottic airway access, all participants received personalized feedback about their performance and hands-on instruction in wide-gauge percutaneous cricothyrotomy. Participants were then randomized to return at 6 or 12 months after initial training to repeat the simulated CICV scenario. Time to place the cricothyrotomy was significantly decreased at both 6 and 12 months after initial teaching. This finding was contrary to the earlier results of Kuduvali et al. (2008), who reported that the technical skill of wide-gauge percutaneous cricothyrotomy decayed at 6 to 8 months after initial training.

Friedman et al. (2008) investigated the impact of model fidelity during task training on performance during wide-gauge percutaneous cricothyrotomy in a randomized controlled trial. After baseline assessment of cricothyrotomy performance on an embalmed cadaver, 11 anesthesia residents performed wide-gauge percutaneous cricothyrotomy twice on a high-fidelity mannequin and 11 performed wide-gauge percutaneous cricothyrotomy on a low-fidelity task trainer constructed of corrugated anesthesia circuit tubing, tape, and silicone membrane. Two weeks after training participants were reassessed during performance of a wide-gauge percutaneous cricothyrotomy on a second embalmed cadaver. Both groups demonstrated similar improvements in time to perform cricothyrotomy and similar success rates.

You-Ten and Wong et al. (2015) investigated the impact of simulation fidelity on technical performance during wide-gauge percutaneous cricothyrotomy. In a randomized crossover design, a sample of 6 anesthesia assistants, 23 emergency medicine residents, and 36 anesthesia residents completed a total of four CICV scenarios requiring placement of a wide-gauge percutaneous cricothyrotomy into a pig trachea secured to a mannequin after a 30-minute lecture and hands-on demonstration of two different percutaneous infraglottic access devices. Two scenarios were conducted under high-fidelity conditions with actors playing an operating team and the mannequin and monitors configured to simulate a CICV situation (once with each device), and two scenarios were conducted under low-fidelity conditions without actors and the mannequin and monitors turned off (again, once with each device). Time to place either device and success rates were not significantly different between low-fidelity and high-fidelity simulation conditions.

Much like studies that investigated the impact of training in infraglottic airway access on adherence to difficult airway guidelines, studies focused on psychomotor performance were small and methodologically heterogeneous. However, these studies provide some evidence to inform programs aimed at sustaining psychomotor performance at infraglottic airway access over time. There is evidence that improvement in psychomotor performance on percutaneous infraglottic airway placement peaks after five repetitions, may be sustained for as long as 1 year, and is not significantly impacted by the fidelity of the model used to practice the repetitious task. This has significant financial implications for initial training and skills sustainment programs, as decisional skills can be honed in high-fidelity simulation, while technical skills can be developed through repetitious practice on low-fidelity and low-cost task trainers.

CONCLUSIONS

An anesthetist may never face a CICV scenario in clinical practice, but if he or she does, it will most likely be unanticipated. Salvaging a patient from a CICV situation requires the anesthetist to recognize that the situation is dire and act rapidly to restore oxygenation and/or ventilation by initiating the placement of an infraglottic airway. There is insufficient data at this point to recommend a particular infraglottic approach as superior to all others, and training and experience will likely contribute more to the successful resolution of a CICV situation than small technical differences between commercial infraglottic access kits. Thus, anesthetists should undergo initial training that involves extensive reinforcement of difficult airway management practice guidelines and at least five repetitions of the skill of infraglottic airway placement. Whether high-fidelity simulation is a necessary component of this initial training is not known. This training should be repeated every 6 to 12 months, but the ideal composition of refresher training, to include the number of task repetitions, is not known. Furthermore, the generalizability of these findings to providers who are not physicians and patients who are not simulated is not known. Future research studies should seek to close these knowledge gaps and identify best practices for gaining and sustaining competence and proficiency in managing the terminal end state of CICV.

REFERENCES

American Board of Anesthesiology. (2011). *Primary certification in anesthesiology: Content outline*. Raleigh, NC: Author.

American Society of Anesthesiologists Task Force on Management of the Difficult Airway. (1993). Practice guidelines for management of the difficult airway. A report by the American Society of Anesthesiologists Task Force on Management of the Difficult Airway. *Anesthesiology*, *78*(3), 597–602.

American Society of Anesthesiologists Task Force on Management of the Difficult Airway. (2003). Practice guidelines for management of the difficult airway: An updated report by the American Society of Anesthesiologists Task Force on Management of the Difficult Airway. *Anesthesiology*, *98*(5), 1269–1277.

Apfelbaum, J. L., Hagberg, C. A., Caplan, R. A., Blitt, C. D., Connis, R. T., Nickinovich, D. G., et al. (2013). Practice guidelines for management of the difficult airway: An updated report by the American Society of Anesthesiologists Task Force on Management of the Difficult Airway. *Anesthesiology*, *118*(2), 251–270. http://dx.doi.org/10.1097/aln.0b013e31827773b2

Assmann, N. M., Wong, D. T., & Morales, E. (2007). A comparison of a new indicator-guided with a conventional wire-guided percutaneous cricothyroidotomy device in mannequins. *Anesthesia & Analgesia*, *105*(1), 148–154. http://dx.doi.org/10.1213/01.ane.0000266439.43797.9e

Boet, S., Borges, B. C., Naik, V. N., Siu, L. W., Riem, N., Chandra, D., et al. (2011). Complex procedural skills are retained for a minimum of 1 yr after a single high-fidelity simulation training session. *British Journal of Anaesthesia*, *107*(4), 533–539. http://dx.doi.org/10.1093/bja/aer160

Borges, B. C., Boet, S., Siu, L. W., Bruppacher, H. R., Naik, V. N., Riem, N., et al. (2010). Incomplete adherence to the ASA difficult airway algorithm is unchanged after a high-fidelity simulation session. *Canadian Journal of Anesthesia/Journal canadien d'anesthésie*, *57*(7), 644–649. http://dx.doi.org/10.1007/s12630-010-9322-4

Brantigan, C. O., & Grow, J. B., Sr. (1976). Cricothyroidotomy: Elective use in respiratory problems requiring tracheotomy. *The Thoracic and Cardiovascular Surgeon*, *71*(1), 72–81.

Cook, T. M., Bigwood, B., & Cranshaw, J. (2006). A complication of transtracheal jet ventilation and use of the Aintree intubation catheter during airway resuscitation. *Anaesthesia*, *61*(7), 692–697. http://dx.doi.org/10.1111/j.1365-2044.2006.04686.x

Cook, T. M., Woodall, N., Frerk, C., & Fourth National Audit Project. (2011). Major complications of airway management in the UK: Results of the Fourth National Audit Project of the Royal College of Anaesthetists and the Difficult Airway Society. Part 1: anaesthesia. *British Journal of Anaesthesia*, *106*(5), 617–631. http://dx.doi.org/10.1093/bja/aer058

Durbin, C. G., Jr. (2005). Techniques for performing tracheostomy. *Respiratory Care*, *50*(4), 488–496.

Eisenburger, P., Laczika, K., List, M., Wilfing, A., Losert, H., Hofbauer, R., et al. (2000). Comparison of conventional surgical versus Seldinger technique emergency cricothyrotomy performed by inexperienced clinicians. *Anesthesiology*, *92*(3), 687–690.

Enterlein, G., Byhahn, C., & American Society of Anesthesiologists Task Force. (2013). Practice guidelines for management of the difficult airway: Update by the American Society of Anesthesiologists task force. *Anaesthesist*, *62*(10), 832–835. http://dx.doi.org/10.1007/s00101-013-2222-6

Ezri, T., Szmuk, P., Warters, R. D., Katz, J., & Hagberg, C. A. (2003). Difficult airway management practice patterns among anesthesiologists practicing in the United States: Have we made any progress? *Journal of Clinical Anesthesia*, *15*(6), 418–422.

Frerk, C., Mitchell, V. S., McNarry, A. F., Mendonca, C., Bhagrath, R., Patel, A., et al. (2015). Difficult Airway Society 2015 guidelines for management of unanticipated difficult intubation in adults. *British Journal of Anaesthesia*, *115*(6), 827–848. http://dx.doi.org/10.1093/bja/aev371

Friedman, Z., You-Ten, K. E., Bould, M. D., & Naik, V. (2008). Teaching lifesaving procedures: The impact of model fidelity on acquisition and transfer of cricothyrotomy skills to performance on cadavers. *Anesthesia & Analgesia*, *107*(5), 1663–1669. http://dx.doi.org/10.1213/ane.0b013e3181841efe

Henderson, J. J., Popat, M. T., Latto, I. P., Pearce, A. C., & Society, D. A. (2004). Difficult Airway Society guidelines for management of the unanticipated difficult intubation. *Anaesthesia*, *59*(7), 675–694. http://dx.doi.org/10.1111/j.1365-2044.2004.03831.x

Hubble, M. W., Wilfong, D. A., Brown, L. H., Hertelendy, A., & Benner, R. W. (2010). A meta-analysis of prehospital airway control techniques part II: Alternative airway devices and cricothyrotomy success rates. *Prehospital Emergency Care*, *14*(4), 515–530. http://dx.doi.org/10.3109/10903127.2010.497903

Hubert, V., Duwat, A., Deransy, R., Mahjoub, Y., & Dupont, H. (2014). Effect of simulation training on compliance with difficult airway management algorithms, technical ability, and skills retention for emergency cricothyrotomy. *Anesthesiology*, *120*(4), 999–1008. http://dx.doi.org/10.1097/aln.0000000000000138

Jackson, C. (1909). Tracheotomy. *The Laryngoscope*, *19*(4), 285–290.

Kuduvalli, P. M., Jervis, A., Tighe, S. Q., & Robin, N. M. (2008). Unanticipated difficult airway management in anaesthetised patients: A prospective study of the effect of mannequin training on management strategies and skill retention. *Anaesthesia*, *63*(4), 364–369. http://dx.doi.org/10.1111/j.1365-2044.2007.05353.x

Langeron, O., Bourgain, J. L., Laccoureye, O., Legras, A., & Orliaguet, G. (2008). [Difficult airway algorithms and management: Question 5. Societe Francaise d'Anesthesie et de Reanimation]. *Annales Françaises d'Anesthésie et de Réanimation*, *27*(1), 41–45. http://dx.doi.org/10.1016/j.annfar.2007.10.025

Langvad, S., Hyldmo, P. K., Nakstad, A. R., Vist, G. E., & Sandberg, M. (2013). Emergency cricothyrotomy–a systematic review. *Scandinavian Journal of Trauma, Resuscitation and Emergency Medicine*, *21*, 43. http://dx.doi.org/10.1186/1757-7241-21-43

Metzner, J., Posner, K. L., Lam, M. S., & Domino, K. B. (2011). Closed claims' analysis. *Best Practice & Research Clinical Anaesthesiology*, *25*(2), 263–276. http://dx.doi.org/10.1016/j.bpa.2011.02.007

National Board of Certification and Recertification for Nurse Anesthetists. (n.d.). *NBCRNA National Certification Examination (NCE) content outline*. Park Ridge, IL: Author.

Norskov, A. K., Rosenstock, C. V., Wetterslev, J., Astrup, G., Afshari, A., & Lundstrom, L. H. (2015). Diagnostic accuracy of anaesthesiologists' prediction of difficult airway management in daily clinical practice: A cohort study of 188 064 patients registered in the Danish Anaesthesia Database. *Anaesthesia, 70*(3), 272–281. http://dx.doi.org/10.1111/anae.12955

Patel, R. G. (1999). Percutaneous transtracheal jet ventilation: A safe, quick, and temporary way to provide oxygenation and ventilation when conventional methods are unsuccessful. *Chest, 116*(6), 1689–1694.

Peterson, G. N., Domino, K. B., Caplan, R. A., Posner, K. L., Lee, L. A., & Cheney, F. W. (2005). Management of the difficult airway: A closed claims analysis. *Anesthesiology, 103*(1), 33–39.

Quick, J. A., MacIntyre, A. D., & Barnes, S. L. (2014). Emergent surgical airway: Comparison of the three-step method and conventional cricothyroidotomy utilizing high-fidelity simulation. *The Journal of Emergency Medicine, 46*(2), 304–307. http://dx.doi.org/10.1016/j.jemermed.2013.08.065

Ross-Anderson, D. J., Ferguson, C., & Patel, A. (2011). Transtracheal jet ventilation in 50 patients with severe airway compromise and stridor. *British Journal of Anaesthesia, 106*(1), 140–144. http://dx.doi.org/10.1093/bja/aeq278

Shetty, K., Nayyar, V., Stachowski, E., & Byth, K. (2013). Training for cricothyroidotomy. *Anaesth Intensive Care, 41*(5), 623–630.

Stothert, J. C., Jr., Stout, M. J., Lewis, L. M., & Keltner, R. M., Jr. (1990). High pressure percutaneous transtracheal ventilation: The use of large gauge intravenous-type catheters in the totally obstructed airway. *The American Journal of Emergency Medicine, 8*(3), 184–189.

Tachibana, N., Niiyama, Y., & Yamakage, M. (2015). Incidence of cannot intubate-cannot ventilate (CICV): Results of a 3-year retrospective multicenter clinical study in a network of university hospitals. *Journal of Anesthesia, 29*(3), 326–330. http://dx.doi.org/10.1007/s00540-014-1847-1

Wong, D. T., Lai, K., Chung, F. F., & Ho, R. Y. (2005). Cannot intubate-cannot ventilate and difficult intubation strategies: Results of a Canadian national survey. *Anesthesia & Analgesia, 100*(5), 1439–1446, table of contents. http://dx.doi.org/10.1213/01.ane.0000148695.37190.34

Wong, D. T., Mehta, A., Tam, A. D., Yau, B., & Wong, J. (2014). A survey of Canadian anesthesiologists' preferences in difficult intubation and "cannot intubate, cannot ventilate" situations. *Canadian Journal of Anesthesia/Journal canadien d'anesthésie, 61*(8), 717–726. http://dx.doi.org/10.1007/s12630-014-0183-0

Wong, D. T., Prabhu, A. J., Coloma, M., Imasogie, N., & Chung, F. F. (2003). What is the minimum training required for successful cricothyroidotomy?: A study in mannequins. *Anesthesiology, 98*(2), 349–353.

You-Ten, K. E., Bould, M. D., Friedman, Z., Riem, N., Sydor, D., & Boet, S. (2015). Cricothyrotomy training increases adherence to the ASA difficult airway algorithm in a simulated crisis: A randomized controlled trial. *Canadian Journal of Anesthesia/Journal canadien d'anesthésie, 62*(5), 485–494. http://dx.doi.org/10.1007/s12630-014-0308-5

You-Ten, K. E., Wong, C., Arzola, C., Cheung, J., Friedman, Z., Perelman, S., et al. (2015). Role of contextualizing a crisis scenario on the performance of a cricothyrotomy procedural task. *Canadian Journal of Anesthesia/Journal canadien d'anesthésie, 62*(10), 1104–1113. http://dx.doi.org/10.1007/s12630-015-0430-z

CHAPTER 2

Anesthetic Implications of Obesity and Obstructive Sleep Apnea

Jennifer Greenwood

ABSTRACT

The incidence of morbid obesity has tripled within the past 25 years in developed countries, with the highest rate of growth noted among people with body mass index (BMI) greater than 50. The physiologic derangements that accompany obesity affect almost every organ system leading to a vast array of comorbid conditions including obstructive sleep apnea (OSA). This review focuses on the unique perioperative management considerations that the nurse anesthetist must address when caring for these patients as well as the impact of obesity and OSA on postoperative complications and mortality rates. Current research is reviewed to highlight best practice recommendations for all phases of anesthetic management including implications for bariatric surgery and office-based practice.

INTRODUCTION

Arguably one of the biggest challenges facing the medical community, and anesthetists in particular, is the epidemic of obesity in the United States. Body mass index (BMI) is the most common measure used to determine the degree of obesity because it is applicable to both men and women regardless of age. BMI is determined by a person's weight in kilograms divided by the square of his or her height in meters. In 1991, the National Institutes of Health classified the population into

http://dx.doi.org/10.1891/0739-6686.35.17

the following categories: normal weight, BMI less than 24.9; overweight, BMI 25–29.9; obesity, BMI 30–39.9; morbid obesity, BMI 40–49; superobesity, BMI greater than 50 (Consensus Development Conference Panel, 1991).

According to the WHO, the incidence of morbid obesity has tripled in developed countries within the past 25 years. The United States has the highest mean BMI among high-income countries, with 35.9% of American adults with a BMI greater than 30, and 69.2% of adults considered overweight or obese (Flegal, Carroll, Kit, & Ogden, 2012). Between 1986 and 2000, the prevalence of obesity (BMI > 30) doubled, the prevalence of morbid obesity (BMI > 40) quadrupled, and the prevalence of supermorbid obesity (BMI > 50) quintupled (Sturm & Hattori, 2013), indicating an exponential trend in obesity rates. Although the rates of obesity are higher among Hispanics and African Americans, the trends in obesity progression are similar among all ethnicities. The proliferation of this disease does not appear to discriminate according to ethnic divides.

The direct and indirect effects of obesity on health outcomes have been the subject of several large-scale studies using data from the National Health and Nutritional Examination Survey (NHANES) and the Framingham Study due to their large and diverse subject enrollment. Not surprisingly, the models used by NHANES demonstrated a substantial increase in risk among all disease categories with increasing values of BMI. For instance, the rates of hypertension and diabetes were three times greater in obese patients than the rates for those diseases in the nonoverweight group (Hammond & Levine, 2010).

High rates of obesity-related diseases are also associated with rising direct medical costs. Over a nine-year period, subjects with BMI greater than 30 had 36% higher average annual health care costs than the healthy-weight group, including 105% higher prescription costs (Thompson, Brown, Nichols, Elmer, & Oster, 2001). Using regression methodology on nationwide samples, a study by Finkelstein, Trogdon, Cohen, and Dietz (2009), showed the estimated cost of obesity was as high as $147 billion in 2008, which amounted to 10% of all medical spending that year. This estimate was up from $78 billion in 1998. The biggest factor explaining the rise in costs was the exponential growth in the number of obese people seeking care. Although no single study has provided a comprehensive picture of the direct and indirect costs of obesity, the aggregate findings of these individual studies suggest that the impact of obesity on the U.S. economy may exceed $215 billion per year (Hammond & Levine, 2010).

PATHOPHYSIOLOGY OF OBESITY

The physiologic derangements related to obesity and morbid obesity are multifactorial. As outlined in a review article by Terkawi and Durieux (2015), lung function is generally decreased in a restrictive pattern in obese patients, evidenced by a decreased forced vital capacity of 25% to 50%, decreased functional residual capacity (FRC), and reduced total lung capacity. These changes, along with increased airway resistance, result in a rapid desaturation after induction or during periods of apnea. Abdominal surgery, laparoscopic techniques, and Trendelenburg position further decrease FRC below closing capacity, resulting in atelectasis and ventilation/perfusion mismatching (Terkawi & Durieux, 2015).

The cardiovascular system of obese and morbidly obese patients is also stressed. Patients tend to have hypertension, concentric left ventricular hypertrophy (LVH), coronary artery disease, and obesity-related cardiomyopathy manifesting as diastolic failure (Terkawi & Durieux, 2015). The degree of failure correlates with the duration of obesity. Obese patients are also at risk for developing arrhythmias, especially atrial fibrillation, related to epicardial fat deposits and hypoxemia due to sleep apnea. Obese patients are at high risk for developing pulmonary hypertension (PH) and chronic pulmonary thromboembolisms, which drastically increases their risk for surgical morbidity and mortality (Ortiz & Kwo, 2015). In one study, Kaw et al. (2012), found that 26% of patients with PH developed complications such as heart failure, respiratory failure, and sepsis compared to only a 2.6% complication rate among patients without PH.

Metabolic syndrome, which is a combination of central obesity, hypertension, dyslipidemia, and insulin resistance, frequently accompanies obesity due to the chronic low-grade inflammatory state induced by excess adipose tissue. This syndrome has been implicated as an independent predictor for postoperative pulmonary and cardiac complications (Ortiz & Kwo, 2015). Type 2 diabetes, gastroesophageal reflux disease, and gastroparesis are also frequently seen in obese patients. Optimal glycemic control is recommended to reduce postoperative infection. A hemoglobin A1c of less than 6.5% has been associated with a decrease in complications (Ortiz & Kwo, 2015). Obese patients are also at a higher risk for venous thromboembolism when the chronic inflammatory nature of the disease is superimposed on relative immobility and venous stasis that accompanies surgery. The American College of Chest Physicians recommends the use of low-dose unfractionated heparin or low molecular weight heparin in addition to elastic stockings and sequential compression devices (Mechanick et al., 2013). Patients should be ambulated early, and chemoprophylaxis should be continued for 10 days after discharge in bariatric patients and those with a history of deep vein thrombosis (Mechanick et al., 2013).

The impact of obesity is not limited to physiologic factors. Patients with elevated BMI are more likely to have mood and anxiety disorders, social phobias, and personality disorders (Ortiz & Kwo, 2015). In addition to the changes outlined earlier in this section, obesity contributes to the development of osteoarthritis, dyslipidemia, and certain forms of cancer (Ortiz & Kwo, 2015). There are many factors for the anesthetist to consider when formulating a comprehensive anesthetic plan for obese patients.

ANESTHETIC CONSIDERATIONS FOR OBESE PATIENTS

Preoperative testing of obese patients presenting for surgery should be based on their overall health and functional status. Ortiz and Kwo (2015) recommend an EKG only if cardiac disease is suspected. Obese patients presenting with a history of PH should have a preoperative EKG and echocardiogram to assess ventricular function and possible continuation of pharmacologic targeted vascular therapy (Kaw et al., 2012). The anesthetist should ensure adequate fasting time, consider pretreatment with H_2 blockers, sodium citrate, and gastric motility agents, as well as modifications to the induction sequence for patients who are considered a full stomach (Domi & Laho, 2012).

Appropriate preoxygenation and positioning of the patient are critical for successful induction and intubation on the first attempt. Due to pathophysiologic changes in the respiratory system of obese patients outlined earlier, rapid desaturation and difficult mask ventilation should be anticipated in this population. It is recommended that patients are preoxygenated with 100% oxygen for 3 minutes in a 25° head up, or "ramped," position. The addition of 5–10 cm H_2O continuous positive airway pressure (CPAP) during preoxygenation will attenuate the decrease in FRC associated with supine position and induction of general anesthesia, thus delaying desaturation during laryngoscopy attempts (Terkawi & Durieux, 2015).

Rapid sequence induction (RSI) is commonly utilized with obese patients to reduce the incidence of pulmonary aspiration. However, cricoid pressure does not reliably prevent aspiration at the time of induction and intubation (Ebert, Shankar, & Haake, 2006). Several studies confirm that it is often applied inappropriately and that esophageal rupture is a possible complication (Ebert et al., 2006). According to a recent study, morbidly obese patients who were treated with metoclopramide 10 mg tablets and ranitidine 150 mg tablets the night before and 2 hours before elective surgery showed no significant difference in gastric volume (p = .663) and gastric pH compared with the normal-weight group (Mahajan, Hashmi, Singh, Samra, & Aneia, 2015). However, the untreated morbidly obese group demonstrated statistically significant higher residual gastric volume ($p < .001$) and gastric pH ($p < .01$) than the normal-weight and the treated morbidly obese group. These results indicate that pretreatment with a histamine type 2 blocker (H2) and a gastric motility agent is an effective strategy to minimize the risk of aspiration at induction (Mahajan et al., 2015).

The concern about aspiration should not be limited to the induction phase of the anesthetic. The misconception that monitored anesthesia care (MAC) is safer than general anesthesia is not supported in the literature, since the most common cause of aspiration is due to "light" anesthesia and an unprotected airway (Ebert et al., 2006). Current practice guidelines discourage deep sedation techniques without a secure airway in obese patients and recommend extubating these patients awake and in the sitting or semi-upright position (ASA Task Force, 2014).

Intraoperative modifications to the anesthetic plan are also important factors for optimal management of obese patients. Non-depolarizing neuromuscular blockers (NMBs), opioids, benzodiazepines, and induction agents should be dosed according to ideal body weight (IBW); however, succinylcholine should be dosed according to total body weight (TBW) (Domi & Laho, 2012). Additionally, a neuromuscular monitor should always be used to evaluate the extent of recovery from neuromuscular blockade. When propofol is used for maintenance of anesthesia, it should be titrated according to TBW (Domi & Laho, 2012). The obese patient has an increased volume of distribution for lipophilic drugs, such as narcotics, which can lead to an increased elimination time and possible overnarcotization with repeated dosing. Similarly, benzodiazepines and barbiturates may also exhibit a prolonged elimination time due to the larger volume of distribution (Domi & Laho, 2012).

One of the most daunting aspects of anesthesia for patients with obesity and sleep apnea is emergence and airway protection after general anesthesia with muscle relaxant. The traditional method for reversing neuromuscular blockade is with the administration of a competitive antagonist of acetylcholinesterase in conjunction with an anticholinergic agent to mitigate untoward side effects. Any degree of residual muscle paralysis can further impair breathing and airway patency, especially in the obese or sleep apnea patient. Approved for use in the United States by the Food and Drug Administration (FDA) in 2015, sugammadex is a rapidly acting reversal agent that acts as a supermolecule, which encapsulates the steroidal NMB to reverse its effect permanently (Welliver, Cheek, Osterbrink, & McDonough, 2015). It can be administered immediately after a dose of NMB, which makes it an ideal choice for reversal after a rapid sequence intubation with a non-depolarizing paralytic agent (Welliver et al., 2015). Sugammadex should be dosed according to TBW due to the risk of underdosing and incomplete reversal when dosing according to IBW. If the patient displays a train of four (TOF) of 1–2/4 twitches, the recommended dose is 2 mg/kg of TBW. If the patient displays a TOF response of 0/4 twitches, the recommended dose increases to 4 mg/kg of TBW (Welliver et al., 2015). Sugammadex can also be used to augment incomplete reversal with a competitive antagonist. This novel agent undergoes renal elimination and does not alter hemodynamics, which makes it an ideal choice for heart failure and other cardiac patients who cannot tolerate the tachycardia that accompanies reversal with anticholinergics (Welliver et al., 2015).

Because of the changes in lung physiology, several mechanical ventilation strategies can be used to improve oxygenation in obese patients. In addition to the use of CPAP during induction, application of positive end-expiratory pressure (PEEP) up to 10 cm H_2O during the maintenance phase results in improved lung volumes, compliance, and oxygenation with lower intra-abdominal pressure (Domi & Laho, 2012). Tidal volume selections should be based on IBW to prevent overdistention and barotrauma. Respiratory rate can be increased to 12–18 breaths per minute with tidal volumes of 6 to 10 ml/kg to keep the peak airway pressure less than 30 to 35 cm H_2O and arterial carbon dioxide levels between 35 and 45 mmHg (Domi & Laho, 2012).

When possible, regional, neuraxial, and local anesthetic techniques should be employed in order to avoid manipulation of the airway, minimize the administration of cardiodepressant drugs, and reduce the amount of systemic opioids for pain control to the lowest acceptable level. Although placement of a regional or neuraxial block may be technically difficult in obese patients, the use of ultrasound has been shown to increase success with these techniques (Domi & Laho, 2012). The anesthetist should be involved with the multidisciplinary approach to developing and implementing comprehensive preoperative treatment pathways for obese patients, including appropriate testing, glucose management, and specialist referrals to ensure the highest quality of care on the day of surgery.

Anesthetic Complications of Obesity

Difficult, and possibly failed, intubation is one of the most potentially devastating complications of anesthesia in the obese patient. Predictive assessments are used to determine the potential risk for difficult tracheal intubation (DTI), such as Mallampati class, thyromental distance, hyomental distance, and neck circumference, but are frequently unreliable (Ebert et al., 2006). BMI is often used as a potential indicator of DTI with mixed predictive ability. In a cohort of 91,332 patients scheduled for general anesthesia with direct laryngoscopy, Lundstrom, Moller, Rosenstock, Astrup, and Wetterslev (2009) used multiple and logistic regression to identify factors associated with DTI. The independent variables consisted of BMI, Mallampati class, gender, age, surgical priority (scheduled or emergent), history of difficult intubation, and use of NMBs. A Mallampati class of III and IV (OR 3.7; CI 3.41–4.0; $p < .001$) and history of difficult intubation (OR 6.48; CI 4.89–8.58; $p < .001$) were strong predictors of DTI. The impact of BMI on DTI increased in a linear fashion, but was only weakly associated with DTI at any level, with BMI greater than 35 producing an odds ratio of 1.17 ($p = .059$).

Obesity complications are not limited to airway-related issues. In a study of 90,045 total knee arthroplasty patients by D'Apuzzo, Novicoff, and Browne. (2015), the impact of morbid obesity as an independent risk factor for complications was apparent. The obese patients were matched one to one with a nonobese patient for adjusted analysis of complications. Morbidly obese patients had a higher risk of postoperative in-hospital infection (0.24% versus 0.17%; OR 1.3; $p = .001$), genitourinary complications (0.6% vs. 0.44%; OR 1.3; $p < .001$), a higher risk of in-hospital death (0.08% vs. 0.02%; OR 3.2; $p < .001$), and a higher transfer rate to a skilled rehabilitation facility (40% vs. 30%; $p < .001$). Total hospital costs, length of stay (LOS), and postoperative anemia were also higher in the morbidly obese cohort; however, investigators deemed the degree of anemia observed to be clinically insignificant. Morbid obesity was not an independent risk factor for increased cardiac, respiratory, thromboembolic events, or hematomas in this study.

BARIATRIC SURGERY

Even with advances in behavioral and dietary approaches to weight loss, the vast majority of patients do not succeed in conventional weight reduction and bariatric surgery is often the only remaining option for life-saving weight loss. In a recent systematic review and meta-analysis of 16 studies including data on 3,076 patients (Ribaric, Buchwald, & McGlennon, 2013), bariatric surgery was found to be superior to conventional weight loss for reduction in BMI, glycosylated hemoglobin, and fasting glucose. Patients were also more likely to experience remission of their type 2 diabetes mellitus (overall $p < .001$). The surgical approach to weight loss continues to grow. Buchwald and Oien (2013) reported that the number of bariatric surgeries worldwide has grown by 132% from 2003 to 2011; however that number seems to have plateaued between 2008 and 2011. The greatest increase for surgical weight loss has been sleeve gastrectomies, which showed a 121% increase in the United States and Canada between 2008 and 2011.

Because of the weight loss potential and comorbid remission as a result of a variety of approaches to weight loss surgery, a trend toward ambulatory, or short-stay, bariatric surgery is evolving. The concept of Enhanced Recovery After Surgery (ERAS) has also been proposed as a means to streamline the anesthetic technique and surgical approach to bariatric surgery to minimize variability and improve outcomes (Hahl, Peromaa-Haavisto, Tarkiainen, Knutar, & Victorzon, 2015). In their protocol, patients were allowed to consume carbohydrate beverages up to 2 hours prior to surgery. They received no anxiolytics and rarely used antithrombotic agents. Intraoperatively, patients received a standardized regimen of short-acting agents: propofol, remifentanil, desflurane, and rocuronium for muscle relaxation. Nonsteroidal agents, such as Toradol, acetaminophen, and fentanyl were given at the end of surgery. All incisions were infiltrated with local anesthetic. Nausea prophylaxis was provided with dexamethasone early in the case and ondansetron at the end of the case. Intravenous fluids were restricted to less than 30 ml/kg/24 hours. Using this protocol, LOS was reduced to 1.1 days with 83% of the patients being discharged within 23 hours (Hahl et al., 2015).

With the increasing trend toward bariatric surgery for treating morbid obesity, anesthetists can expect to encounter patients at very high risk for surgery and anesthesia due to supermorbid obesity status and the accompanying comorbid conditions. In a recent study from the Cleveland Clinic, investigators analyzed a cohort of 44 extremely high-risk patients undergoing either Roux-en-Y gastric bypass (n = 23), adjustable gastric banding (n = 11), or sleeve gastrectomy (n = 10); see Aminian et al. (2015). These patients had a mean BMI of 54.8 ± 5.5, mean age of 67.9 ± 2.7, and between two and six cardiopulmonary comorbidities. During the observation period, there were no intraoperative complications and no conversions to an open procedure. The 30-day mortality of the cohort was 0%, compared with a larger multisite study (n = 4776), which reported a 30-day mortality of 0.3% (Longitudinal Assessment of Bariatric Surgery [LABS] Consortium, 2009). This study successfully demonstrated that extremely high-risk patients should not be excluded from bariatric surgery; however the identification of high-risk patients necessitates an interdisciplinary approach to preoperative preparation, which is essential to minimizing early and late complications (Aminian et al., 2015).

Postbariatric Surgery

Due to the wide acceptance and proliferation of weight loss surgery, anesthetists will frequently encounter patients who have had bariatric surgery and are now presenting for additional surgery. A consequence of surgical weight loss through gastroplasty and gastric banding is the decrease in esophageal-gastric peristalsis and an impairment of lower esophageal sphincter relaxation (Jean et al., 2008). These changes can predispose a patient to chronic esophageal reflux, regurgitation, and possible bronchial aspiration upon induction of general anesthesia. In a retrospective review of 198 plastic surgeries, 52 patients who had previous bariatric surgery were matched with 120 other patients who had no previous bariatric surgery. At the time of the plastic surgery, the mean BMI of the postbariatric group was 29 ± 4 and the comparison group was 25 ± 3. Pulmonary aspiration occurred in four patients (6%) of the postbariatric group, and there were no cases of aspiration in the comparison group ($p < .006$). The four aspirations occurred after the use of muscle relaxants and were not associated with difficult intubation.

Data from much larger retrospective studies reported an overall incidence of pulmonary aspiration as low as 2.5/10,000 for elective surgery and as high as 11.2/10,000 for emergency surgery (Warner, Warner, & Weber, 1993). A study limited to postbariatric surgery patients lacks the generalizability of larger studies, but demonstrated that perioperative pulmonary aspiration appears to be dramatically increased in this population even after significant weight loss. Postbariatric surgery patients should always be considered high risk for aspiration and treated with the necessary prophylactic agents and induction precautions outlined previously (Jean et al., 2008).

OBSTRUCTIVE SLEEP APNEA

Obesity has been linked to many systemic diseases including metabolic syndrome, and it is the most common cause of obstructive sleep apnea (OSA). Studies using MRI confirm the inverse relationship between BMI and pharyngeal area (Minokadeh, Bishop, & Benumof, 2011). When humans sleep, whether naturally or through the administration of anesthetic agents, muscle tone throughout the body is diminished. The loss of pharyngeal muscle tone contributes to pharyngeal collapse, which can be categorized as partial or complete. Partial airway collapse, often called snoring or hypopnea, is defined as a decrease in airflow of more than 50% of the awake volume for more than 10 seconds. Apnea results from complete airway closure or a reduction in airflow of greater than 90% from baseline despite ventilatory effort for longer than 10 seconds (Tsara et al., 2009). OSA is a syndrome characterized by frequent and repeated occlusion of the upper airway during sleep, which results in disrupted or fragmented sleep as well as nocturnal hypoxemia. As shown in studies by Lam et al. and Coughlin et al., these frequent periods of hypopnea and apnea can also result in accompanying episodes of arousal and sympathetic nervous system stimulation, which leads to several systemic problems such as PH, LVH, arrhythmias related to myocardial ischemia, reflux, and sudden death (as cited in Minokadeh et al., 2011, p. 73).

Anesthesia reduces pharyngeal dilator muscle activation, which predisposes the patient to airway obstruction. In addition, upper airway neuromuscular responses are impaired in patients with OSA (Kaw, 2014). Lung volumes are also dramatically different for patients who present with OSA. The passive closing pressure (PCLOSE) in these patients is up to 9 cm H_2O higher than non-OSA patients. This may lead to quick desaturation during induction and direct laryngoscopy (Kaw, 2014). Due to the depressive effects of anesthesia on the respiratory system and the relaxation of pharyngeal airway musculature, patients with OSA are at high risk for respiratory complications in the perioperative period, as well as other systemic complications. Figure 2.1 illustrates the relationship between OSA and systemic sequelae.

The prevalence of sleep apnea in the United States is approaching the proportion of obesity rates, with the disorder affecting 9% to 25% of the general population (Peppard et al., 2013). The prevalence is even higher in the surgical population. In a study by Singh et al. (2013), 69% of patients presenting for surgery without a previous diagnosis of OSA were found to have sleep apnea using polysomnography. The diagnosis was missed by the anesthesia provider 53% of the time among those with severe OSA and 76% of the time for patients with mild OSA. Diagnostic sleep studies in a traditional sleep lab are the gold standard for diagnosis of OSA, but they can be inconvenient and impractical in the perioperative setting (Munish et al., 2012). Anesthetists must become adept at quickly and accurately determining a patient's risk for OSA without preoperative testing.

The classification of degree of OSA is determined according to the Apnea–Hypopnea Index (AHI) outlined in Table 2.1 from Tsara et al. (2009). The results

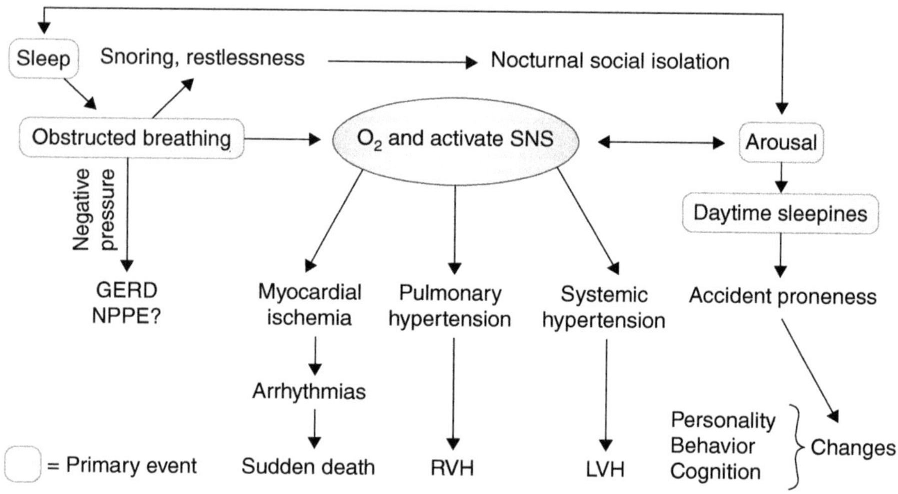

FIGURE 2.1 Systemic pathophysiology of OSA.
Note. GERD = gastroesophageal reflux disease; LVH = left ventricular hypertrophy; NPPE = negative-pressure pulmonary edema; RVH = right ventricular hypertrophy; SNS = sympathetic nervous system. Reprinted with permission from Minokadeh et al. (2011).

TABLE 2.1
Classification of Obstructive Sleep Apnea

Severity of OSA	AHI
None	0–5
Mild OSA	5–15
Moderate OSA	15–30
Severe OSA	>30

of a sleep study classify an OSA patient as mild, moderate, or severe based on the number of apnea or hypopnea episodes per hour of sleep.

When the anesthetist has limited time to perform a preoperative evaluation, questions regarding disease states and medication often take priority. However, a few queries regarding sleep patterns can assist the anesthesia provider in making a decision regarding probable OSA status and treatment of the patient accordingly. The OSA patient and their significant other will frequently report snoring, repeated awakenings, a choking sensation, and witnessed apnea (Minokadeh et al., 2011). Physical exam characteristics of a patient with OSA include a short thick neck, nasal obstruction, tonsillar hypertrophy, narrow oropharynx, retrognathia, and obesity (Minokadeh et al., 2011). For those patients who admit to having sleep apnea, the anesthetist should ask whether or not the patient actually uses the CPAP mask on a nightly basis. Frequent use of the mask has been shown to decrease the incidence of recurrent atrial fibrillation and normalize hemodynamics postoperatively, especially after major vascular surgery (Kaw et al., 2006). It is important to note that patients who have had airway surgery, such as a uvulopalatopharyngoplasty (UPPP), may not snore but still have residual OSA features and require further evaluation and treatment (Kaw et al., 2006).

The STOP-Bang questionnaire was developed in 2008 by Chung et al. and has been validated for use with the surgical population. Consisting of only eight items (Figure 2.2), the STOP-Bang is easy to administer in the preoperative area. Each of the eight items is scored based on Yes/No answers (score 1/0), resulting in a score range from 0 to 8. In a meta-analysis of validation studies using data from over 9,206 patients, Nagappa et al. (2015) found a STOP-Bang score of 0 to 2 had a negative predictive value for assessing likelihood for moderate to severe OSA. Patients with a score 5 or greater had a high probability of having moderate to severe OSA and deserved further attention and intervention. The use of the STOP-Bang tool during the preanesthetic interview can provide the necessary information to identify patients at risk for OSA so that the anesthetic plan and course of hospitalization can be modified to minimize adverse outcomes.

Snoring?

Yes No
O O
Do you **Snore Loudly** (loud enough to be heard through closed doors or your bed-partner elbows you for snoring at night)?

Tired?

Yes No
O O
Do you often feel **Tired, Fatigued, or Sleepy** during the daytime (such as falling asleep) during driving or talking to someone)?

Observed?

Yes No
O O
Has anyone **Observed** you **Stop Breathing** or **Choking/Gasping** during your sleep?

Yes No
O O
Pressure?
Do you have or are being treated for **High blood pressure**?

Yes No
O O
Body Mass Index more than 35 kg/m^2?

Yes No
O O
Age more than 50 years?

Neck size large? (Measured around Adams apple)

Yes No
O O
For male, is your shirt collar 17 inches/43 cm or larger?
For female, is your shirt collar 16 inches/41 cm or larger?

Yes No
O O
Gender = Male?

Answer Yes/No, Score 1/0:

FIGURE 2.2 STOP-bang questionnaire.
Source: Modified from Chung et al. (2008). Reprinted with permission from the University Health Network.

Anesthetic and Perioperative Complications of OSA

Due to the multiple physiological stresses of sleep apnea, the disorder has been found to be an independent risk factor for perioperative complications in noncardiac surgery. OSA is also associated with major adverse events after cardiac surgery including the need for repeat revascularization, stroke, angina, and new onset atrial fibrillation (Memtsoudis et al., 2013; Munish et al., 2012; Kaw et al., 2012; Stundner et al., 2014).

In a study by Munish et al. (2012), 306 high-risk OSA patients were compared as a matched group with 3,286 low-risk patients. Postoperatively, the high-risk group had a higher incidence of hypoxia ($p < .01$), tracheal reintubation ($p < .001$), and CPAP use ($p < .001$). Overall, the incidence of a composite adverse event was 25.4% in the high-risk OSA group and only 17.4% in the low-risk matched group ($p < .01$). Despite the difference in perioperative morbidity, there was no difference in the rates of hospital readmission within 24 hours, intensive care unit (ICU) admission, LOS, or mortality among the two groups.

A meta-analysis of 13 studies regarding OSA and the incidence of postoperative outcomes by Kaw et al. (2012) further supported the role of OSA as an independent predictor of morbidity. In the meta-analysis, OSA was associated with a higher risk of postoperative cardiac events (OR 2.07, $p = .007$), acute respiratory failure (OR 2.43, $p = .003$), higher rates of desaturation (OR 2.27, $p = .01$), and transfer to the ICU (OR 2.81, $p = .002$).

Stundner et al. (2014) analyzed records from 84,655 patients who underwent posterior lumbar fusion to investigate the impact of sleep apnea on postoperative complications. In regression analysis, OSA emerged as an independent risk factor for postoperative mechanical ventilation, pneumonia, non-myocardial-infarction (MI) cardiac complications, acute renal failure, blood product transfusion, postoperative infection, prolonged hospitalization, and the need for critical care services (all $p < .0001$).

Memtsoudis et al. (2013) reviewed claims data on over 530,000 cases for patients undergoing total knee or total hip arthroplasty to determine if there was a difference in postoperative complications among OSA patients. Over the data collection period of 2006 to 2010, there was an increase in the incidence of OSA diagnosis from 6.1% to 10.3%, which confirms the rapid rise of this disease as previously mentioned. Overall, patients with OSA had a 47% increased risk for combined postoperative morbidity. The OSA patients exhibited a higher incidence of aspiration pneumonia, postoperative mechanical ventilation and non-invasive ventilator support, and new onset of atrial fibrillation. A higher level of nursing care such as ICU, telemetry, or step-down unit was utilized for 14.5% of OSA patients compared with only 8.1% of the general surgical population.

The importance of screening for OSA was confirmed by Lockhart et al. (2013). The authors found significant differences in one-year mortality between low-risk and high-risk patients screened using the STOP-Bang questionnaire (4.13% vs. 7.45%, $p < .0001$). This finding demonstrates the importance of using a validated tool to risk stratify patients, which will guide planning and coordination to minimize complications.

Recommendations for Management of Patients With OSA

Management of patients with OSA is similar to that for obese patients. Proper positioning with the use of a ramp for induction will reduce the number of passively closed airways and delay the onset of desaturation related to apnea during laryngoscopy. Pharyngeal airway closure can be prevented by application of 10 cm H_2O of PEEP during induction and ventilation (Kaw & Gay, 2015). Rapid induction and possible awake intubation is recommended, especially if a difficult intubation is anticipated.

The use of short-acting agents such as desflurane and propofol is preferred. Regional and neuraxial techniques have been shown to reduce postoperative complications, especially in the orthopedic population. When possible, a multimodal approach to pain management should be utilized. This includes the use of nonsteroidal anti-inflammatory drugs, paracetamol, tramadol, ketamine, pregabalin, and COX-2 inhibitors to minimize the use of opioids (Kaw & Gay, 2015). Intubated patients should be extubated awake, sitting upright, with full reversal of the neuromuscular blockade.

Postanesthetic management should be guided by the severity of the OSA, type of surgery being performed, narcotic analgesic needs, and the clinical course in the recovery room. Any outpatient procedure can be converted to an inpatient encounter if continued monitoring is required secondary to highly invasive surgery, high opioid requirement, underlying severe OSA, or witnessed episodes of apnea and episodic desaturation in the recovery room (Kaw et al., 2006). ICU admission is rarely needed except with patients exhibiting coexisting cardiopulmonary disease, difficult airway, or refractory postoperative pain (Kaw & Gay, 2015).

Patients who have their own CPAP machine should be instructed to bring it on the day of surgery so it can be used during the perioperative period. Although many institutions have developed protocols for CPAP use during the recovery phase, empirical data is lacking on the true impact of this practice for LOS and prevention of cardiorespiratory complications. Practice guidelines for management of patients with OSA had been recommending CPAP support in the early postoperative period since they were first published in 2006 (ASA Task Force, 2014); however, the data from Memtsoudis et al. (2013) showed only a modest increase in the use of ventilator resources for this patient population. They speculate that there has been a low rate of implementation of the recommendations of the task force, and it is possible that few departments have instituted policies to implement the changes for ventilator support of OSA patients. Further research is needed to evaluate that claim.

Optimal Inhalation Agent

Frequently implicated as a contributing factor for influencing postoperative recovery is the choice of inhalation agent used for the maintenance of anesthesia. The two most commonly used agents, desflurane and sevoflurane, have slightly different blood:gas and blood:fat solubility coefficients (0.45 vs. 0.65 and 15 vs. 41 respectively). This difference in fat solubility has a significant effect on the accumulation of agent in obese patients with a large vessel--poor compartment, which contributes to a prolonged terminal elimination (Lockwood, 2010).

Rapid emergence, transfer to the Post Anesthesia Care Unit (PACU), and timely discharge from PACU have become increasingly important to facilities in an effort to minimize cost, increase patient turnover, and improve resource utilization. In a review article by Jakobsson (2012), studies did not reveal differences in PACU time or post operative nausea and vomiting frequency between patients receiving up to 3 hours of sevoflurane or desflurane. However, a meta-analysis cited in the review found that patients receiving desflurane consistently had faster emergence times, followed commands more quickly, were extubated sooner, and were oriented to place and time earlier than those who had received sevoflurane or propofol.

In obese patients, the anesthetist is frequently concerned about the patients' ability to maintain their airway, manage secretions without intervention, and avoid aspiration if there were to be emesis after the endotracheal tube has been removed. Several studies in the review by Jakobsson (2012) agreed that patients anesthetized with desflurane had a faster return of cognitive function and were able to swallow a small amount of water sooner than patients anesthetized with sevoflurane.

Not all of the experts agree that one agent is superior to the other. Arain, Barth, Shankar, and Ebert (2005) found that there were no differences in emergence and recovery times among morbidly obese patients who received desflurane and sevoflurane when the anesthetic concentration was titrated to a defined BIS level intraoperatively. Jakobsson (2012) concludes that there are studies that refute the superiority of desflurane; however, the majority of studies, especially in the obese surgical population, have demonstrated the important characteristics of rapid emergence and extubation, early cognitive recovery, and improved postoperative ventilation and oxygenation compared to sevoflurane.

THE FUTURE OF ANESTHETIZING LOCATIONS

With the advancement of minimally invasive surgical techniques and the safety profile of the anesthetics in use today, an increasing number of surgical cases are moving out of the traditional hospital setting and into ambulatory surgery centers and office-based surgical suites. According to the American Hospital Association (AHA), the number of Medicare-certified Ambulatory Surgery Centers increased from 4,955 in 2008 to 5,364 in 2015, indicating a shift toward out-of-hospital services (AHA, 2015). Due to the variety of accrediting bodies for office-based practices, it is difficult to quantify the number of office-based surgeries; however, the AHA estimated that number doubled from 1995 to 2005 to approximately 10 million surgeries (AHA, 2008). This number has surely risen since that report was issued. Several mortality studies demonstrate the safety of office-based anesthesia compared to the hospital setting; however, the anesthetist should remain especially vigilant to the potential for disaster in this setting. Current conservative recommendations for patient selection in the office setting include limiting access for patients with an unstable physical status 3 or higher, recent MI in the past 6 months, BMI greater than 35, severe chronic obstructive pulmonary disease or OSA, end-stage renal disease, recent stroke within past 3 months, and lack of an adult escort (Twersky & Mohammad, 2013). The paucity of airway rescue devices, lack of availability of CPAP, and limited personnel to assist in an emergency should encourage a conservative approach to patient selection to promote quality outcomes and patient safety.

CONCLUSION

Although presented as separate conditions with unique anesthetic implications, obesity and OSA are frequently encountered together. The prevalence of OSA in obese or morbidly obese patients is nearly double the prevalence observed in normal-weight adults (Romero-Corral, Caples, Lopez, & Somers, 2010). The interaction among the two conditions is complex. Many times obesity, including obesity limited to the abdominal area, can increase the risk of OSA. However, OSA in the normal-weight patient can lead to obesity over time due to the interrupted sleep cycles and psychological changes related to sleep deprivation (Romero et al., 2010). In a study by Peppard et al. (2000), a modest weight gain of 10% resulted in a six-fold increase in the likelihood for moderate to severe OSA ($p < .001$). Conversely, a 10% weight loss can result in a 26% improvement in AHI score, reducing the impact and severity of OSA ($p < .001$).

As the incidence of obesity and sleep apnea continues to grow at a phenomenal pace, anesthetists are constantly challenged to remain educated regarding new agents and techniques as well as practice guideline recommendations to provide the highest quality of care. The reduction in 30-day mortality among these high-risk populations of obese and OSA patients to that of the normal-weight controls, despite the increases in postoperative complications cited in several studies (Munish et al., 2012), is a testament to the timely interventions and adjustments in treatment regimens on the part of the anesthetists caring for these patients. Preparation, anticipation, and clinical assessment skills will continue to be the hallmark of excellent care and patient safety.

ACKNOWLEDGMENT

The STOP-Bang Tool is proprietary to the University Health Network. Any reproduction and/or use of the STOP-Bang Tool without written permission from the University Health Network is strictly prohibited. For additional information, see online (www.stopbang.ca).

REFERENCES

American Hospital Association. (2008). Trendwatch Chartbook 2008—Chart 2.5 Percent of outpatient surgeries by facility type, 1981–2005. Retrieved from http://www.aha.org/research/reports/tw/chartbook/2008/08chapter2.pdf

American Hospital Association. (2015). Trendwatch Chartbook 2015—Chart 2.5 Number of Medicare-certified Ambulatory Surgical Centers, 2009–2014. Retrieved from http://www.aha.org/research/reports/tw/chartbook/ch2.shtml

American Society of Anesthesiologists Task Force on Perioperative Management of Patients with Obstructive Sleep Apnea. (2014). Practice guidelines for the perioperative management of patients with obstructive sleep apnea. *Anesthesiology, 120*(2), 1–19.

Aminian, A., Jamal, M., Andalib, A., Batayyah, E., Romero-Talamás, H., Chand, B., et al. (2015). Is laparoscopic bariatric surgery a safe option in extremely high-risk morbidly obese patients? *Journal of Laparoendoscopic & Advanced Surgical Techniques. Part A, 25*(9), 707–711.

Arain, S., Barth, C., Shankar, H., & Ebert, T. (2005). Choice of volatile anesthetic for the morbidly obese patient: Sevoflurane or desflurane. *Journal of Clinical Anesthesia, 17*, 413–419.

Buchwald, H., & Oien, D. (2013). Metabolic/Bariatric surgery worldwide 2011. *Obesity Surgery, 23*, 427–436.

Chung, F., Yegneswara, B., Liao, P., Chung, S., Vairavanthan, S., Islam, S., et al. (2008). STOP questionnaire. *Anesthesiology, 108*(5), 812–821.

Consensus Development Conference Panel. (1991). Gastrointestinal surgery for severe obesity. *Annals of Internal Medicine, 115*(12), 956–961.

D'Apuzzo, M., Novicoff, W., Browne, J. (2015). The John Insall Award: Morbid obesity independently impacts complications, mortality, and resource use after TKA. *Clinical Orthopaedics and Related Research, 473*(1), 57–63.

Domi, R., & Laho, H. (2012). Anesthetic challenges in the obese patient. *Journal of Anesthesia, 26*(5), 758–765.

Ebert, T., Shankar, H., & Haake, R. (2006). Perioperative considerations for patients with morbid obesity. *Anesthesiology Clinics, 24*(3), 621–636.

Finkelstein, E., Trogdon, J., Cohen, J., & Dietz, W. (2009). Annual medical spending attributable to obesity: Payer and service-specific estimates. *Health Affairs, 28*(5), 822–831.

Flegal, K., Carroll, M., Kit, B., & Ogden, C. (2012). Prevalence of obesity and trends in the distribution of body mass index among US adults, 1999–2010. *The Journal of the American Medical Association, 307*(5), 491–497.

Hahl, T., Peromaa-Haavisto, P., Tarkiainen, P., Knutar, O., & Victorzon, M. (2015). Outcome of laparoscopic gastric bypass (LRYGB) with a program for enhanced recovery after surgery (ERAS). *Obesity Surgery, 26*, 505–511.

Hammond, R., & Levine, R. (2010). The economic impact of obesity in the united states. *Diabetes, Metabolic Syndrome and Obesity: Targets and Therapy, 3*, 285–295.

Jakobsson, J. (2012). Desflurane: A clinical update of a third-generation inhaled anaesthetic. *Acta Anaesthesiologica Scandinavica, 56*(4), 420–432.

Jean, J., Compere, V., Fourdriner, V., Marguerite, C., Auquit-Auckbur, I., Milliez, P., et al. (2008). The risk of pulmonary aspiration in patients after weight loss due to bariatric surgery. *Anesthesia & Analgesia, 107*(4), 1257–1259.

Kaw, R. (2014). Perioperative complications in patients with obstructive sleep apnea. *Current Anestheisology Reports, 4*, 37–41.

Kaw, R., Chung, F., Pasupuleti, V., Mehta, J., Gay, P., & Hernandez, A. (2012). Meta-analysis of the association between obstructive sleep apnoea and postoperative outcome. *British Journal of Anaesthesia, 109*(6), 897–906.

Kaw, R., & Gay, P. (2015). Perioperative management of obstructive sleep apnea. *Current Sleep Medicine Reports, 1*, 251–256.

Kaw, R., Michota, F., Jaffer, A., Ghamande, S., Auckley, D., & Golish, J. (2006). Unrecognized sleep apnea in the surgical patient-implications for the perioperative setting. *Chest, 129*(1), 198–205.

Lockhart, E., Willingham, M., Abdallah, A., Helsten, D., Bedair, B., Thomas, J., et al. (2013). Obstructive sleep apnea screening and postoperative mortality in a large surgical cohort. *Sleep Medicine, 14*(5), 407–415.

Lockwood, G. (2010). Theoretical context-sensitive elimination times for inhalation anaesthetics. *British Journal of Anaesthesia, 1973*(45), 282–293.

Longitudinal Assessment of Bariatric Surgery (LABS) Consortium. (2009). Perioperative safety in the longitudinal assessment of bariatric surgery. *New England Journal of Medicine, 361*(5), 445–454.

Lundstrom, L., Moller, A., Rosenstock, C., Astrup, G., & Wetterslev, J. (2009). High body mass index is a weak predictor for difficult and failed tracheal intubation. *Anesthesiology, 110*, 266–274.

Mahajan, V., Hashmi, J., Singh, R., Samra, T., & Aneya, S. (2015). Comparative evaluation of gastric pH and volume in morbidly obese and lean patients undergoing elective surgery and effect of aspiration prophylaxis. *Journal of Clinical Anesthesiology, 27*(5), 396–400.

Mechanick, J., Youdim, A., Jones, D., Timothy, W., Hurley, D., Molly, M., et al. (2013). Clinical practice guidelines for the perioperative nutritional, metabolic, and nonsurgical support of the bariatric surgery patient–2013 Update. *Endocrine Practice, 9*(2), 337–372.

Memtsoudis, S., Stundner, O., Rasul, R., Sun, X., Chiu, Y., Fleischut, P., et al. (2013). Sleep apnea and total joint arthroplasty under various types of anesthesia: A population-based study of perioperative outcomes. *Regional Anesthesia and Pain Medicine, 38*(4), 274–281.

Minokadeh, A., Bishop, M., & Benumof, J. (2011). Obstructive sleep apnea, anesthesia, and ambulatory surgery. *Anesthesiology News Guide to Airway Management*, 72–78.

Munish, M., Sharma, V., Yarussi, K., Sifain, A., Porhomayon, J., & Nader, N. (2012). The use of practice guidelines by the American Society of Anesthesiologists for the identification of surgical patients at high risk for sleep apnea. *Chronic Respiratory Disease, 9*(4), 221–230.

Nagappa, M., Liao, P., Wong, J., Auckley, D., Ramachandran, S., Memtsoudis, S., et al. (2015). Validation of the STOP-bang questionnaire as a screening tool for obstructive sleep apnea among different populations: A systematic review and meta-analysis. *PLoS One, 10*(12), 1–21.

Ortiz, V., & Kwo, J. (2015). Obesity: Physiologic changes and implications for preoperative management. *BMC Anesthesiology, 15*(97), 1–12.

Peppard, P. E., Young, T., Barnet, J. H., Palta, M., Hagen, E. W., & Hla, K. M. (2013). Increased prevalence of sleep-disordered breathing in adults. *American Journal of Epidemiology, 177*, 1006–1014.

Peppard, P., Young, T., Palta, M., Dempsey, J., & Skatrud, J. (2000). Longitudinal study of moderate weight change and sleep-disordered breathing. *The Journal of the American Medical Association, 284*(23), 3015–3021.

Ribaric, G., Buchwald, J., McGlennon, T. (2013). Diabetes and weight in comparative studies of bariatric surgery vs. conventional medical therapy: A systematic review and meta-analysis. *Obesity Surgery, 24*, 437–455.

Romero-Corral, A., Caples, S., Lopez-Jimenez, F., Somers, V. (2010). Interactions between obesity and obstructive sleep apnea. Implications for treatment. *Chest, 137*(3), 711–719.

Singh, M., Liao, P., Kobah, S., Wijeysundera, C., Shapiro, C., & Chung, F. (2013). Proportion of surgical patients with undiagnosed sleep apnea. *British Journal of Anaesthesia, 110*(4), 629–636.

Stundner, O., Chiu, Y., Sun, X., Ramachandran, S., Gerner, P., Vougioukas, V., et al. (2014). Sleep apnoea adversely affects the outcome in patients who undergo posterior lumbar fusion: A population-based study. *The Bone & Joint Journal, 96-B*(2), 242–248.

Sturm, R., & Hattori, A. (2013). Morbid obesity rates continue to rise rapidly in the United States. *International Journal of Obesity, 37*(6), 889–891.

Terkawi, A., & Durieux, M. (2015, April). Perioperative anesthesia care for obese patients. *Anesthesiology News*, 1–12.

Thompson, D., Brown, J., Nichols, G., Elmer, P., & Oster, G. (2001). Body mass index and future healthcare costs. *Obesity Research, 9*(3), 210–218.

Tsara, V., Amfilochiou, A., Papagrigorakis, M., Georgopolous, D., & Liolios, E. (2009). Guidelines for diagnosis and treatment of sleep-related breathing disorders in adults and children. Definition and classification of sleep related breathing disorders in adults. Different types and indications for sleep studies (Part 1). *Hippokratia, 13*(3), 187–191.

Twersky, R., & Mohammad, S. (2013). Office based anesthesia: Challenges and successes. *Anesthesia and Analgesia, 41*(1), 125–134.

Warner, M., Warner, M., & Weber, J. (1993). Clinical significance of pulmonary aspiration during the perioperative period. *Anesthesiology, 78*, 56–62.

Welliver, M., Cheek, D., Osterbrink, J., & McDonough, J. (2015). Worldwide experience with sugammadex sodium: Implications for the United States. *AANA Journal, 83*(2), 107–115.

CHAPTER 3

Lung-Protective Ventilation

Rex A. Marley and Kaycee Simon

ABSTRACT

Historically, mechanical ventilation of the lungs utilizing relatively large tidal volumes was common practice in the operating room and intensive care unit (ICU). The rationale behind this treatment strategy was to yield better patient outcomes, that is, fewer pulmonary complications, and a reduction in morbidity and mortality. As evidence-based practice has evolved, potential harmful effects of traditional, nonphysiological mechanical ventilation (ventilation with larger tidal volumes and the tolerance of high airway pressures) even in short-term treatment have been shown to correlate with systemic inflammation and the development of ventilator-associated lung injury. Lung-protective ventilation principles using more physiological tidal volumes, avoiding high inspiratory plateau pressures, along with appropriate levels of positive end-expiratory pressure have been shown to decrease pulmonary complications and improve outcomes in patients with acute respiratory distress syndrome requiring ongoing ventilatory support in the ICU. In addition, current research is beginning to validate the benefit of providing more physiologic ventilator support in the operating room, particularly for high-risk patients undergoing major abdominal surgery, in minimizing acute lung injury. A review of lung-protective ventilation measures including benefits and potential side effects is presented. Additional treatment modalities and therapeutic considerations are offered for inclusion in optimal patient management.

http://dx.doi.org/10.1891/0739-6686.35.37

INTRODUCTION

Pulmonary complications, such as acute lung injury, atelectasis, pneumonia, and infection, associated with mechanically ventilated patients, remain a major contributor to increased patient morbidity and mortality (Esteban et al., 2013; Gu, Wang, & Liu, 2015). Significant postoperative pulmonary complications, occurring in approximately 5% of patients (Canet et al., 2010) are the second most common perioperative problem following wound infection (Khuri et al., 2005). Consequences of these pulmonary complications are an increased length of hospital stay, morbidity, and mortality (Canet et al., 2010; Mazo et al., 2014). The contributory role of mechanical ventilation to negative patient outcomes has been reassessed to determine whether modification in our traditional ventilatory management of the patient might translate into realized benefits and improved patient care. Conventional ventilatory parameters consisted of employing relatively large tidal volumes (V_T), in the range of 12 to 15 mL/kg of predicted body weight (PBW), with the belief that these larger breaths were safe, would prevent atelectasis, improve ventilation–perfusion mismatch, and reduce the need for high inspired oxygen concentrations. Positive end-expiratory pressure (PEEP) was not used routinely out of worry for impaired hemodynamic function. Concern over acute lung injury and ventilator-induced pulmonary infection led to questioning the role that the mechanical breath had in contributing to these pathologic conditions. Clinical evidence with supportive meta-analysis showed that relative alveolar overdistension (volutrauma) and high end-inspiratory plateau pressures (barotrauma) are key contributory elements in the development of mechanical ventilatory-induced pulmonary complications (Gu, Wang, & Liu, 2015; Serpa Neto et al., 2012; Serpa Neto, Schultz, & Gama de Abreu, 2015).

The body of scientific evidence now demonstrates that protective lung ventilation is beneficial in reducing acute lung injury, pulmonary infection, prolonged ventilator days, intensive care unit (ICU) stays, and mortality in ventilated patients with acute respiratory distress syndrome (ARDS). In addition, there is increasing evidence that patients without lung injury requiring mechanical ventilation will benefit from protective ventilation measures (Brower, Matthay, Morris, Schoenfeld, & The Acute Respiratory Distress Syndrome Network, 2000; Serpa Neto et al., 2012). Currently accepted ventilatory techniques, referred to as protective lung ventilation, tailored to minimize the negative pulmonary effects include delivering a reduced tidal volume breath thus lowering the mean airway pressure, maintaining appropriate PEEP level, safely limiting the inspired oxygen concentration, employing repeated lung recruitment maneuvers, and utilizing measures to reduce the potential for pulmonary infection (Table 3.1).

TABLE 3.1
Definition of Terms

Abbreviations or Acronym	Definition
PBW (predicted body weight)	Males: 106 pounds (48 kg) plus 6 pounds (2.7 kg) for every inch (2.54 cm) over 5 feet (1.5 m). Females: 100 pounds (45 kg) plus 5 pounds (2.3 kg) for every inch over 5 feet (1.5 m).
V_T (tidal volume)	Lung volume representing the normal volume of air displaced between normal inhalation and exhalation when extra effort is not applied.
f_b (frequency of breathing; respiratory rate)	The number of breaths taken during 1 minute.
$\dot{V}_E$ (minute ventilation)	Volume of air that is exhaled from the lungs in 1 minute. Product of tidal volume and respiratory frequency; V_T (mL) × f_b.
F_IO_2 (fractional concentration of inspired oxygen)	Inspired oxygen percentage expressed as a fraction, for example, inspired room air has an F_IO_2 of 0.21.
PEEP (positive end-expiratory pressure)	The pressure in the lungs (alveolar pressure) above atmospheric pressure that exists at the end of expiration following a mechanically delivered breath.
P_{plat} (end-inspiratory plateau pressure)	End-inspiratory airway pressure, which is reflective of peak alveolar pressure; should be kept as low as possible to prevent lung overdistension. Principal cause of ventilator-induced lung injury is an increased alveolar distending pressure.

MECHANICAL VENTILATION: HISTORICAL PERSPECTIVE

The polio epidemic of the 1950s led to the first widespread use of intermittent positive-pressure ventilation in humans to manage ventilatory failure. A standard method of patient management was via manual bag ventilation since mechanical ventilation was not readily available at this time (Lassen, 1953). Intermittent positive-pressure mechanical ventilation to manage polio patients in the United States was described in 1948 by interfacing the Bennett valve with a standard tank respirator (Bower, Bennett, Dillon, & Axelrod, 1950). As a result of the polio epidemic, the need for a reliable means, to consistently ventilate afflicted patients, was realized. The Engstrom ventilator, one of the first volume-cycled respirators, was beneficial in the long-term care of the polio patient (Engström, 1954). While normal spontaneous tidal volumes range between 6 and 8 mL/kg PBW (Remmers & Tenny, 1963), early consideration for V_T settings with volume-cycled ventilators recommended 12 to 15 mL/kg PBW. The rationale for such large V_T settings in the perioperative period was based on the belief that oxygenation and compliance is increased when peak airway pressure was higher, presumably from increasing end-expiratory lung volume and thus minimizing atelectasis (Bendixen, Whyte, & Laver, 1963). A management goal of normalizing patient acid–base status via augmentation of minute volume was believed achievable by these larger V_T settings. Oftentimes, this was achievable, but at the cost of requiring undesirably high peak inspiratory pressures.

Not appreciated during this early age of mechanical ventilation were the pathophysiologic changes these relatively larger V_T values produced in the lung. In recent years, research has focused on the potential deleterious affect positive airway pressure has on contributing to ventilator-associated lung injury (VALI). Ventilator-associated lung injury involves a complex interaction of regional overdistension of aerated lung tissue during inspiration (volutrauma), increased transpulmonary pressure (barotrauma), cyclic opening of atelectatic lung tissue during inspiration and the subsequent closing of the same alveoli during expiration (atelectotrauma), and the activation of inflammatory mediators (biotrauma); see Dos Santos and Slutsky (2000); Lionetti, Recchia, and Ranieri (2005).

VENTILATOR-ASSOCIATED LUNG INJURY

Pathophysiologic pulmonary changes, as evidenced by diffuse alveolar damage, are known to occur with the lung stress and strain associated when relatively large V_T values and or high peak inspiratory pressures are used to ventilate ARDS patients (Carrasco Loza, Villamizar Rodríguez, & Medel Fernández, 2015) as well as patients free of acute lung injury (Sutherasan, Vargas, & Pelosi, 2014). Clinical and animal studies have demonstrated that VALI symptoms develop in as little as 1.5 hours and up to 12 hours after initiation of conventional mechanical ventilation involving higher V_T values (12–15 mL/kg PBW) as evidenced by induced pulmonary and systemic biochemical and histologic changes involving reduced immunity and increased inflammation in previously healthy subjects without acute lung injury. Protective lung ventilation (6–8 mL/kg PBW) has been shown to minimize the pathophysiologic changes (Pinheiro de Oliveira, Hetzel, dos Anjos Silva, Dallegrave, & Friedman, 2010; Vroom et al., 2006).

The historically higher V_T (>10 mL/kg PBW) delivered via a mechanical ventilator is associated with localized lung inflammation in animal models (De Prost et al., 2013; Wellman et al., 2014), and in patients without preexisting lung injury (Jia, 2008; Pinheiro de Oliveira et al., 2010; Vroom et al., 2006; Wolthuis, 2008). The sustained mechanical stretch of hyperinflation, contributing to volutrauma, barotrauma, and biotrauma, may cause high stress leading to direct cell injury resulting in capillary damage and pulmonary edema (Spieth et al., 2014a), localized tissue inflammation, sustained increase in the local and systemic release of lung borne inflammatory markers (cytokines, interleukins, tumor necrosis factor-a) as well as procoagulant changes in alveolar fluid (Rocco, Dos Santos, & Pelosi, 2012). Polymorphonuclear leukocyte recruitment and activation appear to be key components of the mechanical-stretch-induced inflammatory response (Lionetti, Recchia, & Ranieri, 2005). Nonprotective lung mechanical ventilation for as short as 5 hours will promote localized bronchoalveolar inflammatory changes and activate coagulation in patients without preexisting lung injury (Wolthuis, 2008). The biotrauma invoked by the pulmonary proinflammatory markers can also create a systemic inflammatory response and induce or make worse systemic organ, that is, kidney and small intestine, dysfunction (Plötz, Slutsky, van Vught, & Heijnen, 2004).

In poorly aerated lung tissue areas, the mechanical stretch from cyclical alveolar opening and closing, known as atelectotrauma, creates an inflammatory reaction in alveolar and vascular endothelial cells contributing to VALI (Borges et al., 2014; Slinger, 2015). Repetitive overdistension of alveoli will contribute to surfactant inactivation, which increases surface tension and leads to atelectasis (De Prost & Dreyfuss, 2012). A role of PEEP in protective lung ventilation is to stabilize the alveoli by increasing the end-expiratory lung volume and thus avoid derecruitment.

High inspired oxygen concentrations over time may induce acute lung injury by increasing oxidative stress via increased levels of reactive oxygen-derived free radicals, leading to a release of inflammatory mediators, endothelial cell injury, and increased capillary permeability (Kallet & Matthay, 2013). In subjects with preexisting lung inflammation and alterations in permeability as a result of lung injury, including VALI, there is an increased risk of oxygen toxicity (Aggarwal & Brower, 2014).

Ventilator-associated pneumonia (VAP) is a nosocomial pulmonary infection that occurs in tracheally intubated patients requiring mechanical ventilation for longer than 48 hours (Bassi, Ferrer, Marti, Comaru, & Torres, 2014), largely in part due to the reduced immunity and increased inflammatory response of mechanical ventilation on the lung. VAP occurs at a rate of 17.2 per

1,000 ventilator days (Rosenthal et al., 2012a), and is responsible for prolonged need for mechanical ventilation, increased length of ICU and hospital stay, and increased cost and morbidity (Borgatta & Rello, 2014).

PROTECTIVE LUNG VENTILATION MANAGEMENT

Patient management strategies designed to minimize the deleterious effects of positive-pressure ventilation on the lung have evolved such that goals of perioperative protective lung ventilatory strategies include maintaining:

- Physiologically low V_T ventilator settings to minimize volutrauma
- Moderate levels of PEEP along with periodic lung recruitment maneuvers to prevent atelectotrauma
- Low end-inspiratory plateau pressure to avoid barotrauma (Coppola, Froio, Chiumello, 2014; Futier, Marret, & Jaber, 2014; Goldenberg, Steinberg, Lee, Wijeysundera, & Kavanagh, 2014)
- Low inspired oxygen concentrations to prevent oxygen toxicity and absorption atelectasis
- Measures to reduce the chance for ventilator-associated infection

Lung-protective measures should be initiated early in the ventilatory process since deleterious effects of mechanical ventilation are, in part, dependent on the duration of mechanical ventilation.

In the intensive care setting, lung-protective ventilation principles have been shown to minimize VALI in subjects with ARDS (Brower et al., 2000; Samary et al., 2015), and in those without ARDS (Pinheiro de Oliveira et al., 2010; Serpa Neto et al., 2012). In ICU patients, a reduction in pulmonary complications of 28% was noted in patients who received protective lung ventilation when compared with patients who were ventilated with higher V_T values (Serpa Nato et al., 2015). A comprehensive approach to patient lung-protective ventilatory management, in the operating room and ICU, will minimize biotrauma and the resultant inflammatory process with an end result of reduced pulmonary complications, and morbidity and mortality (Serpa Nato et al., 2012; Serpa Nato, Schultz, & Gama de Abreu, 2015). Several management challenges of protective ventilation have been identified primarily from the hemodynamic effects secondary to positive pressure inhibiting venous return to the heart, or from a patient acceptance of the various ventilatory parameters (Table 3.2; Rubenfeld, Cooper, Carter, Thompson, & Hudson, 2004; Villar & Slutsky, 2010).

TABLE 3.2
Potential Side Effects of Protective Ventilation

Treatment Measure	Adverse Outcome
PEEP and recruitment maneuvers	Hemodynamics Impairment: reduction in right ventricular preload and an increase in right ventricular afterload leading to lower stroke volume, reduction in cardiac output; hypotension requiring the use of fluids and vasopressors Barotrauma risk at high PEEP levels
Low tidal volume	Patient discomfort and increased feeling of dyspnea leading to increased use of sedatives and muscle relaxants Increased ICU delirium, secondary to use of sedatives/muscle relaxants Increased ICU weakness, secondary to use of sedatives/muscle relaxants Increased duration of mechanical ventilation

Source: Modified from Rubenfeld, Cooper, Carter, Thompson, and Hudson (2004), Villar and Slutsky (2010).

Tidal Volume

Tidal volume settings should be limited to 5 to 8 mL/kg PBW with consideration in patients with ARDS to limit breaths to less than 6 mL/kg PBW to ensure less mechanical stress on the alveolar–capillary membrane and thus prevent alveolar overdistension, and improvement of alveolar stability (Gu, Wang, & Liu, 2015; Ogbu, Martin, & Murphy, 2015). Tidal volume limits of 6 mL/kg or less and plateau pressures less than or equal to 30 cm H_2O in patients with ARDS have shown a reduction in patient mortality, and is considered the standard of ventilatory care (Brower et al., 2000; Lionetti, Recchia, & Ranieri, 2005; Ogbu, Martin, & Murphy, 2015; Serpa Nato et al., 2015).

PEEP

Atelectasis is recognized as an important component in the pathogenesis of postoperative pulmonary complications, such as hypoxemia, pulmonary infections, and local inflammatory response (Tusman, Bohm, Warner, & Sprung, 2011). Absorption atelectasis occurs with the induction of anesthesia, especially when high fractional concentration of inspired oxygen (F_IO_2) is employed leading to increased ventilation–perfusion mismatching. When low V_T breaths are given, atelectasis from alveolar collapse and atelectotrauma is likely to occur with the cyclic opening and closing of alveoli with each breath (Slutsky & Ranieri, 2013). PEEP is beneficial with atelectotrauma *by* maintaining the protective lung ventilation strategy of utilizing smaller V_T, by minimizing alveolar unit stability during the entire breathing cycle. The best PEEP level in concert with protective lung ventilation strategy remains undetermined and challenging in patients with ARDS secondary to the differences in regional lung ventilation. A relatively higher PEEP level may be required to stabilize alveoli and prevent derecruitment with each breath in the dependent zones, yet hyperinflation with the potential for volutrauma and barotrauma may present in the nondependent lung regions.

Plateau Pressure (P_{plat})

There is a dose–response relationship between plateau pressure and major respiratory complications. Maintaining an end-inspiratory plateau pressure of less than 30 cm H_2O is desirable to minimize the barotrauma associated with mechanical ventilation (Ogbu, Martin, & Murphy, 2015). The current plateau pressure thresholds considered protective in critically ill patients with lung injury (<30 cm H_2O) may not be low enough for patients with uninjured lungs, and maintaining plateau pressure to no more than 20 cm H_2O has been suggested (Slutsky & Ranieri, 2013). In ARDS patients, further reduction in V_T even with maintaining P_{plat} less than 30 cm H_2O has been shown to have beneficial effects (Brower et al., 2000). Making adjustments to the ventilator driving pressure, that is, modifying the inspiratory-to-expiratory ratio, to reduce plateau pressure is associated with increased patient survival in ARDS patients (Amato et al., 2015).

Permissive Hypercapnia

With protective lung ventilation and accompanying reduction in lung stretch and stress, a tolerance for hypoventilation and a higher $PaCO_2$ is often accepted as one of the ARDS treatments that might improve patient survival in appropriate settings (Contreras, Masterson, & Laffey, 2015; Gu, Wang, & Liu, 2015). Elevated $PaCO_2$ may exhibit adverse effects in certain clinical situations, for example, in patients with increased intracranial pressure or pulmonary vascular resistance, and may not be an appropriate treatment measure. Moderate hypercapnia, in conjunction with reduced plateau pressure, has been shown to protect against VALI, mechanical stretch injury, and the promotion of the inflammatory cascade (Otulakowski et al., 2014), yet conclusive evidence is currently lacking to allow generalized recommendations.

Inspired Oxygen Concentration

Hyperoxia is a condition of excess oxygen in body tissues, and over time may induce pathophysiologic changes (Thomson & Paton, 2014). Pulmonary oxygen toxicity results from longer exposure (at 90% inspired oxygen, it may take 4–22 hours to manifest symptoms of pulmonary oxygen toxicity; Bitterman, 2009) to elevated partial pressures of oxygen over time. A risk factor for the development of postoperative pulmonary complications is the use of a high F_IO_2 during anesthesia (Güldner et al., 2015). For that reason, the lowest acceptable F_IO_2 required to maintain the target P_aO2 should be utilized. Toxic effects of inspired oxygen on the lungs have been shown at inspired oxygen concentrations as low as 50% (Aggarwal & Brower, 2014).

Lung Recruitment Maneuvers

Lung recruitment maneuvers transiently apply increasing airway pressure during mechanical ventilation with the goal of reopening collapsed alveolar regions, improving pulmonary mechanics (increase functional residual capacity, maintain respiratory system elastance), and increase oxygenation (Santos, Silva, Pelosi, & Rocco, 2015). Although PEEP is not capable of opening closed alveoli, adequate ongoing PEEP is important to maintain the open alveoli and prevent recollapse in conjunction with lung recruitment maneuvers (Coppola, Froio, & Chiumello, 2014). A 6% reduction in mortality was documented when recruitment maneuvers were part of the comprehensive care of mechanically ventilated patients with moderate to severe ARDS (Suzumura et al., 2014).

Three common alveolar recruitment maneuvers have been advocated: (a) the sigh (high V_T in controlled mode up to a specific plateau pressure level for a select number of sighs per minute, e.g., three consecutive sighs at 45 cm H_2O), (b) sustained inflation (increase in airway pressure to 40 cm H_2O and maintained for 40 seconds), and (c) stepwise increases of PEEP and/or airway inspiratory pressure (slowly increasing transpulmonary pressure instead of rapidly increasing with sustained inflation; Santos et al., 2015). It is important to monitor patients during recruitment maneuvers for undesired side effects, that is, hemodynamic instability, hypoxemia, or problematic cardiac arrhythmias. The optimal lung recruitment maneuver based on clinically important outcomes is not well established and needs further evaluation (Santos et al., 2015).

Pulmonary Infection Considerations

VAP refers to pneumonia occurring 48 to 72 hours following endotracheal intubation (Bailey & Kalil, 2015). The incidence of VAP approximates 16% of intubated and mechanically ventilated patients and is the most frequent infection occurring in the ICU (Rosenthal et al., 2012b). Endotracheal intubation and subsequent ongoing airway management via the endotracheal tube increases patient susceptibility for VAP via several modalities: (a) aspiration of oropharyngeal secretion during endotracheal intubation, (b) decreased mucosal integrity and mucociliary clearance of secretions subsequent to tracheal wall trauma, (c) microaspiration of secretions around the inflated endotracheal tube, and (d) bacterial colonization and biofilm formation within the endotracheal tube lumen (Deem & Treggiari, 2010).

Additional risk factors for the development of VAP secondary to increasing prevalence of multidrug-resistant (MDR) pathogens include recent prolonged hospitalization, multiple comorbidities, recent broad-spectrum antibiotic therapy, poor functional status, prior infection with MDR organisms, and high disease severity at presentation (Bailey & Kalil, 2015). Currently VAP management is hindered by the lack of a diagnostic gold standard to differentiate airway contamination or colonization versus infection (Borgatta & Rello, 2014). Treatment options and recommendations for reducing the incidence of VAP are listed in Table 3.3 (Deem & Treggiari, 2010; Price et al., 2014; Pugh, Grant, Cooke, & Dempsey, 2015; Society et al., 2005; Tokmaji et al., 2015).

TABLE 3.3

Treatment Regime for Ventilator-Associated Pneumonia

Avoid endotracheal intubations and reintubations when possible
Silver-coated endotracheal tubes may be beneficial in reducing VAP based on limited data; larger studies required for conclusive data
Oropharyngeal hygiene including the application of poorly absorbable antibiotics only to the oropharynx
Utilize noninvasive ventilation whenever appropriate
Orotracheal intubation and orogastric tubes are preferred over nasotracheal intubation and nasogastric tubes to prevent nosocomial sinusitis
Continuous aspiration of subglottic secretions should be used
Endotracheal tube cuff pressure should be maintained at greater than 20 cm H_2O to prevent leakage of bacterial pathogens around the cuff and into the lower respiratory tract
Contaminated condensate should be carefully emptied from ventilator circuits and condensate should be prevented from entering either the endotracheal tube or inline medication nebulizers

(Continued)

TABLE 3.3
Treatment Regime for Ventilator-Associated Pneumonia (Continued)

Passive humidifiers or heat–moisture exchangers decrease ventilator circuit colonization, but have not consistently reduced the incidence of VAP, and thus they cannot be regarded as a pneumonia prevention tool
Reduced duration of intubation and mechanical ventilation may prevent VAP and can be achieved by protocols to improve the use of sedation and to accelerate weaning
Maintain semirecumbent position (30–45 degrees) rather than supine to prevent aspiration, especially when receiving enteral feeding
Antibiotic treatment for VAP • Initiate short-course (7–8 days) broad-spectrum antibiotic treatment early. May reduce antibiotic exposure in the critically ill, with reduced emergence of resistant organisms, and potential for reduction in antibiotic-associated morbidity and cost savings, but is unlikely to be appropriate for all patients with VAP secondary to nonfermenting Gram-negative bacilli • Pending cultures, which should be collected from all patients prior to initiation of antibiotic therapy, empirical antibiotic treatment against likely pathogens (local hospital and intensive care unit microbiological susceptibilities) • Once microbiological tests confirm presenting microorganisms, change to appropriate antibiotic if indicated, and deescalate per microbiological culture results and when patient response is satisfying

Source: Modified from Deem and Treggiari (2010), Price et al. (2014), Puch, Grant, Cooke, and Dempsey (2015), Society et al. (2005), Tokmaji et al. (2015).

Note. VAP = ventilator-associated pneumonia.

EVIDENCE FOR SHORT-TERM VENTILATION UNDER GENERAL ANESTHESIA

Numerous factors, including the use of anesthetic and neuromuscular blocking agents, contribute to a loss of respiratory muscle tone, reduction in lung volume, alteration in diaphragmatic position, further ventilation–perfusion mismatching, pulmonary surfactant alteration, and the promotion of atelectasis and acute lung injury in patients receiving general anesthesia for surgery (Spieth et al., 2014b). The induction of general anesthesia contributes to a reduction in lung volume and the development of atelectasis leading to gas exchange and respiratory mechanic impairment (Hedenstierna & Edmark, 2005). Nearly 90% of patients undergoing general anesthesia for surgery will develop some degree of increasing atelectasis (Duggan & Kavanagh, 2005). Low tidal volume ventilation in conjunction with PEEP has been accepted practice in anesthesia for many years in patients undergoing one-lung ventilation for thoracic procedures. However, the traditional intraoperative two-lung ventilation technique of tidal volumes greater than 10 mL/kg PBW without PEEP remains commonplace (Bender et al., 2015) with even relatively higher tidal volumes seen in the female, obese, or patients of short stature (Fernandez-Bustamante, Wood, Tran, & Moine, 2011). A large multicenter observational study of more than 2,900 patients undergoing general anesthesia showed that 18% of patients were ventilated with a V_T greater than 10 mL/kg PBW and 81% without PEEP (Jaber et al., 2012). In U.S. academic centers, a substantial reduction in delivered tidal volume has evolved to the point where approximately 50% of anesthetics with endotracheal intubation for general surgery utilize lower tidal volumes in combination with PEEP (Wanderer et al., 2015). There is now sufficient evidence to suggest the benefit of the protective ventilatory strategy for short-term management of those having general anesthesia. The benefits include improved pulmonary function and postoperative arterial oxygenation, reduced postoperative pulmonary complications through incorporation of lung-protective ventilation strategy to include maintaining a low peak inspiratory pressure along with a P_{plat} goal of 16 cm H_2O or less, PEEP of 2 to 5 cm H_2O, and use of lung recruitment maneuvers (Canet et al., 2015; Filho & Serpa Neto, 2015; Futier et al., 2013; Gu, Wang, & Liu, 2015; Ladha et al., 2015; Serpa Neto et al., 2012; Serpa Neto, Schultz, & Gama de Abreu, 2015; Serpa Neto, Schultz, & Slutsky, 2015; Severgnini et al., 2013; Staehr-Rye & Eikermann, 2015).

Lung-protective ventilation should be considered routine care in the presence of pulmonary disease, prolonged anesthesia, in high-risk patients, or for high-risk surgery, such as in patients undergoing major abdominal procedures (Coppola, Froio, & Chiumello, 2014; Park, 2016). A reduction in postoperative mortality was shown when intraoperative lung-protective ventilation of lower tidal volumes (6–8 mL/kg PBW) with PEEP was used, compared with ventilating patients with intermediate to high risk of pulmonary complications after major abdominal surgery with a larger tidal volume (10–12 mL/kg PBW) and no PEEP (Futier et al., 2013).

CONCLUSION

Minimizing lung injury as a result of mechanical ventilation is a desirable goal in the operating room and ICU. The best practice ventilation management model for avoiding acute lung injury in this population continues to evolve while additional scientific support is gathered to justify individualized best patient management options. Overall, lung-protective ventilation measures, which are already a standard of patient care in the ICU, are now considered desirable for high-risk patients and/or surgeries in the operating room.

REFERENCES

Aggarwal, N. R., & Brower, R. G. (2014). Targeting normoxemia in acute respiratory distress syndrome may cause worse short-term outcomes because of oxygen toxicity. *Annals of the American Thoracic Society, 11*(9), 1449–1453. http://dx.doi.org/10.1513/annalsats.201407-297ps

Amato, M. B. P., Meade, M. O., Slutsky, A. S., Brochard, L., Costa, E. L. V., Schoenfeld, D. A., et al. (2015). Driving pressure and survival in the acute respiratory distress syndrome. *The New England Journal of Medicine, 372*(8), 747–755. http://dx.doi.org/10.1056/nejmsa1410639

Bailey, K. L., & Kalil, A. C. (2015). Ventilator-associated pneumonia (VAP) with multidrug-resistant (MDR) pathogens: Optimal treatment? *Current Infectious Disease Reports, 17*(8), 1–6. http://dx.doi.org/10.1007/s11908-015-0494-5

Bassi, G. L., Ferrer, M., Marti, J. D., Comaru, T., & Torres, A. (2014). Ventilator-associated pneumonia. *Seminars in Respiratory and Critical Care Medicine, 35*(4), 469.

Bender, S. P., Paganelli, W. C., Gerety, L. P., Tharp, W. G., Shanks, A. M., Housey, M, et al. (2015). Intraoperative lung-protective ventilation trends and practice patterns: A report from the multicenter perioperative outcomes group. *Anesthesia & Analgesia, 121*(5), 1231–1239. http://dx.doi.org/10.1213/ane.0000000000000940

Bendixen, H. H., Whyte, H., & Laver, M. B. (1963). Impaired oxygenation in surgical patients during general anesthesia with controlled ventilation: A concept of atelectasis. *The New England Journal of Medicine, 269*(19), 991–996. http://dx.doi.org/10.1056/nejm196311072691901

Bitterman, H. (2009). Bench-to-bedside review: Oxygen as a drug. *Critical Care (London, England), 13*(1), 205–205. http://dx.doi.org/10.1186/cc7151

Borgatta, B., & Rello, J. (2014). How to approach and treat VAP in ICU patients. *BMC Infectious Diseases, 14*(1), 211–211. http://dx.doi.org/10.1186/1471-2334-14-211

Borges, J. B., Okamoto, V. N., Matos, G. F. J., Caramez, M. P. R., Arantes, P. R., Barros, F., et al. (2006). Reversibility of lung collapse and hypoxemia in early acute respiratory distress syndrome. *American Journal of Respiratory and Critical Care Medicine, 174*(3), 268–278. http://dx.doi.org/10.1164/rccm.200506-976oc

Bower, A. G., Bennett, V. R., Dillon, J. B., & Axelrod, B. (1950). Investigation on the case and treatment of poliomyelitis patients. *Annals West Medicine Surgery*, *4*, 561–715.

Brower, R. G., Matthay, M. A., Morris, A., Schoenfeld, D., & The Acute Respiratory Distress Syndrome Network. (2000). Ventilation with lower tidal volumes as compared with traditional tidal volumes for acute lung injury and the acute respiratory distress syndrome. *The New England Journal of Medicine, 342*(18), 1301–1308. http://dx.doi.org/10.1056/nejm200005043421801

Canet, J., Gallart, L., Gomar, C., Paluzie, G., Vallès, J., Castillo, J., et al. (2010). Prediction of postoperative pulmonary complications in a population-based surgical cohort. *Anesthesiology, 113*(6), 1338–1350. http://dx.doi.org/10.1097/aln.0b013e3181fc6e0a

Canet, J., Sabaté, S., Mazo, V., Gallart, L., de Abreu, M. G., Belda, J., et al. (2015). Development and validation of a score to predict postoperative respiratory failure in a multicentre European cohort: A prospective, observational study. *European Journal of Anaesthesiology*, *32*(7), 458. http://dx.doi.org/10.1097/eja.0000000000000223

Carrasco Loza, R., Villamizar Rodríguez, G., & Medel Fernández, N. (2015). Ventilator-induced lung injury (VILI) in acute respiratory distress syndrome (ARDS): Volutrauma and molecular effects. *The Open Respiratory Medicine Journal*, *9*(Suppl. 2: M6), 112–119. http://dx.doi.org/10.2174/1874306401509010112

Contreras, M., Masterson, C., & Laffey, J. G. (2015). Permissive hypercapnia: What to remember. *Current Opinion in Anaesthesiology, 28*(1), 26–37. http://dx.doi.org/10.1097/aco.0000000000000151

Coppola, S., Froio, S., & Chiumello, D. (2014). Protective lung ventilation during general anesthesia: Is there any evidence? *Critical Care, 18*(2), 210. http://doi.org/10.1186/cc13777

De Prost, N., Costa, E. L., Wellman, T., Musch, G., Tucci, M. R., Winkler, T., et al. (2013). Effects of ventilation strategy on distribution of lung inflammatory cell activity. *Critical Care (London, England), 17*(4), R175–R175. http://dx.doi.org/10.1186/cc12854

De Prost, N., & Dreyfuss, D. (2012). How to prevent ventilator-induced lung injury? *Minerva Anestesiologica, 78*(9), 1054.

Deem, S., & Treggiari, M. M. (2010). New endotracheal tubes designed to prevent ventilator-associated pneumonia: Do they make a difference? *Respiratory Care, 55*(8), 1046.

Dos Santos, C. C., & Slutsky, A. S. (2000). Cellular responses to mechanical stress: Invited review: Mechanisms of ventilator-induced lung injury: A perspective. *Journal of Applied Physiology, 89*(4), 1645.

Duggan, M., & Kavanagh, B. P. (2005). Pulmonary atelectasis: A pathogenic perioperative entity. *Anesthesiology, 102*(4), 838–854. http://dx.doi.org/10.1097/00000542-200504000-00021

Engström, C. (1954). Treatment of severe cases of respiratory paralysis by the engstrom universal respirator. *The British Medical Journal, 2*(4889), 666–669.

Esteban, A., Frutos-Vivar, F., Muriel, A., Ferguson, N. D., Peñuelas, O., Abraira, V., et al. (2013). Evolution of mortality over time in patients receiving mechanical ventilation. *American Journal of Respiratory and Critical Care Medicine, 188*(2), 220.

Fernandez-Bustamante, A., Wood, C. L., Tran, Z. V., & Moine, P. (2011). Intraoperative ventilation: Incidence and risk factors for receiving large tidal volumes during general anesthesia. *BMC Anesthesiology, 11*(1), 22–22. http://dx.doi.org/10.1186/1471-2253-11-22

Filho, R. R., & Serpa Neto, A. (2015). One more brick in the wall of protective ventilation in surgical patients. *Annals of Translational Medicine, 3*(21), 339.

Futier, E., Constantin, J., Paugam-Burtz, C., Pascal, J., Eurin, M., Neuschwander, A., et al. (2013). A trial of intraoperative low-tidal-volume ventilation in abdominal surgery. *The New England Journal of Medicine, 369*(5), 428.

Futier, E., Marret, E., & Jaber, S. (2014). Perioperative positive pressure ventilation: An integrated approach to improve pulmonary care. *Anesthesiology, 121*(2), 400–408. http://dx.doi.org/10.1097/aln.0000000000000335

Goldenberg, N. M., Steinberg, B. E., Lee, W. L., Wijeysundera, D. N., & Kavanagh, B. P. (2014). Lung-protective ventilation in the operating room: Time to implement? *Anesthesiology, 121*(1), 184–188. http://dx.doi.org/10.1097/aln.0000000000000274

Gu, W., Wang, F., & Liu, J. (2015). Effect of lung-protective ventilation with lower tidal volumes on clinical outcomes among patients undergoing surgery: A meta-analysis of randomized controlled trials. *Canadian Medical Association Journal, 187*(3), E101–E109. http://dx.doi.org/10.1503/cmaj.141005

Güldner, A., Kiss, T., Serpa Neto, A., Hemmes, S. N. T., Canet, J., Spieth, P. M., et al. (2015). Intraoperative protective mechanical ventilation for prevention of postoperative pulmonary complications: A comprehensive review of the role of tidal volume, positive end-expiratory pressure, and lung recruitment maneuvers. *Anesthesiology, 123*(3), 692–713. http://dx.doi.org/10.1097/aln.0000000000000754

Hedenstierna, G., & Edmark, L. (2005). The effects of anesthesia and muscle paralysis on the respiratory system. *Intensive Care Medicine, 31*(10), 1327–1335. http://dx.doi.org/10.1007/s00134-005-2761-7

Hegeman, M. A., Hemmes, S. N. T., Kuipers, M. T., Bos, L. D. J., Jongsma, G., Roelofs, J. J. T. H., et al. (2013). The extent of ventilator-induced lung injury in mice partly depends on duration of mechanical ventilation. *Critical Care Research and Practice, 2013*, 1–11. http://doi.org/10.1155/2013/435236

Jaber, S., Coisel, Y., Chanques, G., Futier, E., Constantin, J., Michelet, P., et al. (2012). A multicentre observational study of intra-operative ventilatory management during general anaesthesia: Tidal volumes and relation to body weight. *Anaesthesia, 67*(9), 999–1008. http://dx.doi.org/10.1111/j.1365-2044.2012.07218.x

Jia, X. (2008). Risk factors for ARDS in patients receiving mechanical ventilation for > 48 h. *Chest, 133*(4), 853–861. http://dx.doi.org/10.1378/chest.07-1121

Kallet, R. H., & Matthay, M. A. (2013). Hyperoxic acute lung injury. *Respiratory Care, 58*(1), 123–141. http://dx.doi.org/10.4187/respcare.01963

Khuri, S. F., Henderson, W. G., DePalma, R. G., Mosca, C., Healey, N. A., Kumbhani, D. J., & Participants in the VA National Surgical Quality Improvement Program. (2005). Determinants of long-term survival after major surgery and the adverse effect of postoperative complications. *Transactions of the . . . Meeting of the American Surgical Association, 242*(3), 326–348. http://dx.doi.org/10.1097/01.sla.0000179621.33268.83

Ladha, K., Vidal Melo, M. F., McLean, D. J., Wanderer, J. P., Grabitz, S. D., Kurth, T., et al. (2015). Intraoperative protective mechanical ventilation and risk of postoperative respiratory complications: Hospital based registry study. *BMJ (Clinical Research Ed.), 351*, h3646.

Lassen, H. C. A. (1953). A preliminary report on the 1952 epidemic of poliomyelitis in Copenhagen with special reference to the treatment of acute respiratory insufficiency. *The Lancet, 261*(6749), 37–41. http://dx.doi.org/10.1016/s0140-6736(53)92530-6

Lionetti, V., Recchia, F. A., & Ranieri, V. M. (2005). Overview of ventilator-induced lung injury mechanisms. *Current Opinion in Critical Care, 11*(1), 82–86. http://dx.doi.org/10.1097/00075198-200502000-00013

Mazo, V., Sabaté, S., Canet, J., Gallart, L., de Abreu, M. G., Belda, J., et al. (2014). Prospective external validation of a predictive score for postoperative pulmonary complications. *Anesthesiology, 121*(2), 219–231. http://dx.doi.org/10.1097/aln.0000000000000334

Ogbu, O. C., Martin, G. S., & Murphy, D. J. (2015). A few milliliters of prevention: Lung-protective ventilation decreases pulmonary complications. *Critical Care Medicine, 43*(10), 2263–2264. http://dx.doi.org/10.1097/ccm.0000000000001234

Otulakowski, G., Engelberts, D., Gusarova, G. A., Bhattacharya, J., Post, M., & Kavanagh, B. P. (2014). Hypercapnia attenuates ventilator-induced lung injury via a disintegrin and metalloprotease-17. *The Journal of Physiology, 592*(20), 4507–4521. http://dx.doi.org/10.1113/jphysiol.2014.277616

Park, S. (2016). Perioperative lung-protective ventilation strategy reduces postoperative pulmonary complications in patients undergoing thoracic and major abdominal surgery. *Korean Journal of Anesthesiology, 69*(1), 3–7. http://dx.doi.org/10.4097/kjae.2016.69.1.3

Pinheiro de Oliveira, R., Hetzel, M. P., dos Anjos Silva, M., Dallegrave, D., & Friedman, G. (2010). Mechanical ventilation with high tidal volume induces inflammation in patients without lung disease. *Critical Care (London, England), 14*(2), R39–R39. http://dx.doi.org/10.1186/cc8919

Plötz, F. B., Slutsky, A. S., van Vught, A. J., & Heijnen, C. J. (2004). Ventilator-induced lung injury and multiple system organ failure: A critical review of facts and hypotheses. *Intensive Care Medicine, 30*(10), 1865–1872. http://dx.doi.org/10.1007/s00134-004-2363-9

Price, R., MacLennan, G., Glen, J., SuDDICU Collaboration, & on behalf of the SuDDICU collaboration. (2014). Selective digestive or oropharyngeal decontamination and topical oropharyngeal chlorhexidine for prevention of death in general intensive care: Systematic review and network meta-analysis. *BMJ (Clinical Research Ed.), 348*(mar31 2), g2197–g2197. http://dx.doi.org/10.1136/bmj.g2197

Pugh, R., Grant, C., Cooke, R. P. D., & Dempsey, G. (2015). Short-course versus prolonged-course antibiotic therapy for hospital-acquired pneumonia in critically ill adults. *The Cochrane Database of Systematic Reviews, 8*, CD007577.

Remmers, J. E., & Tenny, S. M. (1963). Comparative quantitative morphology of the mammalian lung: Diffusing area. *Nature, 197*(4862), 54–56. http://dx.doi.org/10.1038/197054a0

Rocco, P. R. M., Dos Santos, C., & Pelosi, P. (2012). Pathophysiology of ventilator-associated lung injury. *Current Opinion in Anaesthesiology, 25*(2), 123–130. http://dx.doi.org/10.1097/aco.0b013e32834f8c7f

Rosenthal, V. D., Bijie, H., Maki, D. G., Mehta, Y., Apisarnthanarak, A., Medeiros, E. A., & INICC members. (2012b). International nosocomial infection control consortium (INICC) report, data summary of 36 countries, for 2004-2009. *American Journal of Infection Control, 40*(5), 396. http://dx.doi.org/10.1016/j.ajic.2011.05.020

Rosenthal, V. D., Rodrigues, C., álvarez-Moreno, C., Madani, N., Mitrev, Z., Ye, G., et al. (2012a). Effectiveness of a multidimensional approach for prevention of ventilator-associated pneumonia in adult intensive care units from 14 developing countries of four continents: Findings of the international nosocomial infection control consortium. *Critical Care Medicine, 40*(12), 3121–3128. http://dx.doi.org/10.1097/ccm.0b013e3182657916

Rubenfeld, G. D., Cooper, C., Carter, G., Thompson, B. T., & Hudson, L. D. (2004). Barriers to providing lung-protective ventilation to patients with acute lung injury. *Critical Care Medicine, 32*(6), 1289–1293. http://dx.doi.org/10.1097/01.ccm.0000127266.39560.96

Samary, C. S., Santos, R. S., Santos, C. L., Felix, N. S., Bentes, M., Barboza, T., et al. (2015). Biological impact of transpulmonary driving pressure in experimental acute respiratory distress syndrome. *Anesthesiology, 123*(2), 423–433. http://dx.doi.org/10.1097/aln.0000000000000716

Santos, R. S., Silva, P. L., Pelosi, P., & Rocco, P. R. (2015). Recruitment maneuvers in acute respiratory distress syndrome: The safe way is the best way. *World Journal of Critical Care Medicine, 4*(4), 278.

Serpa Neto, A., Cardoso, S. O., Manetta, J. A., Pereira, V. G. M., Espósito, D. C., Pasqualucci, Mde. O., et al. (2012). Association between use of lung-protective ventilation with lower tidal volumes and clinical outcomes among patients without acute respiratory distress syndrome: A meta-analysis. *The Journal of the American Medical Association, 308*(16), 1651–1659. http://dx.doi.org/10.1001/jama.2012.13730

Serpa Neto, A., Schultz, M. J., & Gama de Abreu, M. (2015). Intraoperative ventilation strategies to prevent postoperative pulmonary complications: Systematic review, meta-analysis, and trial sequential analysis. *Best Practice & Research Clinical Anaesthesiology*, 29(3), 331.

Serpa Neto, A., Schultz, M. J., & Slutsky, A. S. (2015). Current concepts of protective ventilation during general anaesthesia. *Swiss Medical Weekly, 145*, w14211. http://dx.doi.org/10.4414/smw.2015.14211

Serpa Neto, A., Simonis, F. D., Barbas, C. S. V., Biehl, M., Determann, R. M., Elmer, J., et al. (2015). Lung-protective ventilation with low tidal volumes and the occurrence of pulmonary complications in patients without acute respiratory distress syndrome: A systematic review and individual patient data analysis. *Critical Care Medicine*, *43*, 2155–2163.

Severgnini, P., Selmo, G., Lanza, C., Chiesa, A., Frigerio, A., Bacuzzi, A., et al. (2013). Protective mechanical ventilation during general anesthesia for open abdominal surgery improves postoperative pulmonary function. *Anesthesiology, 118*(6), 1307–1321. http://dx.doi.org/10.1097/aln.0b013e31829102de

Slinger, P. (2015). Perioperative lung protection strategies in one-lung and two-lung ventilation. *ASA Refresher Courses in Anesthesiology, 43*(1), 93–103. http://dx.doi.org/10.1097/asa.0000000000000024

Slutsky, A. S., & Ranieri, V. M. (2013). Ventilator-induced lung injury. *The New England Journal of Medicine, 369*(22), 2126.

Society, A. T., Infectious Diseases Society of America, Infectious Diseases Society of America, & American Thoracic Society. (2005). Guidelines for the management of adults with hospital-acquired, ventilator-associated, and healthcare-associated pneumonia. *American Journal of Respiratory and Critical Care Medicine, 171*(4), 388–416. http://dx.doi.org/10.1164/rccm.200405-644st

Spieth, P. M., Bluth, T., Gama De Abreu, M., Bacelis, A., Goetz, A. E., & Kiefmann, R. (2014a). Mechanotransduction in the lungs. *Minerva Anestesiologica, 80*(8), 933.

Spieth, P. M., Güldner, A., Uhlig, C., Bluth, T., Kiss, T., Schultz, M. J., et al. (2014b). Variable versus conventional lung protective mechanical ventilation during open abdominal surgery: Study protocol for a randomized controlled trial. *Trials, 15*(1), 155–155. http://dx.doi.org/10.1186/1745-6215-15-155

Staehr-Rye, A. K., & Eikermann, M. (2015). Eliminate postoperative respiratory complications: Preoperative screening opens the door to clinical pathways that individualise perioperative treatment. *European Journal of Anaesthesiology, 32*(7), 455.

Sutherasan, Y., Vargas, M., & Pelosi, P. (2014). Protective mechanical ventilation in the non-injured lung: Review and meta-analysis. *Critical Care (London, England), 18*(2), 211–211. http://dx.doi.org/10.1186/cc13778

Suzumura, E. A., Figueiró, M., Normilio-Silva, K., Laranjeira, L., Oliveira, C., Buehler, A. M., et al. (2014). Effects of alveolar recruitment maneuvers on clinical outcomes in patients with acute respiratory distress syndrome: A systematic review and meta-analysis. *Intensive Care Medicine, 40*(9), 1227–1240. http://dx.doi.org/10.1007/s00134-014-3413-6

Thomson, L., & Paton, J. (2014). Oxygen toxicity. *Paediatric Respiratory Reviews, 15*(2), 120–123. http://dx.doi.org/10.1016/j.prrv.2014.03.003

Tokmaji, G., Vermeulen, H., Müller, M. C. A., Kwakman, P. H. S., Schultz, M. J., & Zaat, S. A. J. (2015). Silver-coated endotracheal tubes for prevention of ventilator-associated pneumonia in critically ill patients. *The Cochrane Database of Systematic Reviews, 8*, CD009201.

Tusman, G., Böhm, S. H., Warner, D. O., & Sprung, J. (2011). Atelectasis and perioperative pulmonary complications in high-risk patients. *Current Opinion in Anaesthesiology, 1*. http://dx.doi.org/10.1097/aco.0b013e32834dd1eb

Villar, J., & Slutsky, A. S. (2010). Is acute respiratory distress syndrome an iatrogenic disease? *Critical Care (London, England), 14*(1), 120–120. http://dx.doi.org/10.1186/cc8842

Vroom, M. B., Schultz, M. J., Choi, G., Poll, v. d., Levi, M. T., Wolthuis, E. K., et al. (2006). Mechanical ventilation with lower tidal volumes and positive end-expiratory pressure prevents alveolar coagulation in patients without lung injury. *Anesthesiology, 105*(4), 689–695. http://dx.doi.org/10.1097/00000542-200610000-00013

Wanderer, J. P., Ehrenfeld, J. M., Epstein, R. H., Kor, D. J., Bartz, R. R., Fernandez-Bustamante, A., et al. (2015). Temporal trends and current practice patterns for intraoperative ventilation at U.S. academic medical centers: A retrospective study. *BMC Anesthesiology, 15*(1), 40. http://dx.doi.org/10.1186/s12871-015-0010-3

Wellman, T. J., Winkler, T., Costa, E. L. V., Musch, G., Harris, R. S., Zheng, H., et al. (2014). Effect of local tidal lung strain on inflammation in normal and lipopolysaccharide-exposed sheep. *Critical Care Medicine, 42*(7), e491–e500. http://dx.doi.org/10.1097/ccm.0000000000000346

Wolthuis, E. (2008). Mechanical ventilation with lower tidal volumes and positive end-expiratory pressure prevents pulmonary inflammation in patients without preexisting lung injury. *Anesthesiology, 108*(1), 46–54. http://dx.doi.org/10.1097/01.anes.0000296068.80921.10

CHAPTER 4

Communication in the Operating Room Setting

Lisa Osborne-Smith and R. Kyle Hodgen

ABSTRACT

Ideal and effective communication consists of a clear, audible, and focused message from a transmitter that is delivered to an attentive, undistracted receiver, and consists of both verbal and nonverbal types. Communication in the health care setting is highly complex and dynamic, involving multiple settings, participants, and unique challenges. Effective communication in the perioperative environment is a requirement for safe patient care delivery and an important element of teamwork. A message must be accurately delivered in a uniquely high-risk and time-sensitive location, beset with numerous distractions, barriers, and challenges. Surgical checklists and time-out procedures have promoted a standardized, "all-hands" approach to addressing some of the challenges to effective communication in the perioperative environment. Postoperative debriefing sessions have demonstrated effectiveness in improving team functioning in the simulated learning environment and hold promise as another strategy to address these challenges, but require further research and development. Other promising strategies to improve effective perioperative communication are focused on team building activities and minimizing distractions at critical time points within patient care delivery, but to date are not substantiated by evidence. Future research is necessary to examine these novel approaches to improving communication in

http://dx.doi.org/10.1891/0739-6686.35.55

the perioperative environment to influence the safety of patient care delivery in this highly challenging health care setting.

> *Wise men speak because they have something to say; Fools because they have to say something.*
>
> —*Plato*

PRINCIPLES OF COMMUNICATION

Communication can best be described as a message, or a piece of information, that is transmitted between a transmitter and a receiver. Effective communication requires that the receiver accurately receives the message, but there are many barriers to this process. The message can be fragmented or completely unreceived when there is a source of interference: for instance, if there is excessive environmental noise, resulting in inadequate volume for the message to be heard. In some instances, there may be multiple messages (or inputs) that are incoming at the same time and the receiver must be able to focus on the message for it to be understandable. Distractions could be represented by external and internal inputs; for instance, the receiver could be distracted by external inputs such as noise or activity, but also could simultaneously be distracted by internal inputs such as personal thoughts.

The receiver must also share the same vocabulary and, ideally, the same mental model as the messenger. If the transmitter and the receiver are not of the same educational background, there is a risk of the message not being fully understood. The use of medical jargon is widespread in the operating room setting and not all members have the same command of this language. There may also be idiosyncratic abbreviations that are used that are unique to a particular group.

The ideal communication consists of a clear, audible, and focused message from the transmitter that is delivered to an attentive, undistracted receiver. Upon receipt of the message, a callback, or repeat of what was heard is a process to verify that the message was received as intended. If the message was not received as intended, the transmitter can then clarify the message, if time and other conditions allow. The callback process also helps to verify sharing of the same mental model.

Communication can be verbal or nonverbal and there are nuances that add a qualitative element. Verbal aspects that add a qualitative component to the message include loudness of the voice, urgency of tone, speed of the speech, and the choice of words. The transmitter sends the message in a particular tone, which influences the meaning. There are many influences on tone, including the culture, the language spoken, and emotional status of the transmitter, to name a few.

Characteristics of the nonverbal type of communication are also important to the qualitative aspect, and combine with verbal communication in the context of metacommunication. This metacommunication process adds an important messaging function to the intended meaning of the message itself through ways such as accent or emphasis, complement, contradiction, regulation, repeating, or substitution (Devito, 2002). Eye contact, facial expression, body position, and hand gestures are examples of important nonverbal communication cues that are utilized by the sender and the receiver to convey a picture of the emotional state surrounding the message, thus serving to elucidate nonverbal meaning in the context of metacommunication (Devito, 2002).

COMMUNICATION IN THE HEALTH CARE SETTING

Communication in the health care setting is a highly complex, dynamic phenomenon (Christian et al., 2006). The health care delivery system includes various individuals such as providers from multiple disciplines, administrators, and patients who interact with each other and the system, but come from vastly different perspectives. Coordination of care is dependent upon effective communication between members of the health care delivery team. The collaboration between these groups at different points of time is challenging and providers may function as independent entities, which results in health care fragmentation, and possibly leads to error (Lancaster, Kolakowsky-Hayner, Kovacich, & Greer-Williams, 2015). Communication must be accurate, clear, available, and timely because it is integral to the care of a patient. Communication is a timely topic as hospitals strive to become high reliability organizations.

Perioperative Communication

Effective communication is fundamental to safe patient care delivery, and the unique operating room environment impacts almost every aspect of the communication process. There are numerous examples of how the translation of communication patterns to the operative setting can create misunderstandings, or complete absence of transfer of information (Christian et al., 2006; Cousely, 2015; Garon, 2012). There are many sources of distraction that are inherent in this setting and important barriers to communication. This section describes the specific challenges of communication in the operative setting.

The operating room environment poses a time-sensitive element, even in the noncrisis situation (Lingard et al., 2006). Communication in this high-risk, time-sensitive environment must be stripped down to the essentials. As in aviation, communication in the operating room is characterized by directness and brevity (Thomas, Sexton, & Helmreich, 2004). This is an effective strategy to improve the opportunity for the receiver to pay attention to the message. However, it also requires the sender to remove explanatory material from the conversation, and allows no opportunity for information related to "why." Without the benefit of knowing "why," the receiver must inherently trust the sender.

Trust is a concept that implies an existing relationship (Kaldheim & Slettebø, 2016). However, in the operating room environment in a large facility, it is not uncommon for members of the team to be working together for the first time, and even unfamiliar with one another's name. This lack of familiarity has the potential to complicate the communication, stemming from the absence of preexisting knowledge and trust, which can lead to misinterpretation and poor team performance (Gillespie, Chaboyer, & Fairweather, 2012).

Lack of familiarity extends to the understanding of the nonverbal forms of communication. Since a large percentage of understanding comes from nonverbal cues, individuals who are unfamiliar with one another will depend on nonverbal cues to a great extent. Unfortunately, the nonverbal communication is significantly constrained in the perioperative setting because all members are likely to be in the midst of multitasking, making things like eye contact lacking, or impossible (Moss & Xiao, 2004). This becomes part of the culture of the operative environment, but it remains as a potential barrier to effective communication. The use of nonverbal cues, such as facial expression, is essential to aid in the understanding of the meaning of verbal communication. If the verbal cues do not match the nonverbal cues, the listener is likely to not believe the verbally stated words according to the verbal–nonverbal consistency principle (Rotenberg, Simourd, & Moore, 1989), and there is a tendency to believe the nonverbal message (Eskritt & Lang, 2003). For instance, if a person states, "that didn't hurt," but the facial expression reflects pain, then the conclusion would be that the person was experiencing pain while not admitting it.

When considering the translation of nonverbal cues to the operating room setting, it is possible to imagine that one's facial expression, and even tone of voice, can be related to the degree of challenge of the task at hand, and less related to the spoken word. This is a potential source of confusion for the receiver who will have a tendency to focus on the nonverbal cue, and assume that the intensity is related to the topic of the spoken word (Eskritt & Lang, 2003). Unfortunately, this can add to misunderstanding of the message, increase the emotional stress that is already present in this setting, and may lead to job dissatisfaction.

The operating room team is a multidisciplinary group that includes members from different educational levels. The structure of this group is hierarchical by nature, which affects the communication patterns. There is evidence from the aviation community that members of the crew are hesitant to question the decisions of the captain, and this reluctance has also been seen in the medical setting

(Makry et al., 2006). In addition to the hierarchical structure, the operating room team comprises members who have different roles during the case, and therefore, have different perspectives. This has been compared to an orchestra, where members who play different instruments experience the musical piece differently as their ability to hear is affected by their position within the orchestra (Lancaster et al., 2015). The difference in perception is relevant to the communication pattern and the perception of the degree of collaboration and teamwork.

Mills, Neily, and Dunn (2008) developed a tool to measure Medical Team Training (MTT) for the Veterans Administration, and used it to identify the pattern differences among providers. These authors report differences in perception of communication clarity and teamwork, especially between surgeons and other team members of the operating room staff. It is interesting that the RNs and anesthesia providers were similar in their perceptions. These results have implications for improvement of communication in the operating room.

Distracters to Effective Perioperative Communication

There are multiple distracters in the operating room that impede communication. In a study to identify the potential sources of interruption during surgery, Antoniadis, Passauer-Baierl, Baschnegger, & Weigl (2014) found that frequent interruptions were related to personnel coming in and going out of the room, incoming pages or phone calls, noise of music playing, and communication unrelated to the case. This demonstrates that communication is highly dynamic and noise is a source of interruption of the surgical procedure.

The noise of an operating room can be significant because there are simultaneous conversations, noisy equipment, and sometimes music that are important barriers to communication (Clark, 2013; Shawagfeh, Korsten, Sawaqed, & Sweiss, 2014). In a study to evaluate the communication patterns related to noise, Keller et al. (2016) found that noisy periods of time were associated with decreased verbal communication, especially communication related to the operative case. Because noise tends to decrease the communication, it is a factor that can impact patient safety. A strategy to improve communication would be to limit unnecessary noise during critical periods of the case (Clark, 2013).

Communication Failure

The Joint Commission has identified communication as a major factor in 70% of sentinel events (Braaf, Manias, Finch, Riley, & Munro, 2012). In an evaluation of closed claim cases, Greenberg et al. (2007) determined that 46% of claims involved information that was never transmitted and 44% of claims involved information that was inaccurately received. Interestingly, the communication failures usually involved verbal communication, most often from a single transmitter to a single receiver (Greenberg, 2007). These findings have implications for determining opportunities for preventing communication in the future, and highlight the need for closed-loop communication.

Braaf et al. (2012) examined perceptions of communication along the entire perioperative pathway and found numerous points of restricted information flow. Hand-offs are the most common sources of information loss and when information loss occurs at one point, there are downstream effects along the pathway (Braaf et al., 2012; Manias, Gerdtz, Williams, & Dooley, 2014). The aviation industry is another example of high-risk communication and the safety principles used to eliminate communication failure have been applied to the operative setting. The use of checklists, the preflight (preprocedure) briefing with the crew, and recognized critical periods are all being incorporated into standard procedures (Awad et al., 2005; Clark, 2013; Thomas et al., 2004).

Surgical Checklist

In 2004 the Joint Commission proposed a process called the Universal Protocol, to address wrong-site and wrong-patient surgery (Joint Commission, Universal Protocol, 2016). This process included presurgical review of the patient identifiers compared to the written documentation at two different time points, one in the preoperative setting and another "time-out" process to be completed just prior to incision. The WHO also proposed a worldwide use of a surgical checklist as part of the Safe Surgery Saves Lives (World Health Organization, Surgical Safety Checklist, 2016). This WHO proposal incorporated the items from the Joint Commission and includes 19 steps that involve the whole surgical team. The surgical checklist is designed to address many of the challenges of perioperative communication that have been identified.

The proper use of the surgical checklist requires that all members of the operative team meet as a group for a briefing, prior to the start of an operation. The briefing provides an opportunity for introduction of team members and establishment of clear roles. This briefing also allows for discussion and clarification of the planned procedure, the patient condition, and other case-relevant information. Since this briefing occurs prior to the case, it allows introduction of members, time for questions, and an opportunity for problem solving prior to the time-sensitive portion of the case.

This briefing allows members to focus on the conversation since the meeting is not conducted while members are engaged in other activities (Clark, 2013). The conversation follows a script to ensure that information is not inadvertently omitted. The checklist is designed to prevent wrong-site and/or wrong-patient surgery, but it also allows for a clarification of special equipment for the procedure. The comparison of written content to the actual patient during the "time-out" procedure verifies the procedure, laterality, patient identification, patient allergies, and desired antibiotics and/or deep vein thrombosis prophylaxis.

Although it seems intuitive that these steps will improve patient outcomes, reduce, or eliminate, wrong-site or wrong-patient surgery, in practice the results are inconclusive (Lyons & Popejoy, 2014; Tang, Ranmuthugala, & Cunningham, 2014). Lyons and Popejoy (2014) conducted a meta-analysis on the effects of the surgical checklist on patient outcomes and found that measures of teamwork and communication increased and a reduction in morbidity and mortality was shown, but these authors suggest that there is more research needed to fully evaluate what moderating variables influence the use of the checklist. Russ et al. (2013) similarly found improvements in perceived team functioning and on measures of patient outcomes, but noted that there was suboptimal performance in groups that did not fully adhere to checklist procedures (Halverson et al., 2011; Russ et al., 2013).

Authors have suggested that incomplete implementation of the procedure is partially responsible for the lack of improvement of outcomes (Halverson et al., 2011; Russ et al., 2013; Treadwell, Lucas, & Tsou, 2013). Barriers to the successful implementation of the checklist procedure appear to be beyond the resistance to change that is often seen when a new process is introduced. Examples of barriers to the use of the surgical checklist include: time, disruption of flow, and emergency situations where 3 minutes makes a difference in patient outcome.

Another problem with the surgical checklist is that while it encourages individual participation, checklist use does not necessarily overcome the hierarchical structure of the operating room team and the associated unwillingness of team members to speak up. The recommended procedure to include input from all members is scripted and may or may not enhance spontaneous input. Although all members of the team are supposed to participate in the time-out procedure, in an observational study of the operating room Halverson et al. (2011) observed that the other members of the group sometimes ignore the call for time-out.

The surgical checklist also does not encompass the vulnerabilities in communication for the entire surgical or perioperative process (Collins, Newhouse, Porter, & Talsma, 2014). Nagpal et al. (2012) examined the communication variables related to the entire surgical or perioperative process and described the communication failures that occur and negatively impact the care environment. Through structured interviews, they were able to identify vulnerable times of communication failure, one of which was the point of transfer of patient care. The hand-off of patient care between providers has been known to be particularly vulnerable to communication failure, and a standardized process is recommended (Papaconstantinou, Smythe, Reznik, Sibbitt, & Wehbe-Janek, 2013).

A significant barrier to the proper use of the surgical checklist is the factor of time. Because the surgical checklist use requires full participation from all members, all other activities should cease for this period of time (Clark, 2013). The production pressures of the operating room are in direct competition for the time that the staff takes to fully address all elements of the surgical checklist. Papaconstantinou et al. (2013) evaluated the impact of use of the checklist at a large medical center and did not find a difference in efficiency. Since they also evaluated cost per procedure, these authors were also able to show that this communication prior to the procedure results in significant cost savings. Although not specifically evaluated in the study, it is possible that the use of the checklist could actually be time-saving by enhancing the ability to anticipate problems, or identify unnecessary equipment prior to opening of the package (Papaconstantinou et al., 2013).

The checklist is estimated to take about 3 minutes to complete, depending on the availability of team members (Collins et al., 2014). However, this seemingly small time expenditure still represents a significant cost since operating room minutes are estimated to be $29 to $80 (Macario, 2010) for an uncomplicated case, and so this remains a barrier to the full implementation of the surgical checklist in this era of cost containment. Further research is needed to completely address the issue of the compliance rate, including participation rate of all of the members and the actual fidelity of the process.

Nontechnical Skills

The nontechnical skills that a provider acquires to become a highly functioning team member include communication skills. The process of imparting these skills to different types of trainees has been a topic of interest (Larsson & Helmström, 2013). However, teaching communication skills for the operating room environment is more complex than simply using existing methods because the environment requires that the trainee understand the adaptation of communication skills for this type of setting (Gillespie, Chaboyer, Longbottom, & Wallis, 2010).

Teaching nontechnical skills must be within a particular context and include communication skills that cross multidisciplinary boundaries. The operating room employs its own social context, so understanding how social norms and communication patterns differ is imperative. The contextual meaning of speaking loudly, repeating aloud what was heard in order to demonstrate understanding, and communicating with directness and brevity, are all aspects of operative communication that are unlike other settings (Penprase, Elstun, Ferguson, Schaper, Tiller, 2010).

The ability to speak up is an important part of provider nontechnical skills. The hierarchical structure of the medical environment has been identified as an impediment to speaking up (Weller et al., 2014). In a qualitative study, Garon (2012) identified factors associated with nurses speaking up: confidence in knowledge, cultural background, and a sense of doing "what is right." This author also found that the ability to speak up impacts job satisfaction. Interviewees reported culture as a factor and indicated that the learned behavior from childhood played a significant part in their professional life. This study is informative to nontechnical skills training because factors such as confidence in knowledge can be cultivated in trainees, which can in turn foster the open communications that are required for delivery of high-quality health care (Garon, 2012).

Lyndon et al. (2012) also found similar results in a study of labor and delivery clinicians, specifically that the likelihood of speaking up was related to level of experience and perceived potential harm to the patient. These authors developed a tool to quantify the likelihood of speaking up, which correlates well with bravery and assertiveness. Importantly, there is a negative correlation between the disruptive behavior scale and likelihood of speaking up. Therefore, this adds to the literature on the consequence of the abusive or toxic individual and the potential for adverse team performance effects and possible patient harm from poor communication (Hartung & Miller, 2013).

The tone of communication is also a nontechnical skill that has cultural influences, and can imply a degree of emotion that may be unintended. Unfortunately, a highly passionate tone was found to be related to communication that was quashed (Garon, 2012), which could be further complicated in the perioperative setting. The tone of the voice can reflect emotions, and the loudness of the voice is perceived as related to increasing emotion. However, in the operating room loud and urgent voices may be the norm due to having to speak over noisy equipment. It could be difficult to distinguish between yelling and speaking loudly, and culture differences in the social appropriateness of raised voices make it even more complicated.

Larsson and Hölstrom (2013) conducted a qualitative study of focus groups to evaluate the personal traits of anesthetists. These authors reported that excellence in anesthesia teamwork was related to the social interaction of provider, strong interpersonal skills, including communication skills that were considered to be highly important. The subjects considered interpersonal skills to be as important to patient safety as the technical skills.

Multidisciplinary Team Building

Teamwork is an integral part of communication in the operative setting, and is closely associated with overall team performance (Fan et al., 2016;

Makary et al., 2006; Mills et al., 2008). Makary et al. developed a measure of teamwork called the Safety Attitudes Questionnaire. In a study to evaluate teamwork, these authors note considerable discrepancies in perceptions of teamwork between different levels of providers. Nurses and physicians did not perceive the same amount of teamwork, and nurses also reported less job satisfaction. The results of this study have implications for team building activities of the multidisciplinary team and demonstrate that hierarchical design of the operating room teams remains a barrier to teamwork and communication.

Cumin, Skilton, and Weller (2016) conducted an observational study of simulated scenarios and found that there are differences in the contribution from members of different levels of education and in different roles. Similarly, Lingard et al. (2004) observed operating room personnel and found that 30% of communication events met criteria for "failed communication." These authors identified that many of the communication failures were the result of systems-process issues, one of which was the hierarchical structure of the operating team. Subsequently, Lingard et al. (2006) observed that the role of the team member affected the pattern of communication and the perceived value of the surgical prebrief portion of actual cases. Surgeons, in general, placed less value on the prebrief than other team members and made negative statements such as, "[the prebrief] involves telling people what they should already know" (Lingard et al., 2006). The finding that team members do not equally share the overall value of the process must be considered in planning for implementation of a prebrief process or other safety initiatives to address the link between teamwork and patient outcomes (Gillespie, Chaboyer, Fairweather, 2012).

Awad et al. (2005) evaluated team training utilizing a specific training method and compared perceived communication pre- and postimplementation of daily briefings. The outcomes of antibiotic administration and deep vein thrombus prophylaxis were used to determine the impact of the implementation on patient care. Although the authors were able to demonstrate improvement of these parameters related to patient care, interestingly the perception of teamwork, particularly from the nurses, did not improve.

Weller et al. (2014) conducted a study to evaluate a tool to aid in the "call-out" of information, called SNAPPI (an acronym for Stop; Notify; Assessment; Plan Priorities; Invite Ideas), which is designed to ensure that all members share information and have the same mental picture of the situation. In this simulation-based study, members had information only known to them, called probes, and the posttest evaluated the successful transfer of this information. Interestingly only 32% of the information was shared during all of the simulated crisis situations, demonstrating that critical information was incompletely communicated between different levels of providers.

Collaboration of groups allows for a level of synergy since different multidisciplinary groups have different perspectives and knowledge. When direct, open communication is utilized, problem solving is enhanced (Lancaster et. al., 2015). However, true collaboration can be difficult in the health care delivery system because the hierarchical structure does not encourage different perspectives and mutual respect. Interdisciplinary educational efforts may aid in this process (Sevdalis et al., 2012). Lancaster et al. (2015) also reported that the multidisciplinary rounds were considered to be an ideal form of communication for team building, and the surgical checklist briefings may be a similar model for team building in the perioperative setting.

Impact of Teamwork

The degree of teamwork and the impact on patient outcomes was assessed by Mazzocco et al. (2009). Teams of observers assessed the teamwork in a perioperative setting and evaluated the patient outcomes at 30 days postoperatively. The authors found a relationship between teamwork and patient outcomes, which has implications for the value of the safety initiatives that include elements of team building.

Although verbal forms of communication are highly relevant to the operative setting, written communication is an important form of transferring and documenting patient care. Jylhä, Bates, and Saranto (2016) evaluated adverse events and near-miss cases in a large tertiary medical center and these authors found that these types of cases were most often related to written forms of communication. The electronic medical record is becoming widely used and though it provides widespread access to patient information, research is needed to assess the impact of electronic medical record use on communication patterns and patient safety. As Lancaster reported, different levels of health care providers tend to act independently, and the electronic medical record may actually encourage this behavior.

CONCLUSIONS

There are many aspects of perioperative communication that make the environment a unique social setting. Time pressures and long-standing hierarchical boundaries hinder effective communication across the whole spectrum of health care providers involved in health care delivery. The use of the surgical checklist and time-out procedure holds promise in promoting an "all-hands" conversation and team building prior to the surgical case. Teamwork training has shown improvements in the completion of tasks, but has not necessarily resulted in a perception of improved teamwork (Vincent, Moorthy, Sarker, Chang, & Darzi, 2004).

The use of the surgical checklist process offers an opportunity for verification of case-relevant information and to cross-check information from members of other disciplines. This is important because no other time point exists for this process to occur.

There is little evidence in the literature about the effect of the postbrief on teamwork and patient outcomes. There is resistance to the postbrief because the end point of the case is different between the providers. In simulation, postsimulation debrief is an important aspect for increased learning and team functioning (Garden, Le Fevere, Waddington, & Welter, 2015); however this is not a common practice after a regular day in the operative setting. Future research is necessary to determine the full impact of the postoperative debrief.

Strategies for controlling the level of distraction within the operative environment may improve communication. Identifying the critical aspects of the case and ensuring the team members are all engaged for these periods is an intuitively useful goal, but there is a lack of evidence to support this claim. While simulation and observational studies are helpful in our understanding of operating room communication, prospective, controlled designs would aid in the understanding of the human factors and the impact on communication and patient safety. Future research is also necessary to fully illuminate the barriers to implementation of these types of safety initiatives. The literature is typically focused on the examination of the contributors to error, but studies of the successful navigation and teamwork of complex operative cases will also add important information.

REFERENCES

Antoniadis, S., Passauer-Baierl, S., Baschnegger, H., & Weigl, M. (2014). Identification and interference of intraoperative distractions and interruptions in operating rooms. *The Journal of Surgical Research, 188*(1), 21–29. http://dx.doi.org/10.1016/j.jss.2013.12.002

Awad, S. S., Fagan, S. P., Bellows, C., Albo, D., Green-Rashad, B., De La Garza, M., et al. (2005). Bridging the communication gap in the operating room with medical team training. *The American Journal of Surgery, 190*, 770–774.

Braaf, S., Manias, E., Finch, S., Riley, R., & Munro, F. (2012). Healthcare service providers perception of organisational commuication across the perioperative pathway: A questionnaire survey. *Journal of Clinical Nursing, 22*, 180–192. http://dx.doi.org/10.1111/j.1365-2702.2012.04228x

Christian, C. K., Gustafson, M. L., Roth, E. M., Sheridan, T. B., Gandhi, T. K., Dwyer, K., et. al. (2006). A prospective study of patient safety in the operating room. *Surgery, 139*(2), 159–173. http://dx.doi.org/10.1016/j.surg.2005.07.037

Clark, J. L. (2013). Strategies for preventing distractions and interruptions in the OR. *AORN Journal, 97*, 702–707.

Collins, S. J., Newhouse, R., Porter, J., & Talsma, A. (2014). Effectiveness of the surgical safety checklist in correcting errors: A literature review applying reason's swiss cheese model. *AORN Journal, 100*(1), 65–79.

Cousely, A. (2015). Vulnerability in perioperative patients: A qualitative study. *Journal of Perioperative Practice, 25*(12), 246–254.

Cumin, D., Skilton, C., & Weller, J. (2016). Information transfer in multidisciplinary operating room teams: A simulation-based observational study. *British Journal of Quality & Safety*. http://dx.doi.org/10.1136/bmjqs-2015-005130 [Epub ahead of print].

Devito, J. A. (2002). *Human communication: The basic course*. Boston, MA: Allyn & Bacon.

Eskritt, M., & Lang, K. (2003). Do actions speak louder than words? Preschool children's use of the verbal-non-verbal consistency principle during inconsistent communications. *Journal of Nonverbal Behavior*, 27(1), 25–41.

Fan, C. J., Pawlik, T. M., Daniels, T., Vernon, N., Banks, K., Westby, P., et al. (2016). Association of safety culture with surgical site infection outcomes. *Journal of the American College of Surgeons, 222*(2), 122–128.

Garden, A. L., Le Fevere, D. M., Waddington, H. L., & Welter, J. M. (2015). Debriefing after simulation-based skill training in healthcare: A systematic review of effective practice. *Anesthesia & Intensive Care, 43*(3), 300–308.

Garon, M. (2012). Speaking up, being heard: Registered nurses' perceptions of workplace communication. *Journal of Nursing Management, 20*, 361–371.

Gillespie, B. M., Chaboyer, W., & Fairweather, N. (2012). Interruptions and miscommunications in surgery: An observational study. *AORN Journal, 95*(5), 576–590. http://dx.doi.org/10.1016/j.aorn.2012.02.012

Gillespie, B. M., Chaboyer, W., Longbottom, P., & Wallis, M. (2010). The impact of organisational and individual factors on team communication in surgery: A qualitative study. *International Journal of Nursing Studies, 47*(6), 732–741. http://dx.doi.org/10.1016/j.ijnurstu.2009.11.001

Greenberg, C. C., Regenbogen, S. E., Studdert, D. M., Lipsitz, S. R., Rogers, S. O., Zinner, M. J., et al. (2007). Patterns of communication breakdowns resulting in injury to surgical patients. *Journal of the American College of Surgeons, 204*(4), 533–540. http://dx.doi.org/10.1016/j.jamcollsurg.2007.01.010

Halverson, A. L., Casey, J. T., Andersson, J., Anderson, K., Park, C., Rademaker, A. W., et al. (2011). Communication failure in the operating room. *Surgery, 149*(3), 305–310. http://dx.doi.org/10.1016/j.surg.2010.07.051

Hartung, S. Q., & Miller, M. (2013). Communication and the healthy work environment: Nurse managers' perceptions. *The Journal of Nursing Administration, 43*(5), 266–273.

Jylhä, V., Bates, D. W., & Saranto, K. (2016). Adverse events and near nisses relating to information managemnt in a hospital. *Healthcare Information Management Journal, 45*(2), 1–9. http://dx.doi.org/10.1177/1833358316641551

Kaldheim, H. K. A., & Slettebø, Å. (2016). Respecting as a basic teamwork process in the operating theatre-A qualitative study of theatre nurses who work in interdisciplinary surgical teams of what they see as important factors in this collaboration. *Nordisk Sygeplejeforskning, 5*(1), 49–64.

Keller, S., Tschan, F., Beldi, G., Kurmann, A., Candinas, D., Semmer, N. K, (2016). Noise peaks influence communication in the operating room. An observational study. *Ergonomics*, 1–12. [Epub ahead of print].

Lancaster, G., Kolakowsky-Hayner, S., Kovacich, J., & Greer-Williams, N. (2015). Interdisciplinary communication and collaboration among physicians, nurses, and unlicensed assistive personnel. *Journal of Nursing Scholarship, 47*(3), 275–284. http://dx.doi.org/10.1111/jnu.12130

Larsson, J., & Holmström, I. K. (2013). How excellent anaesthetists perform in the operating room theatre: A quality study on non-technical skills. *British Journal of Anaethesia, 110*(1), 115–121.

Lingard, L., Espin, S., Whyte, S., Regehr, G., Baker, G. R., Reznick, R., et. al. (2004). Communication failures in the operating room: An observational classification of recurrent types and effects. *Quality & Safety in Health Care, 13*(5), 330–334. http://dx.doi.org/10.1136/qhc.13.5.330

Lingard, L., Whyte, S., Espin, S., Baker, G. R., Orser, B., & Doran, D. (2006). Towards safer interprofessional communication: Constructing a model of "utility" from preoperative team briefings. *Journal of Interprofessional Care, 20*(5), 471–483. http://dx.doi.org/10.1080/13561820600921865

Lyons, L. L., & Popejoy, V. E. (2014). Meta-analysis of surgical safety checklist effects on teamwork, communication, morbidity, mortality, and safety. *Western Journal of Nursing Research, 36*(2), 245–261. http://dx.doi.org/10.1177/0193945913505782

Lyndon, A., Sexton, J. B., Simpson, K. R., Rosenstein, A., Lee, K. A., & Wachter, R. M. (2012). Predictors of likelihood of speaking up about safety concerns in labour and delivery. *British Medical Journal of Quality & Safety, 21*(9), 791–799.

Macario, A. (2010). What does one minute of operating room time cost? *Journal of Clinical Anesthesia, 22*, 233–236.

Makary, M. A., Sexton, J. B., Freischlag, J. A., Holzmueller, C. G., Millman, E. A., Rowen, L., et al. (2006). Operating room teamwork among physicians and nurses: Teamwork in the eye of the beholder. *Journal of the American Colleges of Surgeons, 202*, 746–752.

Manias, E., Gerdtz, M., Williams, A., & Dooley, M. (2014). Complexities of medicines safety: Communicating about managing medicines at transition points of care across emergency departments and medical wards. *Journal of Clinical Nursing, 24*, 69–80.

Mazzocco, K., Petitti, D. B., Fong, K. T., Bonacum, D., Brookey, J., Graham, S., et al. (2009). Surgical team behaviors and patient outcomes. *The American Journal of Surgery, 197*, 678–685.

Mills, P., Neily, J., & Dunn, E. (2008). Teamwork and communication in surgical teams: Implications for patient safety. *Journal of the American College of Surgeons, 206*(1), 107–112. http://dx.doi.org/10.1016/j.jamcollsurg.2007.06.281

Moss, J., & Xiao, Y. (2004). Improving operating room coordination: Communication pattern assessment. *The Journal of Nursing Administration, 34*(2), 93–100.

Nagpal, K., Arora, S., Vats, A., Wong, H. W., Sevdalis, C. V., & Moorthy, K. (2012). Failures in communication and information transfer across the surgical care pathway: Interview study. *British Medical Journal of Quality & Safety, 21*, 843–849. http://dx.doi.org/10.1136/bmjqs-2012-000886

Papaconstantinou, H. T., Smythe, W. R., Reznik, S. I., Sibbitt, S., & Wehbe-Janek, H. (2013). Surgical safety checklist and operating room efficiency: Results from a large multispecialty tertiary care hospital. *The American Journal of Surgery, 206*, 853–860

Penprase, B., Elstun, L., Ferguson, C., Schaper, M., Tiller, C. (2010). Preoperative communication to improve safety: A literature review. *Nursing Management, 41*(11), 18–24. http://dx.doi.org/10.1097/01.numa.0000390370.89205.74

Rotenberg, K. J., Simourd, L., & Moore, D. (1989). Children's use of verbal-nonverbal consistency principle to infer truth and lying. *Child Development, 60*(2), 309–322.

Russ, S., Rout, S., Sevdalis, N., Moorthy, K., Darzi, A., & Vicent, C. (2013). Do checklists improve teamwork and communication in the operating room? *Annals of Surgery, 258*, 856–871. http://dx.doi.org/10.1097/SLA 0000000000000206

Sevdalis, N., Wong, H. W., Arora, S., Nagpal, K., Healey, A., Hanna, G. B., et al. (2012). Quantitative analysis of intraoperative communication in open and laparoscopic surgery. *Surgical Endoscopy, 26*(10), 2931–2938. http://dx.doi.org/10.1007/s00464-012-2287-3

Shawagfeh, M. T., Korsten, P., Sawaqed, R. S., & Sweiss, N. J. (2014). Noise or silence in the operating room? *Journal of the American College of Surgeons, 218*, 150. http://dx.doi.org/10.1016/j.jamcollsurg.2013.09.019.

Tang, R., Ranmuthugala, G., & Cunningham, F. (2014). Surgical safety checklists: A review. *ANZ Journal of Surgery, 84*, 148–154.

The Joint Commission. (2012). *Safe surgery checklist.* Retrieved from http://www.jointcommission.org/safe_surgery_checklist

The Joint Commission. (2016). *Universal protocol.* Retrived from http://www.jointcommission.org/standards_information/up.aspx

The World Health Organization, Safe Surgery Saves Lives. (2016). Retrieved from http://www.who.int/patientsafety/safesurgery/en

Thomas, E. J., Sexton, J. B., & Helmreich, R. L. (2004). Translating teamwork to behaviours from aviation to healthcare: Development of behavioural markers for neonatal resuscitation. *Quality and Safety in Healthcare, 13*(Suppl. 1), i57–i64.

Treadwell, J. R., Lucas, S., & Tsou, A. Y. (2014). Surgical checklists: A systematic review of impacts and implementation. *British Medical Journal of Quality & Safety, 23*, 299–318.

Vincent, C., Moorthy, K., Sarker, S. K., Chang, A., & Darzi, A. W. (2004). Systems approaches to surgical quality and safety: From concept to measurement. *Annals of Surgery, 239*(4), 475–482. http://dx.doi.org/10.1097/01.sla.0000118753.22830.41

Weller, J. M., Torrie, J., Boyd, M., Frengley, R., Garden, A., Ng, W. L., et al. (2014). Improving team information sharing with a structured call-out in anaesthetic emergencies: A randomized controlled trial. *British Journal of Anaesthesia, 112*(6), 1042–1049.

CHAPTER 5

Anesthesia Information Management Systems

Thomas Corey Davis

ABSTRACT

Anesthesia information management systems (AIMS) are rapidly gaining widespread acceptance. Aggressively promoted as an improvement to manual-entry recordkeeping systems in the areas of accuracy, completeness, quality improvement, billing, and vigilance, these systems record all patient vital signs and parameters, providing a legible hard copy and permanent electronic record. With well-documented financial incentives, as well as government subsidies, AIMS are becoming adopted at an unprecedented rate. With the goals of the federal government to enhance the use of the electronic medical record, there is an emerging belief that AIMS may soon be mandated, with more limited choices than currently available. As assessed by, and often in spite of the published evidence, concerns of practitioners still reflect many of the same concerns expressed in the editorial comments of the past.

INTRODUCTION

In the United States, each of the over 50 million anesthetics administered each year generates a detailed record of vital signs, medications, and events of the surgery or procedure (Ishizawa, 2011). Based upon monitoring standards established in 1986, and adopted by both the American Society of Anesthesiologists

http://dx.doi.org/10.1891/0739-6686.35.71

(ASA) and the American Association of Nurse Anesthetists (AANA), anesthesia providers document oxygenation, ventilation, circulation, and temperature (Eichhorn et al., 1986). Initially developed as a means to improve individual practice, the creation of a record of events and techniques of anesthesia has been in existence since 1894 (Beecher, 1920).

As the science of anesthesia delivery advanced, the demands of documentation on the anesthesia provider increased. Electronic means of recordkeeping was proposed as early as 1929 in an effort to reduce the workload of the anesthetist while preserving the accuracy of the record (McKesson, 1934). Such automation of the record did not take precedence over the handwritten record, and only the development of computing technology in the early 1970s brought about a resurgence of interest in an electronically generated anesthesia chart (Drui, Behm, & Martin, 1973).

Throughout the succeeding decades the call for automation of anesthesia documentation increased as computing technology expanded, with claims of enhanced time management (Heinrichs, Monk, & Eberle, 1997), improved data collection for quality improvement (Vigoda, Gencorelli, & Lubarsky, 2006), and superior capture of billing elements (Kheterpal et al., 2007). These claims were met with concerns of potential malpractice liability (Feldman, 2004), significant financial investment (O'Sullivan, Dexter, Lubarsky, & Vigoda, 2007), increased complexity of tasks (Kennedy, Feingold, Wiener, & Hosek, 1976), and decreased vigilance related to a decrease in attentiveness to the patient and monitors (Abenstein, DeVos, Tarhan, & Tarhan, 1992). Studies analyzing vigilance and workload indicated no significant differences between the two methods (Loeb, 1994; Thrush, 1992; Yablok, 1990). Many of these studies had significant flaws, such as small sample size or methodological errors (Loeb, 1994; Thrush, 1992), or failure to account for extraneous variables such as the threat of expectancy (the Hawthorne effect; Loeb, 1994; Weinger, Herndon, & Gaba, 1997). In addition, many experts in the field have branded the adoption of anesthesia information management systems (AIMS) as inevitable (Hamilton, 1990; Levitan, 2008; Vigoda et al., 2006).

In 2005, the U.S. government set a goal to have an electronic medical record for each citizen by 2014, and financial incentives for physicians, medical practices, and hospitals have been included in a recent $19 billion economic stimulus package that includes the use of AIMS (Huslin, 2009). Adoption of AIMS has increased, with an adoption rate of 87% of academic medical centers utilizing or planning to implement such a system in 2014 (Stol, Ehrenfeld, & Epstein, 2014). Driven by financial incentives, and "a need to mitigate increasing reporting requirements imposed by various regulatory bodies" (Ehrenfeld & Rehman, 2011, p. 2) widespread adoption of AIMS is occurring at a rapid pace.

HISTORY OF ANESTHESIA RECORDKEEPING

From the time of development of the first documented use of diethyl ether by Dr. William T.G. Morton in 1842, the safety of anesthesia administration has steadily increased. In large part due to the initial delegation of anesthesia practice to medical students more interested in the study of the surgical procedure, morbidity and mortality associated with anesthesia were at unacceptably high levels by the turn of the 20th century (Gunn, 2005). This role fell to nurses rather than physicians, and the role of the nurse anesthetist was created to fill the need for a provider dedicated to the delivery of anesthesia (Thatcher, 1953). To those few physicians who were conscripted to the role, the near nonchalant attitude toward mortality of patients under anesthesia became unacceptably troubling. Dr. Harvey Cushing and a colleague, Dr. E.A. Codman sought to develop a tool to record their practices of anesthesia delivery, in an attempt to improve their skill and reduce morbidity and mortality (Beecher, 1920). The anesthesia record was born.

Handwritten records prevailed through much of the early 20th century, and even at this early stage, voices were raised in caution, as "too elaborate a record of this kind might take the administrator's mind from his primary job" (Beecher, 1920, p. 690). In defense, Cushing stated, "I feel most emphatically that it keeps his mind on his job" (Beecher, 1920, p. 690). Similar concerns of distraction and reduced vigilance led Dr. E.I. McKesson (1934) to develop a device to record vital signs/parameters in 1929. This device also recorded the first example of "artifact," or erroneous data, as a "notch" indicating a reduction in tidal volume respirations, which was in fact the failure of the anesthetist to maintain a proper mask seal. This artifact was indicated by a handwritten notation on the completed record (McKesson, 1934). McKesson (1934) recognized the value of automatic recordkeeping in the areas of accuracy, enhanced opportunity for vigilance of the practitioner, and improved quality of anesthesia care and patient safety.

By the early 1970s, technology advanced to a point where Dr. McKesson's vision could become a reality. Again, the intent was to examine anesthesia practice with the goal of improving patient care and enhancing safety. The task of manually entering data on a written record, a task that required little knowledge or skill, was determined to occupy a large portion of the anesthesia providers' time. Automation of this task was recommended (Drui et al., 1973). Zollinger, Kreul, and Schneider (1977) compared handwritten records against those generated by "a computerized surveillance system," revealing that the automated system was consistently more accurate, particularly during times of high workload, such as induction. Results indicated that in many cases, providers altered the actual values, "to make the record look smooth" (Zollinger, Kreul, & Schneider, 1977).

Other articles from the 1970s revealed the wide variety of quality of recordkeeping practices in general, indicating a severe lack of standardization and significant deficiency in the ability to review records for their original intent; quality improvement to enhance patient safety (Shaffer, Kaiser, Klingenmaier, & Gordon, 1978). As a result, the call for greater automation of the record was increased, with specific attributes defined (see Table 5.1).

The dawn of the 1980s saw a continued advancement of technology, and increasing optimism toward the development of a fully automated anesthesia record. Apple, Schneider, and Fadel (1982) developed a prototype of such a device and compared its accuracy to that of handwritten records. The device was found to have significantly enhanced accuracy (93.1% for the automated device as compared to 77.4% accuracy in handwritten records), with many blood pressure readings in the handwritten group found to be entered incorrectly or at an incorrect time, indicating later entry from memory (Apple et al., 1982).

By 1986, following the publication of patient monitoring standards at Harvard Medical School (Eichhorn et al., 1986), standards for basic monitoring of patients receiving anesthesia were adopted by the ASA (2005) and the AANA (2007). With the introduction of these standards of monitoring, the search for an automated solution to the task of recordkeeping continued with renewed vigor.

Opinions, however, were polarized on the topic. In a storm of controversy expressed through opposing editorial comments, opponents and proponents of the emerging AIMS technologies traded criticisms and praise. Topics debated included accuracy, vigilance, risk of exposure of medical malpractice claims, and communication between devices both within the same institution as well as different facilities. These concerns continued from the 1980s well into the 1990s, and many persist today.

The first hospital in the United States to adopt AIMS for full use was Burbank Hospital in Fitchburg, Massachusetts in 1988 (Eichhorn & Edsall, 1991). Documenting their experience with over 8,000 records generated from inception to publication, the authors indicated benefits such as the enhancement

TABLE 5.1

Attributes of the Ideal AIMS

Automatic capture of information with the ability to edit inaccurate or erroneous data
Ability to enter data manually through a keyboard, light pen, or graphic display
Reliability of function
Ease of electronic storage and retrieval of information

of timeliness of recordkeeping, quality assurance, and even cost savings from their initial investment due to enhancements in billing and inventory management. Other institutions would soon follow this example.

Abenstein et al. (1992) documented use of AIMS at the Mayo Medical Center in Rochester, Minnesota. With over 24,000 records generated, the authors indicated benefits that included enhanced completeness of the record, improved organization of the record, and greatly improved legibility. Difficulties with the user interface, particularly at times of high task density, were cited as a primary deficiency of the system, and a consistent concern to acceptance of the system (Abenstein et al., 1992). Others echoed such issues overseas, with Zbinden et al. (1992) sharing similar concerns, although the authors reported similar, significant benefits. Computing and automation technologies continued to improve throughout the decade, although concerns regarding the impact of AIMS on vigilance, accuracy of the record, completeness, financial investment, risk of medicolegal complications, and ultimately, quality improvement persisted.

VIGILANCE

By the year 1989, computing technology had advanced to a point where a fully automatic recording of a patient's physiologic parameters and vital signs was widely available. Various systems were beginning to become implemented in academic centers as well as private practice facilities both in the United States and abroad. In many of these facilities, obstacles to complete acceptance and satisfaction continued to surface in the form of concerns about the effect of computerized charting on the overall vigilance of the anesthesia provider (Block, 1989).

Vigilance as affected by the workload of the anesthesia provider has been studied long prior to the advent of the AIMS of the 1990s. A definition is offered for vigilance as a task, "which requires the detection of changes in a stimulus during long monitoring periods when the subject has little or no prior knowledge of the sequence of the changes" (Olmedo & Kirk, 1977, p. 715). In 1981, Paget et al. examined the tasks of the anesthesia provider and the effect of these tasks on the concept of vigilance. Multiple effects were cited as influencing vigilance, both positively and negatively. Multitasking or time sharing, noise, gas pollution, and sleep deprivation were all cited as having a negative impact on vigilance, whereas complex stimuli (complex displays, audio and visual displays of the same alarm), and the approach of the end of the case were found to improve vigilance (Paget, Lambert, & Sridhar, 1981). Furthermore, Kay and Neal in 1986 and Yablok in 1990 documented findings of reduced vigilance when using automated devices.

Methods to assess the impact of AIMS on vigilance have been varied in published research, from the use of accuracy of practitioners' ability to recall

TABLE 5.2
Comparison of Vigilance

Author	Year	Method	Comparison	Vigilance (Outcome)
Kay and Neal	1986	Occlusion of ear piece	Manual vs. automated blood pressure device	Worse with automated
Yablok	1990	Recall accuracy	Handwritten vs. AIMS	Worse with automated
Allard et al.	1995	Recall accuracy	Handwritten vs. AIMS	No difference
Loeb	1995	Vigilance task	Handwritten vs. scribe	No difference
Weinger et al.	1997	Vigilance task	Handwritten vs. AIMS	No difference
Davis et al.	2012	Recall accuracy	Handwritten v.s. AIMS	No difference

vital signs (Davis, Green, Colquhoun, Hage, & Biddle, 2012; Yablok, 1990), "scribes"—providers who only recorded vital signs (Loeb, 1995), or "vigilance tasks" (Loeb, 1995; Weinger et al., 1997). Much of the published literature has suffered from small sample sizes or other threats to validity, such as threats of expectancy (the "Hawthorne effect"). Davis et al. (2012) sought to overcome these limitations, in a large, multicenter study comparing the recall accuracy of practitioners using handwritten records versus AIMS. Ultimately, no differences were found between the two groups, indicating equivalent vigilance of providers, and maintenance of connection to the anesthetic case and patient, regardless of the method of recordkeeping (Davis et al., 2012). A summary of publications, methods, and results of comparison of vigilance of providers with various methods of recordkeeping may be found in Table 5.2.

ACCURACY

A second aspect of the controversy regarding the adoption of AIMS over existing Manual Entry Recordkeeping systems is that of accuracy. With the advent of an alternative method to handwritten recordkeeping during the delivery of an anesthetic, critics called into question the benefits of computerization of the process. Prior to the advent of monitoring standards in 1986, the composition and organization of handwritten records varied by institution and even practitioner. The quality of such records often suffered from poor handwriting, rendering even complete records illegible to all but the practitioner responsible for the chart. Zollinger et al. (1977) compared the composition of 100 records handwritten by anesthesia residents to those generated simultaneously by a computerized

TABLE 5.3
Comparisons of Accuracy

Author	Year	Method	Comparison	Accuracy (Outcome)
Zollinger et al.	1977	Comparison	Handwritten vs. simultaneous generation	Automated
Logas et al.	1987	Comparison	Handwritten vs. NIBP record	Automated
Lerou et al.	1988	Comparison	Handwritten vs. AIMS	Automated
Cook et al.	1989	Comparison	Handwritten vs. NIBP record	Automated
Thrush	1992	Comparison	Handwritten vs. AIMS/scribe	Automated

Note. AIMS = anesthesia information management systems; NIBP = Non–Invasive Blood Pressure.

system. The authors noted that, "Significant changes in data were often underestimated by humans who tended to smooth out a record. In addition, a computerized monitoring recording tends to pick up changes when the anesthesiologist is otherwise occupied" (Zollinger et al., 1977, p. 423). Such discrepancies between computerized and handwritten records would be noted over the course of many comparisons in years to follow.

Other studies of accuracy between handwritten records and AIMS were to follow. In each case, vital signs generated by AIMS were found to be more accurate and timely than handwritten records. In addition, many of these studies indicated significant evidence of late entries, missed values, and "smoothing" of the record. Table 5.3 provides a list of publications addressing comparisons of accuracy.

COMPLETENESS

In 1993, Edsall et al. reviewed concerns of completeness, time spent in recordkeeping tasks, and the overall quality of the anesthetic record. The authors used only a small sample of subjects, with each subject completing an equal number of handwritten and AIMS records. Subjects were videotaped, and subsequently reviewed by the researchers to measure the time spent in recordkeeping activities. Quality of the anesthetic record was determined by the number of illegible or incorrect entries by either method of recordkeeping. Completeness of the anesthetic record was determined by the inclusion of 46 predetermined elements of patient care, including demographic data about the patient, appropriate frequency of notation of vital signs, and narrative data about procedures and events of the anesthetic. The average length of a case was similar for the two groups.

Results of the study indicated that significantly more time was spent in recordkeeping activities with handwritten records (11.9 minutes per case) than with the AIMS (4.95 minutes per case). Frequency of artifact was not significantly different between the two groups, and AIMS records were found to be more complete in both clinical items and vital signs. There were no incidents of missing data in the AIMS group, while the Manual Entry Recordkeeping System group had 71 absences of data. Despite the limitations of a very small sample size, the authors submitted that, "In addition to producing a more complete, accurate, and easily reviewable record for quality assurance and other review purposes, AIMS's require proportionately less time than manual systems for anesthesia record keeping, thereby allowing more time for patient observation and direct patient care" (Edsall et al., 1993).

In accompaniment to the work of Edsall et al. (1993), critical elements for inclusion in the anesthetic record were the subject of a study by Biddle et al. (2001). Based upon the standards of monitoring and recordkeeping of the ASA and AANA, 13 variables were identified as important for inclusion in an anesthetic record. These variables included: patient identification, surgery and/or anesthesia start time, anesthesia provider name(s), heart rate/rhythm, blood pressure, oxyhemoglobin saturation, end-tidal carbon dioxide, FiO_2, or $O_2/N_2O/$ air liter flow, volatile agent concentration, airway management, intravenous fluid, emergence from anesthesia, and surgical positioning (Biddle et al., 2001). Through a multicenter study that included four academic medical centers and five community hospitals, a total of 4,989 anesthesia records were tabulated for missing variables. Results indicated significant lapses in completeness, with only the variable of "patient identification" present on every chart evaluated (Biddle et al., 2001). The authors suggested that the high volume of tasks associated with emergence of anesthesia, coupled with performance pressure for efficient operating room turnover, could have resulted in the unusually high rate of absence of the variable "emergence from anesthesia" (Biddle et al., 2001). These findings are consistent with the findings of Edsall (1993), and serve to support the findings that periods of high workload may have a significant effect on recordkeeping.

FINANCIAL INCENTIVES/RETURN ON INVESTMENT

Many proponents of electronic recordkeeping have cited improved capture of billing elements associated with anesthesia delivery as a distinctive benefit (Edsall et al., 1993; Lubarsky et al., 1997). In 1997, Lubarsky et al. examined use of the AIMS to perform and implement cost containment practices within the anesthesia department at the Duke University Medical Center in Durham, North Carolina. This work was an expansion of previous research by the authors who cited in an abstract a cost saving of approximately one million dollars per year by introducing practice guidelines for pharmaceutical use (Edsall et al., 1993; Lubarsky et al., 1996). In this research, total costs of muscle relaxants, induction agents, anxiolytics, opioid analgesics, fluids, and volatile anesthetics, were studied to determine usage practices and total costs, with 99% accuracy (Lubarsky et al., 1997). Results were considered by five "best practice committees," which examined the results of the study and created suggestions for cost containment. As a result of this research, practice guidelines were implemented at the facility to reduce pharmaceutical costs. In particular, individual pharmaceutical costs were calculated, and this information shared with each provider. A reward program was instituted to provide practitioners with financial incentive in the form of an educational expense account for practitioners with high degrees of compliance. In this way, the authors felt certain to enhance or at least maintain cost savings through practice guidelines created through the use of the extensive database complied by the AIMS (Lubarsky et al., 1997).

Thys (1998) cited enhanced capture of billing elements as one of several benefits that substantiate the claim that the use of AIMS was "essential" (Thys, 1998). Enhanced billing services included more accurate documentation of services provided to the patient, more accurate accounting of costs with the ability to produce cost containment through practice guidelines, and improved utilization of resources to improve efficiency and limit waste of time and materials.

Reich et al. (2006) explored the possibilities of improved efficiency through use of AIMS, developing a program to obtain billing elements directly from the computerized anesthesia record at the time of service, rather than at a later time by billing personnel using paper vouchers. The program examined every record generated by the anesthesia department on a daily basis, and identified any missing elements that would be required for payment of services rendered. Billing elements included electronic signatures for all anesthesia personnel, patient demographic information and diagnosis, anesthetic technique and placement of invasive monitors, and surgical procedure performed. Use of this program reduced "charge lag" (time elapsed from date of service to submission of charges to the payer) by 7.3 days, and direct collection of billing elements eliminated the need for a full-time employee assigned to anesthesia charge reconciliation, a cost saving determined to be $32,000 per year. Further cost savings were realized by decreased costs for printing, transporting, and filing of records, a reduction of an additional $10,000 per year. The authors cited the cost savings, enhanced accuracy of billing elements, and reduction of charge lag, as justification for the purchase, implementation, and maintenance of AIMS (Reich et al., 2006).

The concept of accuracy of documentation of all elements necessary for acceptance and reimbursement from third-party payers was further explored by

Spring et al. in 2007. The authors developed software that would examine each anesthetic record for completeness, and automatically notify practitioners by e-mail of missing elements in need of correction. Over the course of this research, cases that could not be billed were reduced from 3.4% of all cases to 0.04% of all cases. Time elapsed from identification to correction of these billing elements was reduced from an average of 33 days to 3 days. Time to release an anesthetic bill to the payers was reduced from an average of 3.1 days to an average of 1.1 days. Overall, more than 90% of anesthesia providers found the system easy to use. The authors stated that calculations of cost savings indicated, "…the time to return on investment was one half year" (Spring et al., 2007, p. 162).

This "return on investment" concept was further refined by O'Sullivan et al. in 2007. The authors identified four areas of benefits unique to AIMS recordkeeping that enhanced billing and reimbursement, justifying the initial cost of investment in the system. These benefits included the reduction of pharmaceutical costs, reduction of anesthesia staffing costs through enhanced efficiency of scheduling of staff and cases, enhanced capture of billing elements, and more accurate documentation of diagnosis and procedure charge coding. In addition to a reduction in pharmaceutical costs, the authors suggested that use of prelabeled, bar-coded syringes could also enhance patient safety by the reduction or elimination of medication errors.

Findings from O'Sullivan et al. (2007) were cited by Egger Halbeis and Epstein (2008) as arguments to present to hospital facilities reluctant to provide initial financial outlay for purchase and implementation of AIMS, despite similar utilization by other services within the facility (radiology or pharmacy; Egger Halbeis & Epstein, 2008). Potential impediments to the purchase of AIMS offered by hospital administrators were cited as lack of understanding of benefit to the institution, despite clear evidence of benefit to the anesthesia department. In many facilities, anesthesia services are provided by a private group contracted for service to the hospital, a fact indicated as a cause for such beliefs by the institution. These four benefits, particularly that of enhanced accuracy of billing elements for the hospital, were cited by Egger Halbeis and Epstein (2008) as part of a "value proposition" to administrators who failed to recognize many of the potential benefits of AIMS over more traditional handwritten anesthesia records (Egger Halbeis & Epstein, 2008).

ENHANCED MEDICOLEGAL PROTECTION

The concept of enhanced medicolegal protection of the practitioner by use of automated anesthesia recordkeeping systems has been likened to the use of cockpit data recorders in the airline industry (Gibbs, 1989). Comparisons between the delivery of anesthesia and piloting a commercial airliner have long been illustrated. Similarities between the two industries have been linked through safety checklists (preflight versus anesthesia machine checkout), the intensity of workload at the beginning and end of the case or flight (takeoff and landing versus induction and emergence from anesthesia), and the paucity of stimulation during routine operations and the requirement for intense vigilance to enable swift response to any unexpected event (Gibbs, 1989). The benefit of AIMS to serve as a flight data recorder for an anesthetic was illustrated by Gibbs (1989), and almost immediately refuted. In an editorial to the *Journal of Clinical Monitoring*, Gaba (1990), an author known for work with human error and patient safety, countered the arguments presented by Gibbs (1989). Gaba (1990) suggested that AIMS were limited by the accuracy of man-made and frequently noninvasive devices monitoring a human patient, while flight data recorders directly documented the functions of mechanical and electronic systems of a mechanical airframe. The potential for erroneous data recording by AIMS of the human patient would limit the accuracy of any documentation produced (Gaba, 1990). The concern of artifact has long been a common theme among practitioners considering the risks and benefits of AIMS. Concerning the medicolegal aspects of AIMS, Gaba (1990) stated, "Paradoxically, were it not for the medico-legal environment, the profession [anesthesiology] might have more quickly adopted many aspects of automated recordkeeping, with all its current limitations and flaws, because it would have benefits with few risks" (Gaba, 1990, p. 338).

An illustration of actual data omitted by AIMS was made in 1994. Through three case studies, Feingold et al. (1994) cited episodes of severe bradycardia in the form of sinus pauses of up to 5 seconds requiring treatment with atropine for correction that were not recorded by the AIMS in use at the time. These omissions were noted to be due to the fact that data was recorded by the AIMS at a maximum frequency of 30 seconds (Feingold, Galindo, & Feingold, 1994). In one case, placement of a permanent cardiac pacemaker was required due to recurrences of significant and symptomatic bradycardia (Feingold et al., 1994). The authors cited the omissions noted in these three cases as examples of significant risk of automated recordkeeping systems and the need for sustained vigilance on the part of the anesthesia provider assigned to the case (Feingold et al., 1994).

Continued concerns of accuracy and potential exposure to medical malpractice claims prompted a survey of anesthesia departments utilizing AIMS in 2004. Of particular concern were two scenarios, (a) documentation of actual data that is both innocuous and self-limiting and (b) documentation of erroneous data or artifact by the AIMS. In each scenario, the author contended that most practitioners would choose not to record this data, relying on professional judgment that such data was of little benefit to the case (Feldman, 2004). Such data, as recorded by AIMS, could serve as potentially damaging, albeit erroneous, data in the event of a poor outcome for the patient and subsequent medicolegal proceedings (Feldman, 2004).

The opposing viewpoint illustrates that anesthesia records generated by AIMS would be more timely, more complete, and more legible than the equivalent report generated on a handwritten record. To research the validity of each point, the author developed and distributed a survey to anesthesia departments utilizing AIMS for anesthesia recordkeeping (Feldman, 2004). Results of the survey indicated that in no case was the anesthetic record generated by the AIMS determined to serve as a hindrance to the defense of practitioners. Comments attached to the survey results indicated that in some cases, practitioners using AIMS felt that the system served to prevent malpractice claims. The practitioners felt that AIMS could reveal unsafe practices prior to a critical incident that could result in a lawsuit (Feldman, 2004). Other comments also indicated that although the objectivity and legibility of an AIMS record serve to benefit the defense, in some cases the record implicated the practitioner's obvious lack of vigilance, resulting in a settlement with the plaintiff (Feldman, 2004). As a tool for defense of anesthesia practitioners, results of this survey indicated that such a record was most accurately described as objective; exonerating the innocent and implicating the guilty.

Despite the benefits of AIMS records in medical malpractice lawsuits, concerns of artifact and missing data prevailed. In 2006, Vigoda and Lubarsky documented a case report in which a significant failure of the AIMS to capture patient data resulted in the implication of the anesthesia provider managing the case in a medical malpractice suit. Over the course of a craniotomy for a patient with a brain tumor, some 90 minutes of data was not captured by the AIMS. This AIMS contained software that allowed multiple "windows" of data to be displayed. Each window occupied the entire display screen, yet only the "home" screen displayed incoming data from the patient monitors. The loss of data capture was unrecognized by the anesthesia provider, who had a "summary" window displayed, and was unable to view incoming data. Upon recognition of this issue as a result of a change of anesthesia providers, the problem was rapidly corrected, but the data was not entered manually. Upon emergence, there was complete loss of motor function of the extremities. Over the course of the lawsuit, the anesthesia provider assigned to the case was charged with negligence due to the lack of proper monitoring of the patient, and the recording of data at five-minute intervals as required by the monitoring standards of the ASA (Vigoda & Lubarsky, 2006a). Loss of data was determined to be due to the simple disconnection of a single cable between the patient monitors and the AIMS. Also unique to this lawsuit was the evidence of documentation by the attending anesthesiologist of physical presence on emergence; this documentation was determined to have been entered within minutes of the beginning of the case, rather than at the end of the case, as would be appropriate. By entering this data immediately after induction of anesthesia, the anesthesiologist cast doubt as to whether or not he or she was actually physically present on emergence from anesthesia. While there was evidence that indicated that the anesthesia provider displayed vigilance in patient care and was aware of vital signs that were unrecorded, the lack of documentation of vital signs and evidence of inappropriately timed documentation of other elements were "difficult to defend". The outcome of this case resulted in significant changes in documentation practices at the facility as well as a modification of the AIMS software by the manufacturer to add a "pop-up" window that would indicate the loss of incoming data (Vigoda & Lubarsky, 2006a).

Timeliness of documentation was examined by Vigoda and Lubarsky in an article published just 1 month later in 2006. The difficulty in the maintenance of the timeliness of required documentation when an anesthesiologist is supervising the anesthesia delivery of more than one operating room was illustrated, and differences in electronic and manual records were examined. The identification of an "audit trail," or the electronic record of the time of entry of documentation in an AIMS record, by medical malpractice lawyers has resulted in a significant reduction of "prospective charting"—documentation of events that have yet to occur—by anesthesia providers. Due to the lack of accurate determination of the timing of entries made on a handwritten anesthetic record, such prospective charting was, "according to private communications, not uncommon in many practices." Through educational sessions, e-mail contact of performance/compliance, and subsequent e-mail "copy notification" to the department chairman, documentation timing accuracy improved to 99.5% at the authors' facility. Through such actions, prospective charting—a practice potentially damaging to the integrity of the anesthesia care team—was virtually eliminated (Vigoda & Lubarsky, 2006b).

QUALITY IMPROVEMENT

With the development of electronic medical records, the potential advantages of computerized database systems over traditional handwritten records were quickly recognized. Directed review of a medical record by query entries showed the potential to improve the speed and quality of analysis of a patient's entire medical history (Whiting-O'Keefe, Simborg, Epstein, & Warger, 1985). Automation of an anesthetic record could also carry the added benefit of increased data through shorter sampling intervals, rather than the standard 5-minute documentation of vital signs. In addition to reducing the workload of the anesthesia provider by eliminating the need to manually record each value, an automated system could be programmed to record values much more frequently than could be feasibly recorded on a handwritten record. For some rapidly changing vital signs, such enhancement could result in a more accurate record of events of anesthesia and surgery (Gravenstein, de Vries, & Beneken, 1989).

Once recorded, the anesthesia record could be consolidated into a large database, where each record produced could be stored electronically for future retrieval. Review of this database could potentially result in recognition of trends of poor or inefficient performance, or even the identification of practices that could prove detrimental to patient safety. Once identified, such practices could be examined more carefully, and refined, altered, or eliminated. Individual review of a database of such large volume would be infeasible without electronic means (Edsall, Jones, & Smith, 1992).

Such queries have been shown to reveal potentially detrimental events occurring during the course of anesthesia delivery, with the use of electronic review illustrated to be more sensitive than the practice of voluntary reporting of such incidents. Sanborn et al. (1996) compared deviations from normal and expected values of vital signs (heart rate, blood pressure, oxygen saturation, and temperature) voluntarily reported by anesthesia providers and the same deviations discovered by computerized searching software of anesthesia records collected by AIMS. The electronic scans revealed 434 "incidents," of which only 18 were voluntarily reported by anesthesia providers (Sanborn, Castro, Kuroda, & Thys, 1996).

Identification of errors or potential complications is only the first step in a series of measures that move medical care toward improvement. Once a problem has been identified, the factors that contribute to the negative outcome must be evaluated, with a goal of prevention of complications. AIMS have been utilized to assist the anticipation of potential complications, as illustrated by the use of AIMS for prediction of the need for antiemetic treatment in a postanesthesia care unit (PACU; Junger et al., 2001). AIMS have also been utilized for the identification of more serious complications that may develop over the course of an anesthetic, such as the prediction of hypoxia during one-lung ventilation (Sticher et al., 2002), or for the need for inotropic support for patients undergoing cardiac surgery (Jost et al., 2003). Such predictions were accomplished through complex software analysis of large consolidations of many anesthetic records over many years, made possible by the electronic collection and storage of this data.

Further research supported the development of such large databases through use of AIMS. The physiologic effects of anesthetic agents have been examined, with suggestions for practice guidelines that may result in enhanced patient safety. The physiologic effects of selected induction agents were categorized by

ASA classification of patients, with the outcome of postinduction hypotension measured (Benson et al., 2000). After analysis of over 8,000 anesthetic records, propofol was found to produce the greatest reduction in blood pressure. Further division of patients by ASA classification revealed that hypotension was greater in those patients with a classification of III or higher, and least with those of II or lower. These findings were consistent with the literature specifically analyzing the physiologic effects of these agents, leading the authors to conclude that data analysis of computerized records was valid and reliable (Benson et al., 2000).

Analysis of electronic records may also be focused on the outcomes of specific anesthesia procedures. The incidence of severe bradycardia or asystole following spinal or epidural anesthesia administration was examined by the use of an AIMS database in 2003 by Lesser et al. Over 57,000 records were analyzed, with cases that involved spinal or epidural anesthesia associated with general anesthesia eliminated from analysis. Results of the data analysis revealed that an initial heart rate of less than 60 bpm and male gender were most predictive of severe bradycardia following neuraxial blockade, with spinal anesthesia resulting in a higher incidence of bradycardia than epidural anesthesia administration. These findings were presented to enable anesthesia practitioners to recognize the potential for severe bradycardia in select patients, allowing for alternate anesthesia plans or pretreatment with agents to increase heart rate in susceptible patients. Development of such results served to establish the benefit of an AIMS database to significantly increase the speed and accuracy of analysis of a large volume of records (Lesser, Sanborn, Valskys, & Kuroda, 2003).

Development of results such as those presented by Lesser et al. (2003) and others (Egger Halbeis & Epstein, 2008) encouraged the development of "decision support systems (DSSs)" to identify patients at risk of anesthetic complications and make appropriate adjustments in anesthesia administration and planning to prevent negative outcomes.

Limitations of utilizing data from AIMS to inform decision making and policy formulation were illustrated by Epstein, Dexter, Ehrenfeld, and Sandberg (2009). Delay in entry of automated records into a consolidated database could affect the results of targeted queries that could be influenced by the absence of such late records. Other potential sources of error included the absence of entries, a delay in processing the record from the workstation to the central database, the rounding of timing of events by the AIMS, or by the lack of synchronization of clocks throughout the operating theater. When relying on queries to a large database generated by AIMS, users were cautioned to take delays and latency of entries into account prior to making policy decisions based solely on this data (Epstein et al., 2009).

CONCLUSION

Beginning with the first known account of anesthesia recordkeeping in 1894, handwritten records have sought to improve the safety and efficacy of practitioners in the care of their patients, and provide archival records for subsequent clinical cases and research purposes. With increasing monitoring capabilities, patient safety has improved, at the cost of increasing demands of recordkeeping for anesthesia providers. As early as 1934, Dr. McKesson expressed concern that the number of recordkeeping tasks exceeded the ability of a human practitioner to maintain appropriate vigilance to patient care while creating an accurate and timely anesthesia record.

With these concerns in mind, development of an electronic means to record data from an anesthetic was initiated, although this goal exceeded the capabilities of technology until more modern times. As technology advanced to the point that a complete and accurate recording of multiple patient variables and events of anesthesia and surgery was possible, many experts raised voices of dissension, concerned that removal of the handwritten record would disconnect the practitioner from the flow of data critical to safe patient care (Lees, 1985; Noel, 1986; Rosen & Rosenzweig, 1985; Saunders, 1990). Others made the claim that removal of the human element could produce a record that was more accurate and of higher quality, as data collection could be increased through electronic means that would far exceed the capability of a handwritten chart created by a practitioner also engaged in patient care (Gravenstein et al., 1989). Perhaps the greatest concerns focused on potential for the loss of attentiveness to the patient (Kay & Neal, 1986) and studies to compare the effects of methods of recordkeeping on the vigilance of anesthesia providers sought to respond.

With well-documented financial incentives (Lubarsky et al., 1997; O'Sullivan et al., 2007; Reich et al., 2006), as well as government subsidies (Egger Halbeis et al., 2008; Ehrenfeld & Rehman, 2011), AIMS are becoming adopted at an unprecedented rate (Egger Halbeis et al., 2008). With the goals of the federal government to enhance the use of the electronic medical record, there is an emerging belief that AIMS may soon be mandated (Paradis, 2011), with more limited choices than currently available. As assessed by, and often in spite of the published evidence, concerns of practitioners still reflect many of the same concerns expressed in the editorial comments of the past.

REFERENCES

Abenstein, J. P., DeVos, C. B., Tarhan, A., & Tarhan, S. (1992). Eight year's experience with automated anesthesia record keeping: Lessons learned-new directions taken. *International Journal of Clinical Monitoring and Computing, 9*, 117–129.

Allard, J., Dzwonczyk, R., Yablok, D., Block, F. E., & McDonald, J. S. (1995). Effect of automatic record keeping on vigilance and record keeping time. *British Journal of Anaesthesia, 74*, 619–626.

American Association of Nurse Anesthetists. (2007). *Scope and standards for nurse anesthesia practice.* Retrieved from http://www.aana.com/Resources.aspx?ucNavMenu_TSMenuTargetID=51&ucNavMenu_TSMenuTargetType=4&ucNavMenu_TSMenuID=6&id=783

Apple, H. P., Schneider, A. J., & Fadel, J. (1982). Design and evaluation of a semiautomatic anesthesia record system. *Medical Instrumentation, 16*(1), 69–71.

ASA. (2005). *Standards, guidelines and statements.* Retrieved from http://www.asahq.org/publicationsAndServices/sgstoc.htm

Beecher, H. K. (1920). The first anesthesia records (codman, cushing). *Surgery, Gynecology, and Obstetrics, 71*, 689–693.

Benson, M., Junger, A., Fuchs, C., Quinzio, L., Bottger, S., & Hempelmann, G. (2000). Use of an anesthesia information management system (AIMS) to evaluate the physiologic effects of hypnotic agents used to induce anesthesia. *Journal of Clinical Monitoring and Computing, 16*(3), 183–190.

Biddle, C., Bauer, L., Dosch, M., Dove, C., Nagelhout, J., Waugaman, W., et al. (2001). Analysis of noteworthy indicators on the anesthesia record: A prospective, multiregional study. *AANA Journal, 69*(5), 407–410.

Block, F. E. (1989). Automatic anesthesia record keeping. *Journal of Clinical Monitoring, 5*(4), 284–286.

Cook, R. I., McDonald, J. S., & Nunziata, E. (1989). Differences between handwritten and automatic blood pressure records. *Anesthesiology, 71*(3), 385–390.

Davis, T. C., Green, J. A., Colquhoun, A., Hage, B. L., & Biddle, C. (2012). Anesthesia recordkeeping: Accuracy of recall with computerized and manual entry recordkeeping. *Journal of Clinical Monitoring and Computing, 26*(3), 163–169.

Drui, A., Behm, R., & Martin, W. (1973). Predesign investigation of the anesthesia operational environment. *Anesthesia and Analgesia, 52*, 584–591.

Edsall, D. W., Deshane, P., Giles, C., Dick, D., Sloan, B., & Farrow, J. (1993). Computerized patient anesthesia records: Less time and better quality than manually produced anesthesia records. *Journal of Clinical Anesthesia, 5*(4), 275–283.

Edsall, D. W., Jones, B. R., & Smith, N. T. (1992). The anesthesia database, the automated record, and the quality assurance process. *International Anesthesiology Clinics, 30*(2), 71–92.

Egger Halbeis, C. B., & Epstein, R. H. (2008). The value proposition of anesthesia information management systems. *Anesthesiology Clinics, 26*(4), 665–679, vi.

Egger Halbeis, C. B., Epstein, R. H., Macario, A., Pearl, R. G., & Grunwald, Z. (2008). Adoption of anesthesia information management systems by academic departments in the united states. *Anesthesia and Analgesia, 107*(4), 1323–1329.

Ehrenfeld, J. M., & Rehman, M. A. (2011). Anesthesia information management systems: A review of functionality and installation considerations. *Journal of Clinical Monitoring and Computing, 25*(1), 71–79.

Eichhorn, J. H., Cooper, J. B., Cullen, D. J., Maier, W. R., Philip, J. H., & Seeman, R. G. (1986). Standards for patient monitoring during anesthesia at Harvard medical school. *The Journal of the American Medical Association, 256*(8), 1017–1020.

Eichhorn, J. H., & Edsall, D. W. (1991). Computerization of anesthesia information management. *Journal of Clinical Monitoring, 7*(1), 71–82.

Epstein, R. H., Dexter, F., Ehrenfeld, J. M., & Sandberg, W. S. (2009). Implications of event entry latency on anesthesia information management decision support systems. *Anesthesia and Analgesia, 108*(3), 941–947.

Feingold, A., Galindo, A., & Feingold, H. E. (1994). Lack of documentation of severe transient bradycardia by an automated anesthesia record. *Journal of Clinical Monitoring, 10*(6), 382–386.

Feldman, J. M. (2004). Do anesthesia information systems increase malpractice exposure? results of a survey. *Anesthesia and Analgesia, 99*(3), 840–843.

Gaba, D. M. (1990). The present and future medicolegal importance of record keeping in anesthesia and intensive care: The case for automation. *Journal of Clinical Monitoring, 6*(4), 338–339.

Gibbs, R. F. (1989). The present and future medicolegal importance of record keeping in anesthesia and intensive care: The case for automation. *Journal of Clinical Monitoring, 5*(4), 251–255.

Gravenstein, J. S., de Vries, A., & Beneken, J. E. (1989). Sampling intervals for clinical monitoring of variables during anesthesia. *Journal of Clinical Monitoring, 5*(1), 17–21.

Gunn, I. P. (2005). Nurse anesthesia: A history of challenge. In J. J. Nagelhout, & K. L. Zaglaniczny (Eds.), *Nurse Anesthesia* (3rd ed., pp. 1–29). St. Louis, MO: Elsevier.

Hamilton, W. K. (1990). The automated anesthesic record is inevitable and valuable. *Journal of Clinical Monitoring, 6*, 333–334.

Heinrichs, W., Monk, S., & Eberle, B. (1997). Automated anesthesia record systems. [Automatische Anasthesieprotokollsysteme]. *Der Anaesthesist, 46*(7), 574–582.

Huslin, A. (2009). Online health data in remission. *Washington Post*, pp. D01. Retrieved from http://www.washingtonpost.com/wp-dyn/content/article/2009/02/15/AR2009021501284.html

Ishizawa, Y. (2011). Special article: General anesthetic gases and the global environment. *Anesthesia and Analgesia, 112*(1), 213–217.

Jost, A., Junger, A., Zickmann, B., Hartmann, B., Banzhaf, A., Quinzio, L., et al. (2003). Potential benefits of anaesthesia information management systems for multicentre data evaluation: Risk calculation of inotropic support in patients undergoing cardiac surgery. *Medical Informatics and the Internet in Medicine, 28*(1), 7–19.

Junger, A., Hartmann, B., Benson, M., Schindler, E., Dietrich, G., Jost, A., et al. (2001). The use of an anesthesia information management system for prediction of antiemetic rescue treatment at the postanesthesia care unit. *Anesthesia and Analgesia, 92*(5), 1203–1209.

Kay, J., & Neal, M. (1986). Effect of automatic blood pressure devices on vigilance of anesthesia residents. *Journal of Clinical Monitoring, 2*(3), 148–150.

Kennedy, P. J., Feingold, A., Wiener, E. L., & Hosek, R. S. (1976). Analysis of tasks and human factors in anesthesia for coronary-artery bypass. *Anesthesia and Analgesia, 55*(3), 374–377.

Kheterpal, S., Gupta, R., Blum, J. M., Tremper, K. K., O'Reilly, M., & Kazanjian, P. E. (2007). Electronic reminders improve procedure documentation compliance and professional fee reimbursement. *Anesthesia and Analgesia, 104*(3), 592–597.

Lees, D. E. (1985). Computerized anesthesia records may have drawbacks. *Anesthesiology, 63*(2), 236–237.

Lerou, J. G., Dirksen, R., van Daele, M., Nijhuis, G. M., & Crul, J. F. (1988). Automated charting of physiological variables in anesthesia: A quantitative comparison of automated versus handwritten anesthesia records. *Journal of Clinical Monitoring, 4*(1), 37–47.

Lesser, J. B., Sanborn, K. V., Valskys, R., & Kuroda, M. (2003). Severe bradycardia during spinal and epidural anesthesia recorded by an anesthesia information management system. *Anesthesiology, 99*(4), 859–866.

Levitan, D. (2008). AIMS poised to revolutionize anesthesia care. *Anesthesiology News, 34*(3), 8–11.

Loeb, R. G. (1994). Monitor surveillance and vigilance of anesthesia residents. *Anesthesiology, 80*(3), 527–533.

Loeb, R. G. (1995). Manual record keeping is not necessary for anesthesia vigilance. *Journal of Clinical Monitoring, 11*, 9–4.

Logas, W. G., McCarthy, R. J., Narbone, R. F., & Ivankovich, A. D. (1987). Analysis of the accuracy of the anesthetic record [Abstract]. *Anesthesia and Analgesia, 66*(2), S107.

Lubarsky, D. A., Gan, T. J., Glass, P. S. A., Dear, G. D., Mythen, M., Dentz, M. et al. (1996). PACU clinical outcomes and financial savings following a pharmaceutical cost containment program in anesthesia using practice guidelines [Abstract]. *Anesthesia and Analgesia,* 82 S285.

Lubarsky, D. A., Sanderson, I. C., Gilbert, W. C., King, K. P., Ginsberg, B., Dear, G. L., et al. (1997). Using an anesthesia information management system as a cost containment tool. description and validation. *Anesthesiology, 86*(5), 1161–1169.

McKesson, E. I. (1934). The technique of recording the effects of gas-oxygen mixtures, pressures, rebreathing and carbon-dioxid, with a summary of the effects. *Anesthesia and Analgesia, 13*(1), 1–7.

Noel, T. N. (1986). Computerized anesthesia records may be dangerous. *Anesthesiology, 60*, 300.

Olmedo, E. L., & Kirk, R. E. (1977). Maintenance of vigilance by non-task-related stimulation in the monitoring environment. *Perceptual and Motor Skills, 44*(3 Pt 1), 715–723.

O'Sullivan, C. T., Dexter, F., Lubarsky, D. A., & Vigoda, M. M. (2007). Evidence-based management assessment of return on investment from anesthesia information management systems. *AANA Journal, 75*(1), 43–48.

Paget, N. S., Lambert, T. F., & Sridhar, K. (1981). Factors affecting an anaesthetist's work: Some findings on vigilance and performance. *Anaesthesia and Intensive Care, 9*(4), 359–365.

Paradis, M. (2011). *Five things every anesthesia provider should know about AIMS*. Retrieved from Surgical Information Systems website: http://www.sisfirst.com/solutions/anesthesia.html

Reich, D. L., Kahn, R. A., Wax, D., Palvia, T., Galati, M., & Krol, M. (2006). Development of a module for point-of-care charge capture and submission using an anesthesia information management system. *Anesthesiology, 105*(1), 179–186; quiz 231–232.

Rosen, A. S., & Rosenzweig, W. (1985). In reply to computerized anesthesia records may have drawbacks. *Anesthesiology, 62*(2), 237.

Sanborn, K. V., Castro, J., Kuroda, M., & Thys, D. M. (1996). Detection of intraoperative incidents by electronic scanning of computerized anesthesia records. comparison with voluntary reporting. *Anesthesiology, 85*(5), 977–987.

Saunders, R. J. (1990). The automated anesthetic record will not automatically solve problems in record keeping. *Journal of Clinical Monitoring, 6*, 334–337.

Shaffer, M. J., Kaiser, P. R., Klingenmaier, C. H., & Gordon, M. R. (1978). Manual record-keeping and statistical records for the operating room. *Medical Instrumentation, 12*(3), 192–197.

Spring, S. F., Sandberg, W. S., Anupama, S., Walsh, J. L., Driscoll, W. D., & Raines, D. E. (2007). Automated documentation error detection and notification improves anesthesia billing performance. *Anesthesiology, 106*(1), 157–163.

Sticher, J., Junger, A., Hartmann, B., Benson, M., Jost, A., Golinski, M., et al. (2002). Computerize anesthesia record keeping in thoracic surgery—suitability of electronic anesthesia records in evaluating predictors for hypoxemia during one-lung ventilation. *Journal of Clinical Monitoring and Computing, 17*(6), 335–343.

Stol, I. S., Ehrenfeld, J. M., & Epstein, R. H. (2014). Technology diffusion of anesthesia information management systems into academic anesthesia departments in the United States. *Anesthesia and Analgesia, 118*(3), 644–650.

Thatcher, V. S. (1953). *History of anesthesia: With emphasis on the nurse specialist*. Philadelphia, PA: Lippincott.

Thrush, D. N. (1992). Are automated anesthesia records better? *Journal of Clinical Anesthesia, 4*(5), 386–389.

Thys, D. M. (1998). *The role of information systems in anesthesia*. Retrieved from http://www.apsf.org/resource_center/newsletter/2001/summer/03Infosys.htm

Vigoda, M. M., Gencorelli, F., & Lubarsky, D. A. (2006). Changing medical group behaviors: Increasing the rate of documentation of quality assurance events using an anesthesia information system. *Anesthesia and Analgesia, 103*(2), 390–395.

Vigoda, M. M., & Lubarsky, D. A. (2006a). Failure to recognize loss of incoming data in an anesthesia record-keeping system may have increased medical liability. *Anesthesia and Analgesia, 102*(6), 1798–1802.

Vigoda, M. M., & Lubarsky, D. A. (2006b). The medicolegal importance of enhancing timeliness of documentation when using an anesthesia information system and the response to automated feedback in an academic practice. *Anesthesia and Analgesia, 103*(1), 131–136, table of contents.

Weinger, M. B., Herndon, O. W., & Gaba, D. M. (1997). The effect of electronic record keeping and transesophageal echocardiography on task distribution, workload, and vigilance during cardiac anesthesia. *Anesthesiology, 87*(1), 144–155.

Whiting-O'Keefe, Q. E., Simborg, D. W., Epstein, W. V., & Warger, A. (1985). A computerized summary medical record system can provide more information than the standard medical record. *The Journal of the American Medical Association, 254*(9), 1185–1192.

Yablok, D. O. (1990). Comparison of vigilance using automated versus handwritten records [Abstract]. *Anesthesiology, 73,* A416.

Zbinden, A. M., Christensen, J., & Kuster, M. (1992). How can a standard software package for data management in anesthesia be achieved? *The Journal of Clinical Monitoring, 8*(4), 315–318.

Zollinger, R. M, Jr., Kreul, J. F., & Schneider, A. J. (1977). Man-made versus computer-generated anesthesia records. *The Journal of Surgical Research, 22*(4), 419–424.

CHAPTER 6

Chronic Postsurgical Pain

Steven R. Wooden

ABSTRACT

Chronic postsurgical pain (CPSP) is defined as a persistent pain state that exists more than 2 months postoperatively and cannot be explained by other causes such as recurrence of disease, apparent inflammation, or other nonsurgical related factors. CPSP is a type of persistent pain condition that often complicates recovery from surgical procedures. It is thought to be caused by surgical nerve injury, but the fact that an identifiable nerve injury can be found in only one-third of CPSP patients suggests that the problem may be far more complex than a simple surgically created nerve injury. Certain surgical procedures report a high incidence of CPSP, helping to isolate likely candidates for this problem, but instituting preventative measures and identifying a treatable source of pain continues to be elusive. Some progress has been made in the areas of prevention and treatment.

INTRODUCTION

Pain comes in many forms and degrees. Its purpose is integrally tied to the human central nervous system (CNS) and the human response to physical threats. However, when pain persists and no longer serves as a survival response, it can cause damage to the nervous system, lost productivity, and disability. Persistent pain is defined in a variety of ways, but is universally recognized as containing negative physical, psychological, and quality of life components

http://dx.doi.org/10.1891/0739-6686.35.91

(Netto & Brites, 2011). Persistent pain has a greater negative impact on the U.S. economy than cancer, heart disease, and diabetes (Gaskin & Richard, 2012).

Persistent pain associated with a distinct uninterrupted period of 3 months or more, which includes a negative sensory and emotional experience, is often referred to as "chronic pain" (Pozek, Beausang, Baratta, & Viscusi, 2016). Other definitions of chronic pain use terms such as "nociceptive pain" or "neuropathic pain." Nociceptive pain is a broader concept than neuropathic pain. Nociceptive pain can be caused by soft tissue damage, tumor expansion, or other non-nerve damaging origins that stimulate a painful sensory event. Neuropathic pain is specific to nerve injury. Both can trigger a dysfunctional response, leading to chronic pain symptoms and treatment challenges.

Chronic pain is also sometimes categorized as psychogenic, inflammatory, or neuropathic in origin, and the defining time period of interrupted pain ranges from 2 to 6 months. The categories of chronic pain are important to understand because each one demonstrates unique characteristics related to spinal cord and sensory neuron changes (Honore et al., 2000). In addition, understanding the neurochemical markers related to the generation of chronic pain in each category may be important in helping to identify treatment options for chronic pain patients. However, chronic pain is a complex phenomenon that often contains elements of all the so-called "chronic pain categories" of emotional, inflammatory, and neuropathic components.

Chronic pain can be physically, psychologically, and socially devastating. It has been linked to divorce, poverty, homelessness, despair, and sometimes suicide (Ilgen et al., 2013). The management of chronic pain is often elusive because the source is not always clear. Assessment and treatment requires a health care professional who can appreciate the physical, psychological, and social aspects of the multidimensional nature of chronic pain. Advanced practice nurses are particularly well suited to address the problems associated with all types of chronic pain, using nursing theory, evidence-based intervention, multidisciplinary collaboration, and their unique skills as a nurse.

THE UNIQUE PROBLEM OF CHRONIC POSTSURGICAL PAIN

Chronic postsurgical pain (CPSP), sometimes called persistent postsurgical pain (PPP), is a particularly troublesome type of chronic pain that has a reported incidence of between 5% and 50%, depending on the particular type of surgical procedure (Kehlet & Rathmell, 2010). Large gaps exist in the knowledge of the origins of CPSP, which when elaborated may help to define and identify the reasons for this syndrome (Cregg, Anwar, & Farquhar-Smith, 2013). Although CPSP appears to be neuropathic in nature, it is not always associated with identifiable nerve injury (Johansen, Schirmer, Nielsen, & Stubhaug, 2016; Steegers, Snik, Verhagen, van der Drift, & Wilder-Smith, 2008). The International Association for the Study of Pain defines CPSP as “a persistent pain state that is apparent more than two months postoperatively that cannot be explained by other causes such as recurrence of disease, apparent inflammation, or others.” This very simplistic and obscure definition does little to help lead to identification and treatment of causative factors.

Much of the research into CPSP has been focused on specialty surgical procedures, but a compilation of studies related to CPSP has identified a group of the most common surgical procedures associated with CPSP, and potential methods to predict and prevent CPSP. Surgical procedures associated with CPSP are those of the thorax, abdomen, and pelvis. Those procedures include mastectomy, thoracotomy, cholecystectomy, nephrectomy, sternotomy, and other chest and upper abdominal procedures. Other common types of surgery that report a high incidence of CPSP are amputation, and inguinal/pelvic surgical procedures such as hernia repair. Nearly one out of four patients who undergo thoracic surgery develop CPSP, but only one-third of them have an identifiable nerve injury (Peng et al., 2014). This would suggest that multiple factors are responsible for CPSP. Even in the absence of evidence that nerve injury is the causative factor, nerve compression, entrapment, and other types of nerve damage are often initially suspected.

Predictors of CPSP do help to isolate likely candidates, but do little to identify a treatable source of pain. Some studies suggest that CPSP is functional (Pinto, McIntyre, Ferrero, Araujo-Soares, & Almeida, 2013), while others point to psychological factors (Yarnitsky et al., 2008). The existence of preoperative pain, which can fall into either a functional or psychological category, appears to be a predictor of CPSP. In at least one study, preoperative pain was the most significant clinical predictor of CPSP (Pinto, McIntyre, Ferrero, Almeida, & Araujo-Soares, 2013). However, other studies indicate multiple predictive factors such as thyroid function, occult wound infection, or even secondary gain as possible contributors to CPSP (Costa et al., 2015). There are a few factors that predict a lower incidence of CPSP, such as young age (Kristensen, Pedersen, Hjortdal, Jensen, & Nikolajsen, 2010) and immunosuppressant therapy. The latter, immunosuppressant therapy, suggests that autoimmune issues may play a role in CPSP because those who are immunosuppressed postoperatively have a significantly lower incidence of CPSP when compared to those whose immune systems are not suppressed, for identical surgical procedures.

It is very apparent that CPSP is complex, and this complexity makes successful treatment very elusive. It is import, as with every type of chronic pain that we have an understanding of the anatomy and physiology of pain, pathophysiology of pain, and how chronic pain is thought to develop. Only then can we begin to understand how to develop a reasonable plan of care for CPSP patients.

ANATOMY, PHYSIOLOGY, AND PATHOPHYSIOLOGY OF PAIN

In order to understand the development, consequences, and possible treatment of CPSP, it is first important to understand the anatomy, physiology, and pathophysiology of pain. The body is under constant sensory stimulation. The inhibitory pain transmission systems, which maintain a balance between sensory input transmission and inhibition, prevent us from being overwhelmed with constant pain. However, the body needs an appropriate amount of sensory information to respond to potential harm.

There are three heuristic subdivisions of painful stimulation: (a) painful stimulation without tissue damage, (b) tissue damage without nerve damage, and (c) nerve damage (Deer, Leong, Buvanendran, & American Academy of Pain Medicine, 2013, pp. 3–19). It is important to understand the normal response of each subdivision of painful stimulation so that treatment can be appropriately targeted.

If we perceive pain, but there is no tissue damage, then we would normally withdraw from the stimulation. This withdrawal should terminate the sensation and resulting response. Under normal circumstances, the painful stimulation is specific to the site of potential injury and does not radiate beyond that site.

If there is tissue injury, pain would persist after removal of the stimulus. The area of injury will exhibit an intensified response to tactile stimulation, and the sensation of pain will spread beyond the local area of injury. The local and extended response is intended to protect the body and promote healing. Tissue damage releases a number of cell types and substances into the internal milieu that activate and support the response system. These substances include red cells, white cells, potassium, clotting factors, peptides, prostaglandins, inflammatory substances that cause vascular leaking and swelling, and other substances that promote neurotransmission through nerve membrane channel activation.

The final subdivision is damage that includes nerve injury. This can be caused by disease, accidental tissue injury involving nerve fibers, or by unintentional or unavoidable nerve injury during a surgical procedure. The extent of nerve injury can be classified into demyelinating or axonal injury. The type of injury to the nerve may indicate the likelihood of return to normal function with treatment (Uncini & Kuwabara, 2015).

Normal activation of neurotransmission is an important part of recognizing injury and limiting further damage. Once stimulated, A-delta and C nociceptive fibers produce an action potential through the release of substance P and other excitatory amino acids appropriate to the intensity and duration of stimulation. The sensory stimulation proceeds though the afferent nervous system to the dorsal horn of the spinal cord. At this point, inhibitory mechanisms play an important role in modulating sensation and response. If the stimulation is sufficient to overcome the inhibitory mechanisms of the spinal neuroanatomy, then the sensory information proceeds to the pain perception centers in the brain. This information is used to provide a motor response, through a flex arc, to pain. The information that passes on to the brain helps to build experience, expectation, and mood (Deer, Leong, Buvanendran, & American Academy of Pain Medicine, 2013, pp. 9–12).

In the event of an injury with associated tissue or nerve damage, chronic pain may emerge through a complex set of circumstances. The origin is not always identifiable, and the outcome is produced by a cascade of events. Chronic pain is not just a localized phenomenon. There are three anatomical regions that are associated with every pain response. The peripheral, spinal, and cerebral structures contribute to various aspects of pain recognition and response. When pain is present for an extended period of time, it can create dysfunctional changes in these three structures that may become irreversible. This dysfunctional activity is the basis for all types of chronic pain, including CPSP. In order to treat chronic pain, it is not always sufficient to simply remove the source of pain. However, successful treatment must start by addressing the source of the pain if it can be identified, which generally is located outside of the CNS created by soft tissue or nerve tissue damage. If the pain has become chronic, inhibitory mechanisms in the peripheral and spinal nervous systems may have become ineffective, and simply removing the original source of pain will be insufficient to eliminate the negative sensation. For that reason, the dysfunctional inhibitory mechanisms in the peripheral and spinal nervous system must also be addressed. Finally, pain perception in the cerebrum is normally a protective mechanism, which allows us to anticipate painful stimulation and avoid it. However, chronic pain may create havoc with these perceptive functions and addressing the dysfunction in this area is an important part of chronic pain management.

Treatment of chronic pain must include all three areas involved in pain transmission and perception. Return to normal function means that the pain generator is removed, the peripheral system is once again able to block innocuous stimulation, the spinal ascending inhibitory system can be returned to balance, and the forebrain perception of stimulation is normalized (Cross, 1994).

TYPES OF CHRONIC PAIN

Psychogenic

The terms psychogenic and psychosomatic are often used interchangeably. Psychosomatic describes a physical problem originating from a psychological component, while psychogenic is used to describe the perception of pain without physical findings. Many pain practitioners feel psychogenic is a meaningless term because all pain experiences have a psychological component. Psychosomatic pain is thought to exist by some groups of practitioners, but the phenomenon appears to be very rare and difficult to validate. Using either description may only stigmatize the patient and perhaps ignore the real possibility that an occult physical condition has contributed to some sort of psychopathology (Covington, 2000).

Inflammatory

Tissue damage in the human body results in a cascade of neurochemical responses. These responses are both local, at the site of injury, and sensory, which involves the peripheral and central nervous system. The localized response serves as a protective mechanism to help prevent further tissue damage, initiates a healing process, and begins a sensory response through the peripheral and central nervous system to create the perception of pain and trigger further protective mechanisms (Morrison, Perini, & Dunham, 2013). The localized response includes the release of inflammatory mediators that produce capillary vasodilatation, smooth muscle contraction, and promote synaptic transmission of pain impulses to the CNS. Those mediators include histamine, bradykinin, and substance P (Rodriguez, 2015). Increase in substance P and substance P receptor (neurokinin-1) activity is specifically associated with inflammatory pain, while diminished or absent in neuropathic and cancer pain respectively (Honore et al., 2000).

The sensory portion of the inflammatory response is often called "nociception." Nociception begins at the point of injury. Inflammatory mediators initiate a neuronal action potential, which is carried to the dorsal horn of the spinal cord, and then ascends to the thalamus where the perception of pain occurs (Rodriguez, 2015).

Neuropathic

When nerves are injured, pain radiates along a dermatome, or sensory pathway supplied by the nerve. Nerve injury often leads to a condition called allodynia (Richner, Bjerrum, Nykjaer, & Vaegter, 2011), which is triggering of a pain response from stimuli that do not normally provoke pain. Individuals with allodynia often have an intense burning sensation with small changes in temperature or light touch, typically along the dermatome of the injured nerve.

Pain and pain response to a normal inflammatory process is distinctly different from neuropathic pain in three ways. First, the pain associated with tissue injury improves within a given period of time, and the inflammatory response resolves. In contrast, neuropathic pain is persistent, even with evidence of tissue healing, and often an apparent or occult inflammatory response continues. The second difference is the presence of allodynia with neuropathic pain, which is absent with normal inflammatory response. The third difference is that neuropathic pain does not respond well to nonsteroidal anti-inflammatory agents (Xu & Yaksh, 2011).

EVOLUTION OF CHRONIC PAIN AND CPSP: WINDUP

Repetitive stimulation from chronic inflammation or nerve damage can lead to a condition referred to as "windup." Windup is a cyclical response to pain that leads to an abnormal pain response and chronic pain sensation, and can be physically and psychologically debilitating. Preventing windup is critical to the prevention of chronic pain and CPSP. Therefore it is critically important to treat the underlying cause of pain, and not ignore pain symptoms. Health care providers often label those who complain about pain as "drug seekers," "chronic complainers," or even "crazy." These types of statements indicate that the provider does not understand the history and physical issues that have placed the patient in a position to find anything possible to stop the pain. Chronic pain is not a psychological condition, but it can lead to psychological dysfunction (Deer, Leong, Buvanendran, & American Academy of Pain Medicine, 2013, pp. 3–16).

Peripheral Nervous System Contribution to Windup

The normal response to potentially traumatic peripheral stimulation is to withdraw. This response is initiated by the transmission of sensory impulses through the afferent peripheral nervous system, to the spinal nervous system, and into the perceptive centers of the brain, which in turn initiate a motor response. The peripheral fibers responsible for this quick response are myelinated fast and moderate acting nociceptors called "A" fibers. These fibers are responsible for sensations of cold temperature, pressure, and sharpness. The unmyelinated afferent peripheral "C" fibers are slow acting and are responsible for secondary sensations such as warmth, burning, itching, and touch. Neuropathic pain is thought to involve dysfunctional activity of both A and C fibers.

Upon normal stimulation of A and C fibers, substance P and excitatory amino acids are released, which activate neurokinins. Neurokinins generate an action potential, which carries sensory impulses up the afferent nerve pathways to the CNS appropriate to the intensity and duration of stimulation. Under normal conditions, N-methyl-D-aspartate (NMDA) receptors remain inactive because of magnesium stability. However, in the presence of chronic pain and CPSP, magnesium is displaced, NMDA receptors are activated, and calcium ions enter the axon terminal causing an exaggerated release of substance P and excitatory amino acids. This dysfunctional activation of NMDA receptors contributes greatly to windup.

Spinal Nerve Contribution to Windup

The spinal neuroanatomy has many complex features. There are similar cross-sectional structures and function at all spinal cord levels. The spinal cord carries sensory information from the body and some from the head to the CNS via afferent fibers, and it performs the initial processing of this information. Motor neurons in the ventral horn project their axons into the periphery to innervate skeletal and smooth muscles that mediate voluntary and involuntary reflexes. The spinal cord contains neurons whose descending axons mediate autonomic control for most of the visceral functions.

Various substances reside in the spinal neuroanatomy and play a role in neurotransmission. Galanin is one of those substances, a neuropeptide that functions as a cellular messenger. Galanin is multifunctional and includes inhibition of action potentials as a protective mechanism. Galanin is also implicated in many dysfunctional physiologic activities, some that may be connected with chronic pain and CPSP, including depression and eating disorders (Kuteeva et al., 2008; Lundstrom, Elmquist, Bartfai, & Langel, 2005).

Cerebral Contribution to Windup

One of the least understood, but no less important areas of pain activity is the brain. Various areas of the brain are involved in pain modulation. The human brain is capable of recognizing prior pain experiences, developing attention and expectations related to those experiences, and creating anticipatory responses that are not always proportional to the situation. In CPSP, prolonged and unexpected postsurgical pain can lead to exaggerated negative perception and dysfunctional responses. Pain experiences and cerebral responses to painful activity affect mood, create anxiety, and can also lead to depression (Bingel & Tracey, 2008).

In order to better understand how cerebral activity plays a role in treatment of chronic pain and CPSP, it is important to recognize the connection between psychology and physiology. One of the most intriguing aspects of pain modulation related to cerebral activity is the placebo effect. What has once been thought to be a purely psychological event appears to actually be associated with neurophysiological responses (Medoff & Colloca, 2015). Placebo analgesia is a prime example of cognitive modulation of pain (Bingel & Tracey, 2008). This cognitive modulation includes the release of endogenous opioids, which may imply that placebo activity is actually a neurochemical event. It is evident that cerebral involvement in pain modulation is a complex system of events that include both psychological and physiological activities resulting in the promotion of protective mechanisms when functioning properly, but detrimental under the conditions of chronic pain.

Another aspect of achieving appropriate treatment of chronic pain and CPSP is the perception of the treating health care providers. It is interesting to note that our own perception of other's pain responses may be related to our individual experiences with pain. Empathy, which is the ability to understand and share the feelings of others, is influenced by the cerebral mechanisms that help to protect us. Studies suggest that firsthand emotional experience with pain is an important aspect of empathetic development, and analgesics may have the unwanted effect of reducing empathy and concern for others (Rutgen et al., 2015). This lack of empathy may delay or distort the treatment plan for an individual who suffers from CPSP.

TREATMENT OF CPSP

Treatment goals for CPSP should be multifaceted. Goals should initially address the removal of the stimulus, which typically is located in a peripheral area, but can originate centrally as well. Once the original source of pain is addressed, or if an original source of pain cannot be identified, then it is important to reset the inhibitory mechanisms of the central spinal area, and address the psychological impact of chronic pain located in the prefrontal cerebral area.

Aggressive postoperative treatment appears to be important in the treatment of recognized CPSP. Antidepressants play an important role in treating CPSP, in addition to short-term opioid use, and selective use of anticonvulsants, topical agents, and NMDA antagonists (Bouman et al., 2014; Chaparro, Wiffen, Moore, & Gilron, 2012).

Finding solutions to CPSP can be very elusive. That is why preventative measures are important. Research has pointed to the benefits of preventative measures that reduce central sensitization. This can be accomplished through the use of regional anesthesia, preoperative doses of anti-inflammatory agents, and administration of other antihyperalgesia medications such as ketamine (Andreae & Andreae, 2012; Lavand'homme & De Kock, 2006; Lavand'homme, De Kock, & Waterloos, 2005).

Pharmacology

In the fight against CPSP we often turn to pharmaceuticals. Some pharmaceuticals are effective in reducing the dysfunctional activity associated with CPSP development, some are effective in helping the body return to normal function after the development of CPSP, and others simply treat pain perception and do little or nothing to reduce the dysfunctional cycle of CPSP.

Non-Steroidal Anti-Inflammatory Drugs

The category of drugs referred to as non-steroidal anti-inflammatory drugs (NSAIDs) have properties well suited to help reduce the development of CPSP, and to treat ongoing pain symptoms. Drugs in this category have antipyretic, anti-inflammatory, and analgesic properties. Their primary mechanism of action is the acetylation of cyclooxygenase (COX), which prevents the synthesis of prostaglandins from arachidonic acid. Arachidonic acid is present in cellular tissue and is released when the cellular membranes are disrupted by injury or disease. Prostaglandins are short-lived localized hormones that are responsible for inflammatory activity (vasodilatation, erythema, edema, and fever), and nociceptor sensitization, among other things (Atkinson et al., 2013; Haeggstrom, Rinaldo-Matthis, Wheelock, & Wetterholm, 2010). Elevated levels of prostaglandins, consistent with the intensity of tissue damage, are related to trauma and surgery (Eisenach, Curry, Rauck, Pan, & Yaksh, 2010) A prolonged elevation of prostaglandins may be found in patients with CPSP due to occult inflammatory activity and related processes.

Although acetaminophen is often included in this category, it is not a true NSAID because it lacks any significant anti-inflammatory properties. Acetaminophen does have inhibitory COX activity, but it is thought to provide this inhibition in the CNS rather than peripherally. This explains the lack of anti-inflammatory activity, while pain relief is thought to be provided by reduction in nociceptor activity in the CNS (Hinz, Cheremina, & Brune, 2008).

There are two types of COX enzymes in the human body. The first is referred to as COX-1, which is a constitutive enzyme continually produced to protect gastric mucosa, reduce gastric acid secretions and pepsin content, and promote platelet aggregation. The other enzyme, COX-2 is activated by tissue damage and is responsible for inflammation, fever, some anticoagulation activity, modulation of cell proliferation, and pain sensation (Fitzgerald, 2004; Sobolewski, Cerella, Dicato, Ghibelli, & Diederich, 2010).

Understanding the pharmacokinetics of NSAIDs is critical to a long-term treatment plan. Distribution and elimination of any drug plays an important role in effectiveness, side effects, and toxicity. Oral NSAIDs are absorbed in the stomach and small intestines. Most NSAIDs peak in 1–4 hours, are delayed by food consumption, and taking NSAIDs with food does not reduce the negative gastric mucosa effects. This class of drugs is weakly acidic, highly plasma bound, and lipophilic; and only the unbound portion of the drug is effective. Elimination is accomplished primarily through hepatic oxidation and conjugation. Less than 10% is eliminated through renal activity. Some of these drugs have active metabolites. Generally, NSAIDs have very similar targets of action, but their therapeutic profiles are different. Some are more COX selective than others, peak plasma times differ, distribution profiles vary, and elimination profiles may impact individuals with kidney and liver disease differently.

NSAIDs are the most widely used analgesics in the United States, with over 30 million users. They may be a useful adjunct in the prevention and treatment of CPSP. They are reasonably safe when used as intended, but serious side effects still exist. The most significant side effects of long-term NSAID use include nephrotoxicity, cardiothrombotic events, peptic ulceration, and bleeding. The anti-inflammatory effects of NSAIDs make them ideal for back pain related to neuraxial inflammation, but their distribution profile requires maximum recommended doses to be effective. Ibuprofen, for example, has an over-the-counter (OTC) dosing limitation of six tablets (1,200 mg) in a 24-hour period, but some studies indicate that an effective minimum dose of ibuprofen in a 24-hour period for the treatment of inflammatory back pain is 1,600 mg (eight tablets). Even at doses of 1,600 mg per day, the risks associated with ibuprofen are limited.

Acetylsalicylic acid is a nonselective COX inhibitor. It has excellent long-term antipyretic and anti-inflammatory properties, but unlike other NSAIDs, acetylsalicylic acid causes irreversible COX inhibition. The irreversibility may contribute to more serious side effects that cannot be limited by discontinuation of the drug. Acetylsalicylic acid has a significant impact on platelet aggregation that may be prolonged. In small doses, acetylsalicylic acid has been shown to help reduce cardiothrombotic events. Its effectiveness in pain reduction is tempered by its potential side effects and irreversibility.

Acetaminophen has no significant anti-inflammatory activity. For that reason, it is not well suited for treatment of chronic pain related to inflammatory processes. Studies indicate that acetaminophen used for back pain was no more effective than a placebo (Koes & Enthoven, 2014). Like opioids, acetaminophen treats pain symptoms but does little to address the source of the problem. However, unlike opioids, acetaminophen is not addictive and has a reasonably safe therapeutic profile when doses are limited to less than 1 gram per dose or 4 grams per day (Gokhale & Martin, 2012). Because the action of acetaminophen is thought to be the inhibition of prostaglandin production in the CNS, rather than peripherally, many of the serious hematologic side effects associated with NSAIDs are absent in acetaminophen. For that reason, it is thought to be a safe alternative in reduction of pain symptoms for those patients who are at high risk for hematologic or cardiovascular problems.

It should not be ignored that acetaminophen is the leading cause of acute liver failure in the United States because of accidental overdose (Khandelwal et al., 2011). Accidental overdoses are often related to the fact that acetaminophen is combined with many common prescription and OTC drugs. Some individuals do not recognize that they are exceeding the maximum recommended dose by ingesting both prescription and cold medications that contain acetaminophen. Careful monitoring of total acetaminophen intake for chronic pain patients is essential in prevention of liver toxicity.

The side effect profile of NSAIDs is relatively safe, but not inconsequential. At the higher doses and long-term therapy necessary for the treatment of chronic inflammation and chronic pain, side effects can be problematic and need to be considered when designing a chronic pain care plan.

Opioids

Like acetaminophen, opioids act primarily in the CNS. This prevents them from being useful in treating the source of pain, but they are valuable for short-term relief of operative and traumatic injury. They also have value in the treatment of CPSP when used for short-term pain in conjunction with a long-term treatment strategy. Opioids work at specific receptors in the CNS that block nociception. It is helpful to understand the primary receptor site activity of each therapeutic opioid in order to minimize undesirable side effects.

Many of the positive and side effects of opioids can be traced to metabolites and some metabolites can produce hyperalgesia. Morphine is the prototype opioid for which all other opioids are compared (Yekkirala, Kalyuzhny, & Portoghese, 2010). It acts at mu and delta receptors. Oxycodone, one of the most widely prescribed semisynthetic opioids, has significant kappa activity making it highly addictive. Oxymorphone has more mu receptor activity than other semisynthetic opioids, some delta activity, and less kappa activity. Hydromorphone is primarily a mu agonist with significant kappa activity. Hydrocodone produces mu activity and some delta activity. Methadone is an interesting synthetic mu agonist. It is also an NMDA antagonist like ketamine, a mu receptor agonist like morphine, and does not have any metabolites. The unique properties of methadone have generated renewed interest in its use for chronic pain. However, it does have a complicated dosing profile and potential cardiotoxic effects, which make it inappropriate for some outpatient applications.

Opioid therapy for CPSP is not a good long-term solution because of substantial negative side effects and lack of value in treating the source of pain.

In addition to potentially fatal side effects, tolerance develops over time, which reduces the therapeutic value and increases risk.

In consideration of the use of opioids for CPSP patients, it is important to understand their limited value in such situations, the need to develop individualized opioid treatment plans, and the need to use dosing strategies that maximize the value of such drugs. Dosing strategies include the use of nonopioid drugs that help to reduce opioid use by enhancing the positive opioid effects. Rotation of opioids improve analgesia and reduce side effects. Close monitoring of opioid use and effectiveness can help minimize dependence and reduce opioid-related deaths.

Pharmaceutical research continues to pursue development of a pain medication that provides analgesia without the unwanted side effects and dependence of opioids (Majumdar et al., 2012; Varadi et al., 2013). The pursuit of such a drug is allusive. In the meantime, it seems prudent, safer, and less costly to find ways to reduce opioid use for pain.

Antidepressants

Antidepressants can play a very important role in treating chronic pain. Antidepressants should be considered as a first-line treatment for CPSP (O'Connor & Dworkin, 2009). Pain perception is a chemically mediated event in the CNS, and can often be addressed with the addition of antidepressants to the treatment plan in CPSP. Antidepressants can also improve mood, increase treatment compliance, and reduce opioid use. Some of the older tricyclic antidepressants are effective for treating pain, but they have significant side effects that make them unacceptable for pain treatment in many cases. The serotonin and norepinephrine reuptake inhibitors (SNRIs) are effective with more tolerable side effects. Selective serotonin reuptake inhibitors (SSRI) can also be effective, but appear to be less effective in most cases than SNRIs.

Antidepressants can take days or weeks to be effective, so they are not appropriate for acute postoperative pain, nor do they appear to be effective in a preventative strategy for CPSP. Extended release compounds appear to be most effective in the treatment of CPSP. Side effects of SNRIs and SSRIs are generally well tolerated. Antidepressants are sometimes rejected by patients as a treatment for chronic pain because they may feel taking this class of drugs will label them as psychologically impaired. It is important to explain to patients that some drugs designed for one purpose have been found to be beneficial for other purposes, and they should not see the use of SNRIs as a psychological treatment. Viagra is an example of a drug used for purposes beyond its original intent. It was originally designed for treatment of cardiovascular issues, but was found to be beneficial for other physiological purposes (Wang et al., 2014).

Anticonvulsants

The use of anticonvulsants for chronic neuropathic pain, including CPSP is controversial. Some studies have found little to no value in using anticonvulsants for chronic neuropathic pain, while others have demonstrated some efficacy for specific anticonvulsants (Goodyear-Smith & Halliwell, 2009; Wiffen et al., 2005). The anticonvulsants that have been found to provide some efficacy are gabapentin and pregabalin. In a 2014 Cochrane Review, both drugs were found to be associated with modest pain reduction when used for diabetic neuropathy and postherpetic neuralgia when compared to placebo (Moore, Wiffen, & Kalso, 2014). Because of direct to consumer advertising, and provider interest in looking for alternatives for the treatment of chronic pain, pregabalin has become a widely prescribed drug for chronic pain patients. Anticonvulsants probably have little or no place in the treatment of CPSP. Until further evidence exists, anticonvulsants should be limited to the treatment of diabetic neuropathic pain, fibromyalgia, and trigeminal neuralgia.

N-methyl-D-aspartate Receptor Antagonists

The NMDA receptor antagonists have been available for many years. Because of recent research that indicates a significant role of NMDA receptors in the development of chronic pain and CPSP, interest in this drug class is reemerging (Lefevre et al., 2015). It is thought that NMDA receptor systems are involved in the development of chronic pain "windup," and preemptive treatment may be effective in the prevention of postoperative pain hypersensitivity. The mechanisms behind the development of postoperative pain hypersensitivity are poorly understood, but NMDA receptors are thought to support synaptic plasticity, CNS pain processing, and modulation of central pain sensitization induced by incision and tissue damage (De Kock & Lavand'homme, 2007), which may suggest value in the treatment and prevention of CPSP.

Ketamine blocks NMDA receptor site activity, and may be useful in the treatment and prevention of CPSP. Further study is necessary to support such a conclusion, but low-dose ketamine (0.25–0.5 mg/kg) has been used successfully as an adjunct to general anesthesia, reducing central sensitization, and reducing postoperative opioid requirements. Side effects associated with ketamine have concerned providers, but recent research on low dose and postoperative infusion of ketamine in surgical patients do not support these concerns. In fact, a reduction in nausea was common, and other adverse events such as hallucinations and vivid dreams were not reported (Wang et al., 2015).

Muscle Relaxants and Pain Treatment

Many patients with chronic pain are routinely given muscle relaxants. These drugs are not without risk, and should not be routinely prescribed. Relaxation does not provide source treatment, and such drugs become ineffective within a few weeks. They should only be used for short-term symptomatic relief of muscle spasms while the source of pain is treated. The most commonly prescribed muscle relaxant is cyclobenzaprine. It is chemically related to the antidepressant amitriptyline, and its effectiveness begins to decline within four days of therapy. When used alone for pain, it is less effective than ibuprofen. Cyclobenzaprine is best used as an adjunct to NSAIDs. Other muscle relaxants that have been prescribed for chronic pain, such as carisoprodol, have a high potential for dependence, tolerance, and mental impairment. It has been taken off the market in some countries because of its high potential for abuse (Bramness, Furu, Engeland, & Skurtveit, 2007). There have also been some efforts to reclassify the drug in the United States as a controlled substance because of the potential for abuse (Reeves, Burke, & Kose, 2012). Other drugs developed for muscle spasms, such as baclofen, should never be used for muscle spasms related to acute or chronic pain. Baclofen was designed for extreme spasmodic conditions such as cerebral palsy, tetanus, and multiple sclerosis. Withdrawal from baclofen can cause respiratory failure, hemodynamic changes, seizures, and delirium. It is highly toxic, and the benefits do not outweigh the risks in most situations.

Topical Anesthetic Agents

Topical NSAIDs and topical anesthetic agents are an underused tool in the battle of chronic pain and CPSP. Some patients and providers confuse topical agents with drugs that are delivered systemically through a dermal delivery system. Topical agents work without significant systemic absorption, their therapeutic benefit is high, and their safety profile is more favorable than oral comparisons when used in therapeutic doses (Roth & Fuller, 2011). The most common side effect of topical agents is skin irritation. One of the reasons that these drugs may not be more frequently used is because of their relative high cost.

Topical anesthetic agents are effective with CPSP because some chronic pain conditions generate continued peripheral nerve stimulation. Application of anesthetic agents to the source of pain may promote reestablishment of the normal peripheral nociceptive inhibitory systems by temporarily blocking continuous nerve stimulation.

Sleep Aids

Sleep is essential to life and the healing processes. It plays an important part of cellular regulation and regeneration, which is an important part of healing and return to homeostasis after injury (Vyazovskiy, 2015). Chronic pain, including CPSP, disrupts sleep, which in turn impairs cellular regeneration. Lack of sleep can also lead to depression, which also complicates the treatment of chronic pain (Alcantara et al., 2015). The problem of sleep deprivation due to chronic pain can become a vicious cycle. For that reason, promotion of quality sleep is an important part of chronic pain therapy. Current sleep aids are not without risk. Some pharmaceutical sleep aids can actually lower the quality of sleep by disrupting rapid eye movement (REM) sleep. For that reason, treatment of sleep deprivation associated with chronic pain should start with mechanical aids such as better bedding and pillows, proper positions, and white noise.

Polypharmacy in Pain Management

Multiple prescription and nonprescription drugs are often necessary for the treatment of chronic pain. Use of multiple pharmaceutical agents, often called "polypharmacy," has the inherent risk of negative medication interaction, unnecessary duplication of medication, toxicity, disruption of important physiological functions, and an increased mortality rate (Onder et al., 2013) (Ramgoolie & Nichols, 2015). The risk of negative drug interaction ranges from 13% with two medications to 82% with seven or more medications (Fulton & Allen, 2005).

Among medications common to chronic pain, and used in combination with other medications, are anticonvulsants, antidepressants, and NSAIDs. Anticonvulsants present a higher incident of toxicity secondary to competition for metabolic pathways with other drugs. Some antidepressants increase warfarin levels, while those that inhibit the reuptake of serotonin pose a risk of fatal serotonin syndrome when combined with monoamine oxidase inhibitors used to treat atypical depression. Some drugs can inhibit hepatic enzyme activity and increase the risk of elevating serum and tissue levels of other drugs to the point of toxic levels because of diminished hepatic degradation. Adequate renal clearance is critical for many drugs, and competition for renal clearance is maximized when multiple drugs are administered. The competition for renal clearance also increases the blood levels of active metabolites found in many pain medications.

Steroids

Corticosteroids and local anesthetic agents are the most common medications used for the interventional treatment of chronic pain, including CPSP. Interventional treatment for CPSP includes regional block and local infiltration with the goal of blocking pain and reducing inflammation. Local anesthetic agents are beneficial for the immediate reduction or elimination of pain symptoms, as well as identifying proper placement of steroids in the targeted area. Some studies have indicated that local anesthetic agents alone may provide long-term pain relief for certain chronic pain conditions (Meng et al., 2015), which suggest that blocking pain responses for even short periods of time may help to reset inhibitory nociceptor mechanisms in some CPSP patients.

Corticosteroids are thought to support release of anti-inflammatory proteins and repress pro-inflammatory proteins. They are also known to suppress COX activity, which reduces the formation of prostaglandins and reduces pain sensation and response. The most common corticoid steroids used in interventional therapy are moderate to long acting particulate steroids such as triamcinolone, betamethasone, and methylprednisolone. The vehicle, which contains particles, helps to provide localized long acting anti-inflammatory action. However, the particles contained in all of these solutions can lead to catastrophic complications if accidently injected into the vascular system.

Complications of interventional therapy are uncommon when proper technique and precautions are followed. However, even in the best of hands, and with the safest techniques, complications still occur. For that reason, follow-up, recognition of complications, and the ability to manage and treat patients who develop complications are all an important part of the care plan. One of the most common complications include persistent pain from traumatic injection or failure to respond to the therapeutic agent.

Intervention treatment is reasonably safe when administered by competent providers who take care to avoid complications. The benefits are potentially great, while the risks are very low. Proper patient evaluation, safe utilization of equipment, and preparation for the unlikely event of an adverse reaction are all necessary for proper patient care.

AGE-RELATED CONSIDERATIONS

There are significant physiological differences with various age groups. These differences are more pronounced in the very young and the very old. There are physical and functional implications that can create significant barriers to proper assessment, diagnosis, and treatment. For that reason, it is very important to recognize, and incorporate age-related physiology into any plan of care (Colloca, Santoro, & Gambassi, 2010).

The Very Young

Treating the very young can be especially challenging and it must be kept in mind that infants are not simply young adults. They have specific physiologic differences that must be considered when treating pain. One of the more challenging aspects of pain in the very young is identification and as such pain is often ignored in this age group because of their inability to vocalize pain.

Alternative methods for assessing pain in infants are necessary. The most sensitive and reliable method for pain assessment in infants is facial expression as infants in pain do not always cry. Body motion, facial expression, and vital signs are all part of a comprehensive assessment necessary to accurately determine if an infant is in pain. Relying only on one parameter, especially vital signs, may yield inaccurate information, leading to mismanagement of pain treatment. Limited neurological development and illness may constrain response and complicate assessment.

The negative psychological and physical impact of untreated and undertreated pain on the very young should not be ignored. There is evidence that chronic painful stimulation in infants can lead to permanent changes in the CNS and changes in responsiveness of the neuroendocrine and immune systems to stress at maturity (Page, 2004).

The Very Old

Aging is an inconsistent and complex phenomenon that involves the progressive degeneration of organ systems (Nigam, Knight, Bhattacharya, & Bayer, 2012). Aging involves changes in cellular homeostasis, organ function, and functional reserve, which impair an individual's ability to cope with stress, pain, and other health care challenges (Sieck, 2003).

Aging adults report more chronic pain complaints, while studies indicate a reduced tolerance to pain (Cole, Farrell, Gibson, & Egan, 2010). A theory behind this observed increase in pain and reduced tolerance in older adults suggests that aging nerve fibers show damage similar to younger tissue that develop neuropathic pain (Gagliese, 2009). In addition to progressive tissue damage with age, chronic inflammatory responses play a role in increased pain, pain perception (Hughes & Reynolds, 2005), and could make them more likely to develop CPSP.

Health care providers sometimes assume that older adults have reduced pain perception. This misconception and several others about pain in older adults probably stem from several factors. Some, if not most health care providers, assume that pain is a natural part of aging. This notion is not supported in the literature (American Geriatrics Society, 1998). Pain perception may be elevated but pain response is often diminished because of changes in cognitive, communication, and motor functions. In addition to diminished response because of physiologic changes, older adults are often reluctant to report pain because of fears of pathology or negative social issues related to acknowledgment of pain (Herr & Garand, 2001).

Not only is assessment of pain in older adults difficult, but treatment may be difficult as well. Older adults often present with multiple pain generators, or limitations in treatment options based on multiple health issues associated with aging. Therapeutic choices can also be limited by potential interactions with other medications being taken for nonpain issues. Opioids may be considered for short-term pain relief, but should have very limited use in older adults, and be used with extreme caution. Immobility contributes to painful conditions, and also limits options for physical therapies. Conventional treatment that is effective in a younger population is not always an appropriate choice for older adults.

It is important to develop a unique plan of care specific for each elderly patient, understanding how comorbidities, polypharmacy, communication, as well as functional and cognitive impairment may affect assessment and treatment. Treatment of acute and chronic pain in older adults can be challenging, but it is a critical component to improving the quality of life of individuals in this population.

PATIENT-CENTERED APPROACH

Nurses bring a unique philosophical and theoretical approach to patient care and pain management not seen in other disciplines. Nursing care plans often bring in strategies of effective communication, partnership, and health promotion (Constand, MacDermid, Dal Bello-Haas, & Law, 2014).

Patient-centered care is especially important when treating the multidimensional problems associated with CPSP. A patient-centered approach allows for a foundation for creating an assessment and treatment plan based on the physical, psychological, and social needs of the patient, while working to avoid constraints often found in more traditional medical models (Scholl, Zill, Harter, & Dirmaier, 2014).

As part of a patient-centered approach, it is important to utilize expertise from multiple health care resources, incorporating a variety or philosophies, and various treatment regimens. Pathways toward reasonable goals in management of CPSP often require cooperative care, and sometimes unconventional treatment. Reasonable therapeutic goals should include functional improvement in activities of daily living, psychological improvement, rational pharmacologic management of ongoing pain, and return to productive activities. Treatment "teams" should develop a joint plan of care based on unique patient goals, contributing the resources available to help meet those goals, establish primary and secondary treatments plans, identify support systems, and include appropriate spiritual resources as requested by the patient.

A "one size fits all" approach is seldom effective. Consumers, and health care providers alike, have a tendency to compartmentalize their health care problems by seeking a "specialist." This kind of approach often narrowly focuses the treatment and excludes complementary therapies that may enhance, rather than interfere with each other. One example of a cooperative approach is the combination of interventional therapy with physical therapy or chiropractic care.

Evidence exists that this multidisciplinary approach to pain care is often more successful than a single discipline or treatment (Ben-David & Raboy, 1994).

FAILURE TO TREAT

We seldom consider what happens when we fail to treat pain. In fact, it is not unusual to find patients and health care providers who take a "hands-off approach" to chronic pain symptoms and believe that they will resolve themselves without intervention. It is not difficult to find tragic stories of negative consequences associated with failure to treat pain.

Most of the barriers that prevent timely and appropriate treatment of chronic pain are due to patient issues. Those issues usually include lack of access to adequate health care, fear of treatment, misinformation, and cultural barriers. However, provider issues can create barriers as well. Sometimes, preconceived notions play a role in mismanagement of chronic pain. Such misplaced notions can hinder judgment and lead to erroneous assumptions about their patient (Passik, Byers, & Kirsh, 2007). Properly placed empathy, without preconceived judgment, is essential to effective chronic pain management (Tait, 2008).

CONCLUSION

Treatment of CPSP is far more complex than simply addressing a single source of pain. There is no doubt that identification and treatment of the original source of injury is important to the overall goals of pain management, but CPSP includes a vicious cycle of dysfunction, which leads to a breakdown in homeostasis. Return to homeostasis requires addressing peripheral, spinal, and cerebral mechanisms that have broken down due to repetitive painful stimulation. It is important to identify patients who might be predisposed to CPSP, use preemptive treatment when possible, diagnose CPSP as quickly as possible, and aggressively treat the condition. The longer proper treatment is delayed, the more likely the problem will become irreversible or unmanageable. It often requires a significant time commitment from both patients and providers to identify a pathway to functional improvement and return to homeostasis.

REFERENCES

Alcantara, C., Biggs, M. L., Davidson, K. W., Delaney, J. A., Jackson, C. L., Zee, P. C., et al. (2015). Sleep disturbances and depression in the multi-ethnic study of atherosclerosis. *Sleep*, *39*(4), 915–925. Retrieved from http://www.ncbi.nlm.nih.gov/pubmed/26715223

American Geriatrics Society. (1998). The management of chronic pain in older persons: AGS panel on chronic pain in older persons. *Journal of the American Geriatrics Society*, *53*(Suppl. 3), S8–S24. Retrieved from http://www.ncbi.nlm.nih.gov/pubmed/9826952

Andreae, M. H., & Andreae, D. A. (2012). Local anaesthetics and regional anaesthesia for preventing chronic pain after surgery. *Cochrane Database of Systematic Reviews, 10*. http://dx.doi.org/10.1002/14651858.cd007105.pub2

Atkinson, T. J., Fudin, J., Jahn, H. L., Kubotera, N., Rennick, A. L., & Rhorer, M. (2013). What's new in NSAID pharmacotherapy: Oral agents to injectables. *Pain Medicine, 14*(Suppl. 1), S11–S17. http://dx.doi.org/10.1016/j.suronc.2009.11.011

Ben-David, B., & Raboy, M. (1994). Manipulation under anesthesia combined with epidural steroid injection. *Journal of Manipulative and Physiological Therapeutics, 17*(9), 605–609. Retrieved from http://www.ncbi.nlm.nih.gov/pubmed/26715223

Bingel, U., & Tracey, I. (2008). Imaging CNS modulation of pain in humans. *Physiology (Bethesda), 23*, 371–380. http://dx.doi.org/10.1016/j.suronc.2009.11.011

Bouman, E. A., Theunissen, M., Bons, S. A., van Mook, W. N., Gramke, H. F., van Kleef, M., et al. (2014). Reduced incidence of chronic postsurgical pain after epidural analgesia for abdominal surgery. *Pain Practice, 14*(2), E76–E84. http://dx.doi.org/10.1111/papr.12091

Bramness, J. G., Furu, K., Engeland, A., & Skurtveit, S. (2007). Carisoprodol use and abuse in Norway: A pharmacoepidemiological study. *British Journal of Clinical Pharmacology, 64*(2), 210–218. http://dx.doi.org/10.1111/j.1365-2125.2007.02847.x

Chaparro, L. E., Wiffen, P. J., Moore, R. A., & Gilron, I. (2012). Combination pharmacotherapy for the treatment of neuropathic pain in adults. *Cochrane Database of Systematic Reviews*, (7), CD008943. http://dx.doi.org/10.1002/14651858.cd008943.pub2

Cole, L. J., Farrell, M. J., Gibson, S. J., & Egan, G. F. (2010). Age-related differences in pain sensitivity and regional brain activity evoked by noxious pressure. *Neurobiology of Aging, 31*(3), 494–503. http://dx.doi.org/10.1016/j.neurobiolaging.2008.04.012

Colloca, G., Santoro, M., & Gambassi, G. (2010). Age-related physiologic changes and perioperative management of elderly patients. *Surgical Oncology, 19*(3), 124–130. http://dx.doi.org/10.1016/j.suronc.2009.11.011

Constand, M. K., MacDermid, J. C., Dal Bello-Haas, V., & Law, M. (2014). Scoping review of patient-centered care approaches in healthcare. *BMC Health Services Research, 14*(1), 271. http://dx.doi.org/10.1186/1472-6963-14-271

Costa, M. A., Trentini, C. A., Schafranski, M. D., Pipino, O., Gomes, R. Z., & Reis, E. S. (2015). Factors associated with the development of chronic post-sternotomy pain: A case-control study. *Revista Brasileira de Cirurgia Cardiovascular, 30*(5), 552–556. http://dx.doi.org/10.5935/1678-9741.20150059

Covington, E. C. (2000). Psychogenic pain-what it means, why it does not exist, and how to diagnose it. *Pain Medicine, 1*(4), 287–294. Retrieved from http://www.ncbi.nlm.nih.gov/pubmed/26715223

Cregg, R., Anwar, S., & Farquhar-Smith, P. (2013). Persistent postsurgical pain. *Current Opinion in Supportive and Palliative Care, 7*(2), 144–152. http://dx.doi.org/10.1097/spc.0b013e328360b09e

Cross, S. A. (1994). Pathophysiology of pain. *Mayo Clinic Proceedings, 69*(4), 375–383. Retrieved from http://www.ncbi.nlm.nih.gov/pubmed/26715223

De Kock, M. F., & Lavand'homme, P. M. (2007). The clinical role of NMDA receptor antagonists for the treatment of postoperative pain. *Best Practice & Research Clinical Anaesthesiology, 21*(1), 85–98. Retrieved from http://www.ncbi.nlm.nih.gov/pubmed/26715223

Deer, T. R., Leong, M. S., Buvanendran, A., & American Academy of Pain Medicine. (2013). *Comprehensive treatment of chronic pain by medical, interventional, and integrative approaches: The American Academy of Pain Medicine textbook on patient management*. New York, NY: Springer Publishing.

Eisenach, J. C., Curry, R., Rauck, R., Pan, P., & Yaksh, T. L. (2010). Role of spinal cyclooxygenase in human postoperative and chronic pain. *Anesthesiology, 112*(5), 1225–1233. http://dx.doi.org/10.1097/aln.0b013e3181d94dc0

Fitzgerald, G. A. (2004). Coxibs and cardiovascular disease. *New England Journal of Medicine, 351*(17), 1709–1711. http://dx.doi.org/10.1056/nejmp048288

Fulton, M. M., & Allen, E. R. (2005). Polypharmacy in the elderly: A literature review. *Journal of the American Academy of Nurse Practitioners, 17*(4), 123–132. http://dx.doi.org/10.1136%2Fbmjopen-2015-010989

Gagliese, L. (2009). Pain and aging: The emergence of a new subfield of pain research. *The Journal of Pain, 10*(4), 343–353. http://dx.doi.org/10.1016/j.jpain.2008.10.013

Gaskin, D. J., & Richard, P. (2012). The economic costs of pain in the United States. *The Journal of Pain, 13*(8), 715–724. http://dx.doi.org/10.1016/j.jpain.2012.03.009

Gokhale, M., & Martin, B. C. (2012). Prescription-acquired acetaminophen use and potential overuse patterns: 2001-2008. *Pharmacoepidemiology and Drug Safety, 21*(2), 226–230. http://dx.doi.org/10.1002/pds.2235

Goodyear-Smith, F., & Halliwell, J. (2009). Anticonvulsants for neuropathic pain: Gaps in the evidence. *The Clinical Journal of Pain, 25*(6), 528–536. http://dx.doi.org/10.1097/ajp.0b013e318197d4cc

Haeggstrom, J. Z., Rinaldo-Matthis, A., Wheelock, C. E., & Wetterholm, A. (2010). Advances in eicosanoid research, novel therapeutic implications. *Biochemical and Biophysical Research Communications, 396*(1), 135–139. http://dx.doi.org/10.1016/j.bbrc.2010.03.140

Herr, K. A., & Garand, L. (2001). Assessment and measurement of pain in older adults. *Clinics in Geriatric Medicine, 17*(3), 457–478, vi. Retrieved from http://www.ncbi.nlm.nih.gov/pubmed/26715223

Hinz, B., Cheremina, O., & Brune, K. (2008). Acetaminophen (paracetamol) is a selective cyclooxygenase-2 inhibitor in man. *The FASEB Journal, 22*(2), 383–390. http://dx.doi.org/10.1096/fj.07-8506com

Honore, P., Rogers, S. D., Schwei, M. J., Salak-Johnson, J. L., Luger, N. M., Sabino, M. C., et al. (2000). Murine models of inflammatory, neuropathic and cancer pain each generates a unique set of neurochemical changes in the spinal cord and sensory neurons. *Neuroscience, 98*(3), 585–598. Retrieved from http://www.ncbi.nlm.nih.gov/pubmed/26715223

Hughes, K. A., & Reynolds, R. M. (2005). Evolutionary and mechanistic theories of aging. *Annual Review of Entomology, 50(1)*, 421–445. http://dx.doi.org/10.1146/annurev.ento.50.071803.130409

Ilgen, M. A., Kleinberg, F., Ignacio, R. V., Bohnert, A. S., Valenstein, M., McCarthy, J. F., et al. (2013). Noncancer pain conditions and risk of suicide. *JAMA Psychiatry, 70*(7), 692–697. http://dx.doi.org/10.1001/jamapsychiatry.2013.908

Johansen, A., Schirmer, H., Nielsen, C. S., & Stubhaug, A. (2016). Persistent post-surgical pain and signs of nerve injury: The Tromso Study. *Acta Anaesthesiologica Scandinavica, 60*(3), 380–392. http://dx.doi.org/10.1111/aas.12653

Kehlet, H., & Rathmell, J. P. (2010). Persistent postsurgical pain: The path forward through better design of clinical studies. *Anesthesiology, 112*(3), 514–515. http://dx.doi.org/10.1097/aln.0b013e3181cf423d

Khandelwal, N., James, L. P., Sanders, C., Larson, A. M., Lee, W. M., & Acute Liver Failure Study, G. (2011). Unrecognized acetaminophen toxicity as a cause of indeterminate acute liver failure. *Hepatology, 53*(2), 567–576. http://dx.doi.org/10.1002/hep.24060

Koes, B. W., & Enthoven, W. T. (2014). Do patients with acute low-back pain need paracetamol? *The Lancet, 384*(9954), 1556–1557. http://dx.doi.org/10.1016/s0140-6736(14)60978-8

Kristensen, A. D., Pedersen, T. A., Hjortdal, V. E., Jensen, T. S., & Nikolajsen, L. (2010). Chronic pain in adults after thoracotomy in childhood or youth. *British Journal of Anaesthesia, 104*(1), 75–79. http://dx.doi.org/10.1093/bja/aep317

Kuteeva, E., Wardi, T., Lundstrom, L., Sollenberg, U., Langel, U., Hokfelt, T., et al. (2008). Differential role of galanin receptors in the regulation of depression-like behavior and monoamine/stress-related genes at the cell body level. *Neuropsychopharmacology, 33*(11), 2573–2585. http://dx.doi.org/10.1038/sj.npp.1301660

Lavand'homme, P., & De Kock, M. (2006). The use of intraoperative epidural or spinal analgesia modulates postoperative hyperalgesia and reduces residual pain after major abdominal surgery. *Acta Anaesthesiologica Belgica, 57*(4), 373–379. Retrieved from http://www.ncbi.nlm.nih.gov/pubmed/17236639

Lavand'homme, P., De Kock, M., & Waterloos, H. (2005). Intraoperative epidural analgesia combined with ketamine provides effective preventive analgesia in patients undergoing major digestive surgery. *Anesthesiology, 103*(4), 813–820. Retrieved from http://www.ncbi.nlm.nih.gov/pubmed/16192774

Lefevre, Y., Amadio, A., Vincent, P., Descheemaeker, A., Oliet, S. H., Dallel, R., et al. (2015). Neuropathic pain depends upon D-serine co-activation of spinal NMDA receptors in rats. *Neuroscience Letters, 603*, 42–47. http://dx.doi.org/10.1016/j.neulet.2015.07.010

Lundstrom, L., Elmquist, A., Bartfai, T., & Langel, U. (2005). Galanin and its receptors in neurological disorders. *NeuroMolecular Medicine, 7*(1–2), 157–180. http://dx.doi.org/10.1385/nmm:7:1-2:157

Majumdar, S., Subrath, J., Le Rouzic, V., Polikar, L., Burgman, M., Nagakura, K., et al. (2012). Synthesis and evaluation of aryl-naloxamide opiate analgesics targeting truncated exon 11-associated mu opioid receptor (MOR-1) splice variants. *Journal of Medicinal Chemistry, 55*(14), 6352–6362. http://dx.doi.org/10.1021/jm300305c

Medoff, Z. M., & Colloca, L. (2015). Placebo analgesia: Understanding the mechanisms. *Pain Management, 5*(2), 89–96. http://dx.doi.org/10.2217/pmt.15.3

Meng, H., Fei, Q., Wang, B., Yang, Y., Li, D., Li, J., et al. (2015). Epidural injections with or without steroids in managing chronic low back pain secondary to lumbar spinal stenosis: A meta-analysis of 13 randomized controlled trials. *Drug Design, Development and Therapy, 9*, 4657–4667. http://dx.doi.org/10.2147/dddt.s85524

Moore, A., Wiffen, P., & Kalso, E. (2014). Antiepileptic drugs for neuropathic pain and fibromyalgia. *The Journal of the American Medical Association, 312*(2), 182–183. http://dx.doi.org/10.1001/jama.2014.6336

Morrison, I., Perini, I., & Dunham, J. (2013). Facets and mechanisms of adaptive pain behavior: Predictive regulation and action. *Frontiers in Human Neuroscience, 7*, 755. http://dx.doi.org/10.3389/fnhum.2013.00755

Netto, E. C., & Brites, C. (2011). Characteristics of chronic pain and its impact on quality of life of patients with HTLV-1-associated myelopathy/tropical spastic paraparesis (HAM/TSP). *The Clinical Journal of Pain, 27*(2), 131–135. http://dx.doi.org/10.1097/ajp.0b013e3181f195d3

Nigam, Y., Knight, J., Bhattacharya, S., & Bayer, A. (2012). Physiological changes associated with aging and immobility. *Journal of Aging Research, 2012*, 1–2. http://dx.doi.org/10.1155/2012/468469

O'Connor, A. B., & Dworkin, R. H. (2009). Treatment of neuropathic pain: An overview of recent guidelines. *The American Journal of Medicine, 122*(Suppl. 10), S22–S32. http://dx.doi.org/10.1016/j.amjmed.2009.04.007

Onder, G., Liperoti, R., Foebel, A., Fialova, D., Topinkova, E., van der Roest, H. G., et al. (2013). Polypharmacy and mortality among nursing home residents with advanced cognitive impairment: results from the SHELTER study. *Journal of the American Medical Directors Association, 14*(6), 450.e7–450.e12. http://dx.doi.org/10.1016/j.jamda.2013.03.014

Page, G. G. (2004). Are there long-term consequences of pain in newborn or very young infants? *Journal of Perinatal Education, 13*(3), 10–17. http://dx.doi.org/10.1624/105812404x1725

Passik, S. D., Byers, K., & Kirsh, K. L. (2007). Empathy and the failure to treat pain. *Palliative Support Care, 5*(2), 167–172. Retrieved from http://www.ncbi.nlm.nih.gov/pubmed/17578068

Peng, Z., Li, H., Zhang, C., Qian, X., Feng, Z., & Zhu, S. (2014). A retrospective study of chronic post-surgical pain following thoracic surgery: Prevalence, risk factors, incidence of neuropathic component, and impact on qualify of life. *PLoS One, 9*(2), e90014. http://dx.doi.org/10.1371/journal.pone.0090014

Pinto, P. R., McIntyre, T., Ferrero, R., Almeida, A., & Araujo-Soares, V. (2013). Risk factors for moderate and severe persistent pain in patients undergoing total knee and hip arthroplasty: A prospective predictive study. *PLoS One, 8*(9), e73917. http://dx.doi.org/10.1371/journal.pone.0073917

Pinto, P. R., McIntyre, T., Ferrero, R., Araujo-Soares, V., & Almeida, A. (2013). Persistent pain after total knee or hip arthroplasty: Differential study of prevalence, nature, and impact. *Journal of Pain Research, 6*, 691–703. http://dx.doi.org/10.2147/jpr.s45827

Pozek, J. P., Beausang, D., Baratta, J. L., & Viscusi, E. R. (2016). The acute to chronic pain transition: Can chronic pain be prevented? *Medical Clinics of North America, 100*(1), 17–30. http://dx.doi.org/10.1016/j.mcna.2015.08.005

Ramgoolie, P., & Nichols, S. (2015). Polypharmacy and the risk of malnutrition among independently-living elderly persons in trinidad amd tobago. *West Indian Medical Journal*. http://dx.doi.org/10.7727/wimj.2014.285

Reeves, R. R., Burke, R. S., & Kose, S. (2012). Carisoprodol: Update on abuse potential and legal status. *Southern Medical Journal, 105*(11), 619–623. http://dx.doi.org/10.1097/smj.0b013e31826f5310

Richner, M., Bjerrum, O. J., Nykjaer, A., & Vaegter, C. B. (2011). The spared nerve injury (SNI) model of induced mechanical allodynia in mice. *Journal of Visualized Experiments, 54*. http://dx.doi.org/10.3791/3092

Rodriguez, L. (2015). Pathophysiology of pain: Implications for perioperative nursing. *AORN Journal, 101*(3), 338–344. http://dx.doi.org/10.1016/j.aorn.2014.12.008

Roth, S. H., & Fuller, P. (2011). Diclofenac topical solution compared with oral diclofenac: A pooled safety analysis. *Journal of Pain Research, 4*, 159–167. http://dx.doi.org/10.2147/jpr.s20965

Rutgen, M., Seidel, E. M., Silani, G., Riecansky, I., Hummer, A., Windischberger, C., et al. (2015). Placebo analgesia and its opioidergic regulation suggest that empathy for pain is grounded in self pain. *Proceedings of the National Academy of Sciences, 112*(41), E5638–E5646. http://dx.doi.org/10.1073/pnas.1511269112

Scholl, I., Zill, J. M., Harter, M., & Dirmaier, J. (2014). An integrative model of patient-centeredness–a systematic review and concept analysis. *PLoS One, 9*(9), e107828. http://dx.doi.org/10.1371/journal.pone.0107828

Sieck, G. C. (2003). Physiology of aging. *Journal of Applied Physiology, 95*(4), 1333–1334. http://dx.doi.org/10.1152/japplphysiol.00718.2003

Sobolewski, C., Cerella, C., Dicato, M., Ghibelli, L., & Diederich, M. (2010). The role of cyclooxygenase-2 in cell proliferation and cell death in human malignancies. *International Journal of Cell Biology, 2010*, 1–21. http://dx.doi.org/10.1155/2010/215158

Steegers, M. A., Snik, D. M., Verhagen, A. F., van der Drift, M. A., & Wilder-Smith, O. H. (2008). Only half of the chronic pain after thoracic surgery shows a neuropathic component. *The Journal of Pain, 9*(10), 955–961. http://dx.doi.org/10.1016/j.jpain.2008.05.009

Tait, R. C. (2008). Empathy: Necessary for effective pain management? *Current Pain and Headache Reports, 12*(2), 108–112. Retrieved from http://www.ncbi.nlm.nih.gov/pubmed/18474190

Uncini, A., & Kuwabara, S. (2015). Nodopathies of the peripheral nerve: An emerging concept. *Journal of Neurology, Neurosurgery & Psychiatry, 86*(11), 1186–1195. http://dx.doi.org/10.1136/jnnp-2014-310097

Varadi, A., Hosztafi, S., Le Rouzic, V., Toth, G., Urai, A., Noszal, B., et al. (2013). Novel 6beta-acylaminomorphinans with analgesic activity. *European Journal of Medicinal ChemistryChem, 69*, 786–789. http://dx.doi.org/10.1016/j.ejmech.2013.09.031

Vyazovskiy, V. V. (2015). Sleep, recovery, and metaregulation: Explaining the benefits of sleep. *Nature and Science of Sleep, 7*, 171–184. http://dx.doi.org/10.2147/nss.s54036

Wang, L., Johnston, B., Kaushal, A., Cheng, D., Zhu, F., & Martin, J. (2015). Ketamine added to morphine or hydromorphone patient-controlled analgesia for acute postoperative pain in adults: A systematic review and meta-analysis of randomized trials. *Canadian Journal of Anesthesia/Journal canadien d'anesthésie, 63*(7), 311–325. http://dx.doi.org/10.1007/s12630-015-0551-4

Wang, R. C., Jiang, F. M., Zheng, Q. L., Li, C. T., Peng, X. Y., He, C. Y., et al. (2014). Efficacy and safety of sildenafil treatment in pulmonary arterial hypertension: A systematic review. *Respiratory Medicine, 108*(3), 531–537. http://dx.doi.org/10.1016/j.rmed.2014.01.003

Wiffen, P., Collins, S., McQuay, H., Carroll, D., Jadad, A., & Moore, A. (2005). Anticonvulsant drugs for acute and chronic pain. *Cochrane Database of Systematic Reviews*, (3), http://dx.doi.org/10.1002/14651858.cd001133.pub2

Xu, Q., & Yaksh, T. L. (2011). A brief comparison of the pathophysiology of inflammatory versus neuropathic pain. *Current Opinion in Anaesthesiology, 24*(4), 400–407. http://dx.doi.org/10.1097/aco.0b013e32834871df

Yarnitsky, D., Crispel, Y., Eisenberg, E., Granovsky, Y., Ben-Nun, A., Sprecher, E., et al. (2008). Prediction of chronic post-operative pain: Pre-operative DNIC testing identifies patients at risk. *Pain, 138*(1), 22–28 http://dx.doi.org/10.1016/j.pain.2007.10.033

Yekkirala, A. S., Kalyuzhny, A. E., & Portoghese, P. S. (2010). Standard opioid agonists activate heteromeric opioid receptors: Evidence for morphine and [d-Ala(2)-MePhe(4)-Glyol(5)] enkephalin as selective mu-delta agonists. *ACS Chemical Neuroscience, 1*(2), 146–154. http://dx.doi.org/10.1021/cn9000236

CHAPTER 7

Acupuncture and Chronic Pain Management

Ladan Eshkevari

ABSTRACT

According to National Institute of Health Pathways to Prevention Workshop (2014), chronic pain affects an estimated 100 million Americans, with approximately 25 million people experiencing moderate to severe chronic pain, which negatively impacts their ability to function leading to a diminished quality of life. Pain is the primary reason Americans are on disability, which adds to the economic and social burden of suffering for the nation. Chronic pain costs are estimated to be between $560 and $630 billion per year. An estimated 5 to 8 million Americans use opioids for long-term management of chronic pain, which can have deleterious effects on their lives including addiction. Recent evidence suggests that acupuncture, a treatment modality that has been used worldwide for over 2,000 years, may provide a useful pain management option for those who suffer from chronic pain. The investigation into its mechanism of action and efficacy remains elusive, but promising.

INTRODUCTION

Acupuncture History and Prevalence

Acupuncture is the most common treatment modality in traditional Chinese medicine (TCM), and has been dated back to over 2,500 years (Deng et al., 1997).

http://dx.doi.org/10.1891/0739-6686.35.117

According to the WHO, acupuncture is useful as an adjunct in the treatments of over 50 disorders and although it was a modality used only in TCM, it is now used worldwide (Qi & Kelley, 2014). Indeed, 80% of 129 WHO member nations have reported that they now recognize and use acupuncture in a variety of conditions (Qi & Kelley, 2014).

Although acupuncture has been utilized in the world for a very long time, it was not disseminated to the United States until the 1970s when President Richard Nixon traveled to China. Since then acupuncture use has grown in popularity in the United States as a form of complementary and alternative medicine In a 1997 National Institutes of Health (NIH) consensus report acupuncture was recognized as a useful treatment or adjunct for a variety of conditions (NIH, 1997). Further, in a survey of use study by Burke et al., it was found that about 8.19 million Americans had reported lifetime use of acupuncture, with 2.13 million having utilized acupuncture in the previous year (Burke, Upchurch, Dye, & Chyu, 2006).

The general theory of acupuncture is based on the premise that meridians filled with qi (or life energy) traverse the entire human body, and that all the meridians carry this energy from each energetic organ (Figure 7.1). All the organs are thought to possess certain energies, and unlike allopathic medicine they are not thought of as individual and anatomical, rather they are interconnected and

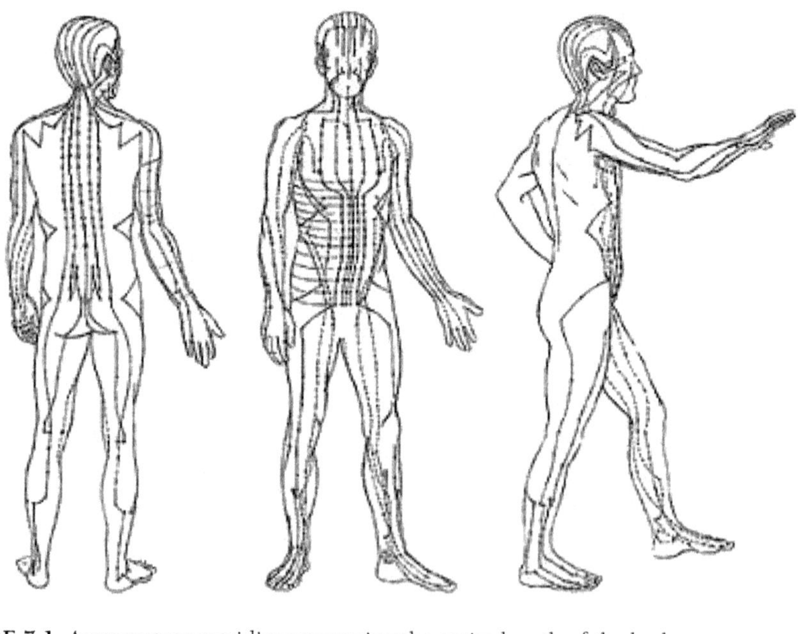

FIGURE 7.1 Acupuncture meridians traversing the entire length of the body.

energetic (Deng et al., 1997). TCM is therefore a more holistic approach to body, mind, and the environment that all intersect in the function of the human body and spirit. In TCM, any disruption of flow of qi is considered to be responsible for causing disease, stress, and/or pain (Deng et al., 1997). In the United States, the licensed acupuncturist inserts sterile stainless steel needles on specific acupoints on the meridians to try to stimulate movement of qi and thereby resolves the underlying pathophysiology that may be occurring as a result of its stagnation. In recent decades the advent of electroacupuncture (EA) has added the benefit of delivering stimulation to several acupuncture points simultaneously, making the treatment more efficient and potentially more beneficial than in the past.

Chronic Pain Physiology and Prevalence

According to the Institute of Medicine (IOM) report on pain, 100 million adults are burdened with chronic pain, with an annual associated cost of approximately six hundred billion dollars (Dzau & Pizzo, 2014). Chronic pain is multifaceted, and encompasses biological, psychosocial, economical, and genetic factors that impact its perception by the sufferer. It is defined as pain lasting 3 months or longer, or lasting beyond the normal time for tissue healing for specific tissue damage (Classification of chronic pain, 1986).

By definition, pain is subjective, a culmination of transduction, and transmission of pain impulse to the spinal cord, which processes the information, and further transmits it to the specialized pathways in the brain that mediate pain-associated behavior (Baliki & Apkarian, 2015). Pain impulses are carried from the peripheral primary afferent neurons to secondary neurons in the spinal cord via the dorsal root ganglion, are modulated and transmitted to the thalamus of the brain via ascending tracts, where they synapse with third-order neurons and send projections to various parts of the cortex, eliciting pain responses (Hu, Cai, Xiao, Luo, & Iannetti, 2014). It has been observed that once pain is detected, both peripheral and central pain pathways display incredible plasticity, enhancing pain signals that can contribute to development of chronic pain, and hypersensitivity (Basbaum, Bautista, Scherrer, & Julius, 2009). At the spinal cord level, numerous molecules such as substance P, and calcitonin-gene-related peptide (CGRP) are responsible for reorganizing neuronal circuitry, causing glial cell changes, and giving rise to central sensitization (Basbaum et al., 2009). Recently, utilizing imaging techniques, the human brain has also been demonstrated to undergo numerous neuroplasticity changes with chronic pain (Apkarian, Hashmi, & Baliki, 2011). It has been further confirmed that in developing chronic pain, some conditions must be met (Baliki & Apkarian, 2015). These conditions include a propensity of the individual brain for being predisposed to synaptic learning that can lead to a maladaptive response to pain (Baliki, Geha, Fields, & Apkarian, 2010), the initial injury that leads to the transition from acute to chronic pain, and the final stage of maintenance of the chronic pain state by the brain (Baliki & Apkarian, 2015). It has been postulated that a genetic or learned predisposition combined with a specific injury causes an amplified, and perhaps maladaptive, nociceptive response that leads to novel neocortical anatomical functional memory creating the chronic pain state (Baliki & Apkarian, 2015). The specifics of the anatomical brain changes that actually occur as a result of chronic pain remain elusive; however growing evidence suggests that regional gray matter decreases with pain, but can partly regenerate with successful chronic pain treatments (Ceko et al., 2015; Gwilym, Filippini, Douaud, Carr, & Tracey, 2010). White matter abnormalities have also been investigated, though they seem to play a more important role as a predisposing risk factor, rather than a consequence of chronic pain associated changes, which thus may be a potential important predictor of development of maladaptive response to pain (Mansour et al., 2013). Further, in animal and human models of pain, and mood disorders such as depression, anxiety, and posttraumatic stress disorder (PTSD), a strong correlation has been observed between these disorders and chronic pain with respect to parallel changes in brain circuitry, whereby there is decreased brain volume in correlating pathways (Baliki & Apkarian, 2015).

Current Treatment Options for Chronic Pain

Opioids

Opioids exert their effects by stimulating endogenous opioid receptors, mu, delta, and kappa, which are located peripherally and centrally along the pain pathways. Once opioids bind to the receptors they cause prevention of presynaptic calcium (Ca^{++}) release, thereby decreasing the release of pronociceptive neurotransmitters such as substance P. Postsynaptic activity causes increased potassium (K^{+}) release leading to hyperpolarization and suppression of nociceptive neurotransmitters, and prevention of propagation of the pain action potential (Nuckols et al., 2014).

Opioids, although effective, have numerous untoward side effects including addiction, overdose, apnea, and depression. In a recent NIH report, it was noted that although numerous treatments are available for chronic pain management, 5 to 8 million Americans use opioids for chronic pain management, and that the number of opioid prescriptions has reached astronomical numbers in the past 20 years (NIH, 2014). In the same report, 40% to 70% of chronic pain patients are not receiving adequate management, leading experts to question the long-term effectiveness of opioids, their risks versus benefits; and what are some evidence-based alternatives to opioid use in chronic pain management (NIH, 2014)?

Nonsteroidal Anti-Inflammatory Drugs

The nonsteroidal anti-inflammatory drugs inhibit cyclooxygenase (COX), the enzyme that catalyzes the transformation of arachidonic acid to prostaglandins and thromboxanes, which in turn cause release of pro-inflammatory cytokines (Kongtharvonskul et al., 2015). Their use is also associated with some side effects such as toxicity, platelet dysfunction, and nephrotoxicity and therefore not recommended for long-term use (Kmietowicz, 2015; Ussai et al., 2015).

Serotonergic Drugs

Serotonin is a neurotransmitter found in the sympathetic nervous system, and acts on 5-hydroxytryptamine (5-HT) receptors within the dorsal horn of the spinal column leading to endogenous pain inhibition (Dogrul, Ossipov, & Porreca, 2009). Drugs that activate 5-HT receptors are also associated with some side effects such as narrowing of coronary arteries and central serotonergic syndrome, with long-term use effects still unclear (Heddini et al., 2014).

Antidepressant and Antiepileptic Drugs

In recent decades antidepressant and antiepileptic drugs have been added to the medications used in chronic pain management as adjuncts to other modalities. Antidepressants work by inhibiting uptake of norepinephrine in the central nervous system (CNS) leading to stimulation of endogenous monoaminergic pain inhibition in the brain and spinal cord (Nekovarova et al., 2014). They are associated with adverse events such as sedation, nausea, dizziness, and sleep disturbances. The antiepileptic agents are used mostly in chronic neuropathic pain and occasionally for migraine headache pain. They are postulated to exert their antinociceptive effects by inhibition of pathologically active sodium, and calcium channels, and enhanced activity of the gamma-amino butyric acid receptors. However, they are also associated with somnolence, dizziness, fatigue, and cognitive and motor impairments (Ghinea, Lipworth, & Kerridge, 2015).

Allopathic Nonsurgical Interventional Methods

The popularity of interventional methods has increased in the past decade; however, most of the methods used are nonevidence-based, and are not curative; rather, they may allay pain thus increasing patient ability to participate in rehabilitation (LeResche, 2005). The most common techniques include injection of local anesthetics, or steroids into facet or zygapophyseal joints or along the medial branch from the posterior ramus of the spinal root. However, there is little convincing evidence that these techniques lead to long-term pain relief (Abdi et al., 2007; Hansen et al., 2012; Rosenow, 2002).

ACUPUNCTURE FOR CHRONIC PAIN

Mechanism of Action–Evidence From Animal Research

Scientists evaluating how acupuncture may work in treatment of pain models have postulated numerous underlying mechanisms of action, and in the past decade preclinical investigators have found mounting evidence in elucidating acupuncture-induced responses in pain models. EA, insertion of needles and delivery of electric impulses, is studied most often, as it allows for uniform stimulation of acupoints in animal studies.

Inflammatory and Neuropathic Models of Pain

Injection of various compounds such as carrageenan causes inflammatory pain similar to osteoarthritis (OA) in humans, thereby providing a useful model for the study of EA in this disease model. This paradigm allows for examination of both peripheral and central mechanisms of pain and the effects that acupuncture may have on the pain pathways, beginning with afferent neurons up to the CNS. Recent studies have found that EA at acupuncture point, Stomach 36 (St36), on the stomach meridian, located near the hind paw of the rat (Figure 7.2) with induced inflammation increases pain threshold. The apparent mechanism for this effect is the release of endogenous opioids such as beta-endorphin from

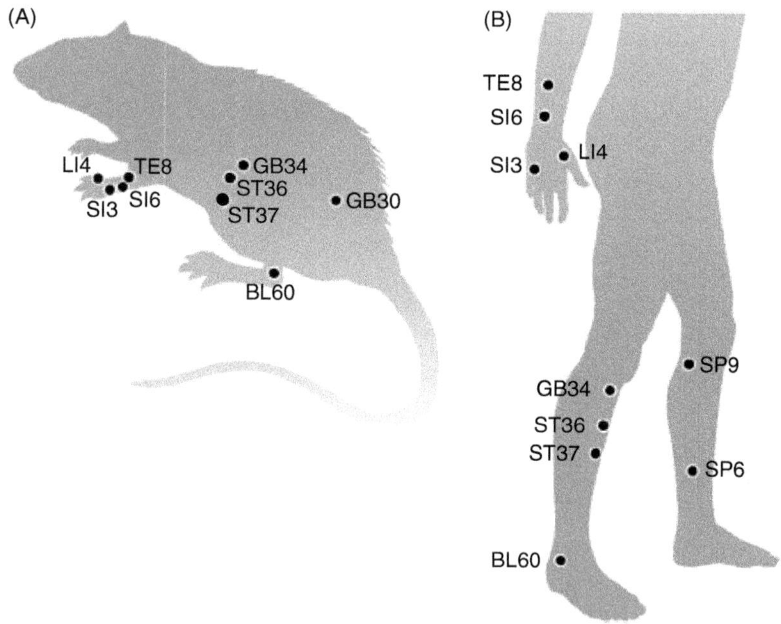

FIGURE 7.2 Rat and human points used in pain studies with permission, Mechanisms of Acupuncture-Electroacupuncture on Persistent Pain (Zhang, Lao, Ren, & Berman, 2014).

lymphocytes, monocytes/macrophages, and granulocytes at the site of inflammation (Cabot et al., 1997; Rittner et al., 2001; Sekido, Ishimaru, & Sakita, 2003; Taguchi, Taguchi, & Kitakoji, 2010).

It has been further elucidated that electrostimulation of acupoints also activates peripheral sympathetic nerve fibers, as well as the cannabinoid system, which in turn increases the levels of opioids at the inflammation site (Kim et al., 2008; Su et al., 2011). Interestingly, EA has also been demonstrated to inhibit cyclooxygenase-2 (COX-2), increasing opioids at the inflammation site, perhaps acting similarly to common anti-inflammatory medications (Lee, Jang, Lee, Choi, & Choi, 2006).

These studies are certainly intriguing and demonstrate that the effects of acupuncture can begin at the local, peripheral site of inflammation. Some researchers have also studied the potential for acupuncture's ability to modulate pain pathways within the CNS, reporting various mechanisms by which acupuncture may exert anti-inflammatory responses both in the spinal cord and in the brain. For example, studies have again demonstrated that in various inflammatory models of pain acupuncture can modulate the effect of opioids via opioid receptors, and can concomitantly activate sympathetic and serotonin neurons to further enhance opioid activity and anti-inflammation (Silva, Silva, & Prado, 2011; Zhang et al., 2012).

Acupuncture analgesia has also been examined in various animal models of neuropathic pain such as cold allodynia, spinal nerve ligation (SNL), and injection of neurotoxic substances into the spinal cord nerves. Using these animal models, researchers have demonstrated that acupuncture can effectively reduce hypersensitivity by modulating the opioid, serotonin, and sympathetic nervous systems predominantly at the spinal cord level (Cidral-Filho et al., 2011; Kim et al., 2005; Pachman, Barton, Watson, & Loprinzi, 2011; Song, Meyerson, & Linderoth, 2011).

Mechanism of Action–Evidence From Clinical Research

Although animal models of chronic pain are useful in elucidating potential underlying mechanisms of acupuncture activity, it is ultimately clinical studies that hone in on its potential as a useful modality and adjunct in the treatment of chronic pain. Therefore, both the underlying mechanism and the efficacy in clinical studies of acupuncture are important if it is to become a mainstay as part of the treatment protocol for chronic pain. Once primary and pain management clinicians are provided with conclusive evidence on the mechanism of action and efficacy of acupuncture, they may be more apt to suggest or prescribe its use to their patients. Therefore, given that 2.1 million visits are made annually to emergency rooms for severe headaches, 5 million women over the age of 18 report fibromyalgia, 26.4% of Americans suffer from low back pain, and 62% of nursing home residents experience arthritic pain (National Academies, 2011), the potential for acupuncture's use as an adjunct in the treatment of chronic pain necessitates a clear understanding of its efficacy and mechanism of action.

Acupuncture for Headache and Migraine

In examining the efficacy of acupuncture as a prophylactic treatment for migraines, Linde et al. (2011) conducted a systematic review of 22 randomized trials, totaling 4,419 patients diagnosed with migraine, comparing the clinical effects of acupuncture with either a control, a sham acupuncture intervention, or another intervention (Linde et al., 2009). They examined outcomes based on data that described frequency, intensity, and medication use related to episodes of headache. The findings of the review were dichotomous; in one respect the evidence demonstrated that acupuncture was an effective adjunct to standard care, and at least as effective as prophylactic treatment with medications in management of pain (Linde et al., 2009). However, the study also showed that verum acupuncture was no better than sham acupuncture in its effects. The authors postulated that acupuncture itself is a "placebo," that sham acupuncture may have some underlying mechanism in itself treating migraine headache pain, or that given the lack of blinding in the studies comparisons may be biased (Linde et al., 2009).

A more recent study of effectiveness of acupuncture for use in migraine symptoms, which also examined functional magnetic resonance imaging (fMRI) of various brain regions associated with migraine headaches, shed some light on the potential physiological effects that could explain the contradictory results from the Linde et al. study (L. Zhao et al., 2014). In this randomized controlled trial, the researchers compared the difference in resting brain activation in 80 migraine patients elicited by acupuncture and sham acupuncture points using fMRI. They also compared possible correlation between their fMRI results and clinical efficacy utilizing a visual analogue scale (VAS) of 0 to 10, number of headache days per month, and duration of pain. The headache impact test (HIT-6) was also used to measure impact of migraines on quality of life (Zhao et al., 2014). The researchers found that both acupuncture and sham acupuncture were as effective after 2 months of therapy significantly reducing migraine symptoms and improving quality of life. Additionally, they found that acupuncture was better than sham at reducing pain intensity. These findings were congruent with their fMRI data in that both acupuncture and sham acupuncture increased activity at the anterior cingulate cortex (ACC), middle frontal gyrus, and middle temporal gyrus areas of the brain, and this activity negatively correlated with VAS pain scores. In essence, these brain areas were activated and led to lower

VAS pain scores, and better efficacy of pain relief, with the ACC being the major region involved in cognitive and affective aspects of pain perception (Zhao et al., 2014). However, the fMRI data also demonstrated that acupuncture versus sham acupuncture was also significant in evoking activity in other brain areas such as bilateral insula, thalamus, cerebellum, and the thalamus. This correlated with acupuncture's ability to significantly reduce pain intensity compared to sham. They hypothesized that acupuncture could potentially alleviate migraine intensity by modulating the afferent network of pain to a physiological rather than maladaptive state (Zhao et al., 2014).

In a more recent systematic review of 10 trials with 997 subjects with a history of migraine headaches that compared acupuncture with sham acupuncture, it was demonstrated that both sham and acupuncture reduced pain intensity, frequency, and duration (Yang, Que, Ye, & Zheng, 2015). However, there was a significant reduction in the rate of migraine occurrence in the acupuncture group (Yang et al., 2015).

The effectiveness of acupuncture has also been examined in other types of headache pain with some promising results. A large randomized, blind study of chronic headache patients found that acupuncture effectively decreased headache days and improved quality of life compared to control groups (Endres et al., 2007). Furthermore, a military study in a similar population of individuals suffering from chronic daily headaches had results mirroring the Endres group's results (Plank & Goodard, 2009).

Collectively, these studies suggest that acupuncture may provide utility as an adjunct in various headache diseases. Furthermore, acupuncture can potentially reduce the amount of medication use, and increase health-related quality of life in this patient population.

Acupuncture for Back Pain

Chronic back pain is a major public health issue and is a leading cause of disability in the United States in patients aged 45 and younger, with 60% to 80% of the adult U.S. population suffering from the disease (Mannion, Balague, Pellise, & Cedraschi, 2007; Strine & Hootman, 2007). Numerous researchers have conducted clinical studies in various settings to determine the effects of acupuncture in symptom management for this prevalent disease.

A systemic review of acupuncture and dry needling (a technique similar to acupuncture used by physical therapists) for low back pain concluded that in chronic low back pain, acupuncture is more effective than no treatment or sham acupuncture in relieving pain and improving functionality, but the results were short term. The results of the review indicated that acupuncture may be useful as an adjunct to chronic management of low back pain (Furlan et al., 2005). A study comparing acupuncture to local anesthetic injection for low back pain demonstrated that although both groups had significantly improved VAS pain scores, the acupuncture cohort had significantly lower pain scores when compared to the local injection group, and that the acupuncture group had sustained effects (Inoue, Hojo, Nakajima, Kitakoji, & Itoi, 2009). In a systematic review of four robust studies of acupuncture for low back pain, Trigkilidas (2010) concluded that acupuncture could be an effective modality in managing patients with low back pain, especially in patients who have a positive view of acupuncture as part of their management therapy (Trigkilidas, 2010). This is intriguing with respect to the placebo effects associated with acupuncture, since a positive view of the treatment correlated with better pain outcomes.

In another more recent systematic review and meta-analysis of auricular acupuncture (AA) for chronic pain, including back pain, the authors concluded that AA therapy could be a "promising technique for chronic pain relief." However, they stated that a definitive conclusion could not be reached due to poor research methodologies such as unclear randomization and lack of blinding of treatment arms (Zhao, Tan, Wang, & Jin, 2015).

Finally, Liu et al. (2015) concurred with Zhao et al. (2015) in a future need for higher quality randomized control trials to determine response to acupuncture treatment in the chronic back pain patient population. They did, however, ascertain that acupuncture is more clinically effective and improves functionality in chronic low back pain than no treatment or standard treatment only, and that acupuncture alone or in conjunction with usual care should be considered for treatment of low back pain (Liu et al., 2015).

Acupuncture for Musculoskeletal Pain

Fibromyalgia

Fibromyalgia is a debilitating disease that affects 5 million adults in the United States, with almost 90% of cases occurring in females of childbearing age (Lawrence et al., 2008). The disease is characterized by generalized musculoskeletal pain, often accompanied by insomnia, exhaustion, and psychiatric mood disorders. Many treatment modalities and a variety of practitioners are frequently necessary to manage the syndrome, including acupuncture, with one in five fibromyalgia patients having used acupuncture as a treatment modality (Deare et al., 2013). However, the evidence of effectiveness remains unclear with many studies underpowered or poorly designed. A recent Cochrane database systematic review examined the benefits of acupuncture as a treatment option by reviewing nine trials involving 395 patients, and found "low to moderate level evidence" that acupuncture improved pain (Deare et al., 2013). Although promising, these results demonstrate that future well-designed randomized controlled trials must be conducted to evaluate the utility of acupuncture in the comprehensive care of fibromyalgia sufferers.

Arthritis

Arthritis is prevalent in the United States, with more than 50 million adults suffering from the inflammatory pain and loss of function of joints that are hallmarks of the disease (Lawrence et al., 2008). There are currently no good treatment options for arthritis symptoms, with most medications having untoward side effects. To that end, acupuncture, a low-risk option with few side effects, may be an attractive option to the arthritis pain sufferer, and acupuncture is indeed used often by patients with arthritis. However, evidence from a systematic review of randomized clinical trials of acupuncture treatments for rheumatoid arthritis patients revealed that there is currently insufficient data to definitively suggest acupuncture as an effective treatment option (Lee, Shin, & Ernst, 2008). Conversely, in a more recent and comprehensive (114 trials) meta-analysis examining the effectiveness of acupuncture and other physical treatments in arthritic knee pain, the authors concluded that acupuncture can be considered as one of the more effective treatments for this patient population (Corbett et al., 2013). In this study, researchers compared eight interventions, including pulsed electrical stimulation, aerobic exercise, sham acupuncture, and acupuncture (Corbett et al., 2013).

Upper Extremity Pain

Chronic shoulder, elbow, arm and hand pain can pose challenges to patients with respect to function in activities of daily living and thus affect health-related quality of life. These patients, like other chronic pain patients can become dependent on medications that often have side effects and can themselves affect functionality and quality of life. Acupuncture use and efficacy has been evaluated in these patients with mixed results. A multicenter study of 424 patients compared acupuncture to sham acupuncture and conventional therapy for shoulder pain and found that acupuncture, but not sham was an effective alternative treatment to standard care (Molsberger, Schneider, Gotthardt, & Drabik, 2010). An overview of 30 systematic reviews using acupuncture to treat rheumatic conditions, including shoulder and elbow pain, demonstrated that although acupuncture is effective for both, the evidence for the value of acupuncture treatment for elbow pain is much stronger than in shoulder pain (Ernst & Lee, 2010). The researchers concluded that these results were mostly due to lack of quality of some of the studies they included in their analysis (Ernst & Lee, 2010). Similarly, Zhang et al. (2016) examined the role of acupuncture in treatment of chronic shoulder pain when added to conventional physiotherapy (Zhang et al., 2016). This group found acupuncture as an adjunct to physical therapy significantly reduced pain and improved function and mobility (Zhang et al., 2016).

Lower Extremity Pain

Several researchers have attempted to elucidate acupuncture's efficacy related to osteoarthritic knee pain and have had mixed results. Plaster, Vieira, Alencar, Nakano, and Liebano. (2014) examined the effects of manual versus EA in 60 randomized patients and found that both groups had significant reduction in pain intensity ($p < .001$) with no differences between their groups (Plaster et al., 2014). In a meta-analysis study comparing acupuncture to other physical treatments for the relief of OA pain of the knee, the researchers concluded that "that acupuncture can be considered as one of the more effective physical treatments for alleviating OA related knee pain in the short-term" (Corbett et al., 2013). This study confirmed results from a prior systematic review with similar design that also demonstrated that acupuncture provided significantly better pain relief and functional improvement when compared to standard care or sham acupuncture in OA-related knee pain (Cao, Zhang, Gao, & Jiang, 2012). Acupuncture has also been shown to improve pain and functional rehabilitation postoperatively after knee arthroplasty, which makes it an attractive adjunct to the rehabilitation regimen for this patient population (Chen et al., 2015; Liu, Xue, Sun, & Li, 2015; Tzeng et al., 2015; Xue, Sun, Li, & Liu, 2015). Given the recent national concerns regarding prescription of narcotics and their addiction potential for acute painful procedures such as knee arthroplasty it seems prudent to utilize acupuncture, which has been demonstrated to be a useful adjunct in treatment for this very painful procedure. This adjunctive treatment modality can alleviate many opioid-related side effects allowing for reduction in dosing, and can further improve joint function and health-related quality of life. In the case of knee pain, there is mounting evidence for effectiveness of addition of acupuncture in pain management, though additional research is warranted in determining which types of patients are best suited for receiving adjunct acupuncture as part of their treatment protocol.

CONCLUSION

Acupuncture is the main treatment modality in Chinese medicine, which has been used for over 2,000 years. It has survived the test of time, but has been scrutinized anew in the context of modern medicine seeking evidence and validation for its use. Acupuncture is known to be commonly used for a wide range of pain syndromes, including headaches, OA, low back pain, and systemic pain such as fibromyalgia. The primary mechanisms of its action are proposed to be via release of endogenous pain modulators such as endorphin in the CNS, and to a certain extent an inhibitory control over noxious stimuli. However, both the clinical efficacy and the mechanism are still a matter of debate. Numerous systematic reviews have been conducted in the recent past, with many of them focusing on acupuncture as a pain relieving modality. However, although these reviews have attempted to clarify and offer evidence, they have conversely caused a great level of contradiction. The most interesting finding from these reviews is that acupuncture is very useful for certain types of pain, but not all types of pain are managed with the same efficiency, and some do not respond to this modality at all. For example, several Cochrane and systematic reviews of acupuncture have found it to provide significant benefits to those suffering from joint OA and headache pain, whereas rheumatoid arthritis type pain is less responsive to its effects (Casimiro et al., 2005; Linde et al., 2009; Manheimer et al., 2010).

Pain is certainly an area where practitioners could use all the treatment options available in managing their patients' symptoms. Given the lack of good, available pharmacological pain therapies that have minimal side effects, it is then incumbent on practitioners to turn to alternatives and adjuncts that may provide some relief to their patients. It is with great hope in the interest of our patients, that we forge ahead in finding more evidence in the Western medicine context for a modality that has a rich history but remains to find its place in common practice.

REFERENCES

Abdi, S., Datta, S., Trescot, A. M., Schultz, D. M., Adlaka, R., Atluri, S. L., et al. (2007). Epidural steroids in the management of chronic spinal pain: A systematic review. *Pain Physician, 10*(1), 185–212. Retrieved from http://www.ncbi.nlm.nih.gov/pubmed/17256030

Apkarian, A. V., Hashmi, J. A., & Baliki, M. N. (2011). Pain and the brain: Specificity and plasticity of the brain in clinical chronic pain. *Pain, 152*(Suppl. 3), S49–S64. http://dx.doi.org/10.1016/j.pain.2010.11.010

Baliki, M. N., & Apkarian, A. V. (2015). Nociception, pain, negative moods, and behavior selection. *Neuron, 87*(3), 474–491. http://dx.doi.org/10.1016/j.neuron.2015.06.005

Baliki, M. N., Geha, P. Y., Fields, H. L., & Apkarian, A. V. (2010). Predicting value of pain and analgesia: Nucleus accumbens response to noxious stimuli changes in the presence of chronic pain. *Neuron, 66*(1), 149–160. http://dx.doi.org/10.1016/j.neuron.2010.03.002

Basbaum, A. I., Bautista, D. M., Scherrer, G., & Julius, D. (2009). Cellular and molecular mechanisms of pain. *Cell, 139*(2), 267–284. http://dx.doi.org/10.1016/j.cell.2009.09.028

Burke, A., Upchurch, D. M., Dye, C., & Chyu, M. A. (2006). Acupuncture use in the United States: Findings from the National Health Interview Survey. *The Journal of Alternative and Complementary Medicine, 12*(7), 639–648.

Cabot, P. J., Carter, L., Gaiddon, C., Zhang, Q., Schafer, M., Loeffler, J. P., et al. (1997). Immune cell-derived beta-endorphin. Production, release, and control of inflammatory pain in rats. *Journal of Clinical Investigation, 100*(1), 142–148. http://dx.doi.org/10.1172/jci119506

Cao, L., Zhang, X. L., Gao, Y. S., & Jiang, Y. (2012). Needle acupuncture for osteoarthritis of the knee. A systematic review and updated meta-analysis. *Saudi Medical Journal, 33*(5), 526–532. Retrieved from http://www.ncbi.nlm.nih.gov/pubmed/22588814

Casimiro, L., Barnsley, L., Brosseau, L., Milne, S., Robinson, V. A., Tugwell, P., et al. (2005). Acupuncture and electroacupuncture for the treatment of rheumatoid arthritis. *Cochrane Database of Systematic Reviews,* (4), CD003788. http://dx.doi.org/10.1002/14651858.cd003788.pub2

Ceko, M., Shir, Y., Ouellet, J. A., Ware, M. A., Stone, L. S., & Seminowicz, D. A. (2015). Partial recovery of abnormal insula and dorsolateral prefrontal connectivity to cognitive networks in chronic low back pain after treatment. *Human Brain Mapping, 36*(6), 2075–2092. http://dx.doi.org/10.1002/hbm.22757

Chen, C. C., Yang, C. C., Hu, C. C., Shih, H. N., Chang, Y. H., & Hsieh, P. H. (2015). Acupuncture for pain relief after total knee arthroplasty: A randomized controlled trial. *Regional Anesthesia Pain Medicine, 40*(1), 31–36. http://dx.doi.org/10.1097/aap.0000000000000138

Cidral-Filho, F. J., da Silva, M. D., More, A. O., Cordova, M. M., Werner, M. F., & Santos, A. R. (2011). Manual acupuncture inhibits mechanical hypersensitivity induced by spinal nerve ligation in rats. *Neuroscience, 193*, 370–376. http://dx.doi.org/10.1016/j.neuroscience.2011.07.076

Classification of chronic pain. Descriptions of chronic pain syndromes and definitions of pain terms. Prepared by the International Association for the Study of Pain, Subcommittee on Taxonomy. (1986). *Pain Supplement, 3*, S1–S226. Retrieved from http://www.ncbi.nlm.nih.gov/pubmed/3461421

Corbett, M. S., Rice, S. J., Madurasinghe, V., Slack, R., Fayter, D. A., Harden, M., et al. (2013). Acupuncture and other physical treatments for the relief of pain due to osteoarthritis of the knee: Network meta-analysis. *Osteoarthritis Cartilage, 21*(9), 1290–1298. http://dx.doi.org/10.1016/j.joca.2013.05.007

Deare, J. C., Zheng, Z., Xue, C. C., Liu, J. P., Shang, J., Scott, S. W., et al. (2013). Acupuncture for treating fibromyalgia. *Cochrane Database System Reviews,* (5), CD007070. http://dx.doi.org/10.1002/14651858.cd007070.pub2

Deng, L., Yijun, G., Shuhui, H., Xiaoping, J., Yang, L., Rufen, W., et al. (1997). *Chinese acupuncture and moxibustion* (2nd ed.). Beijing: Foreign Languages Press.

Dogrul, A., Ossipov, M. H., & Porreca, F. (2009). Differential mediation of descending pain facilitation and inhibition by spinal 5HT-3 and 5HT-7 receptors. *Brain Research, 1280*, 52–59. http://dx.doi.org/10.1016/j.brainres.2009.05.001

Dzau, V. J., & Pizzo, P. A. (2014). Relieving pain in America: Insights from an Institute of Medicine committee. *Journal of the American Medical Association, 312*(15), 1507–1508. http://dx.doi.org/10.1001/jama.2014.12986

Endres, H. G., Bowing, G., Diener, H. C., Lange, S., Maier, C., Molsberger, A., et al. (2007). Acupuncture for tension-type headache: A multicentre, sham-controlled, patient-and observer-blinded, randomised trial. *The Journal of Headache and Pain, 8*(5), 306–314. http://dx.doi.org/10.1007/s10194-007-0416-5

Ernst, E., & Lee, M. S. (2010). Acupuncture for rheumatic conditions: An overview of systematic reviews. *Rheumatology (Oxford), 49*(10), 1957–1961. http://dx.doi.org/10.1093/rheumatology/keq180

Furlan, A. D., van Tulder, M., Cherkin, D., Tsukayama, H., Lao, L., Koes, B., et al. (2005). Acupuncture and dry-needling for low back pain: An updated systematic review within the framework of the cochrane collaboration. *Spine (Phila Pa 1976), 30*(8), 944–963. Retrieved from http://www.ncbi.nlm.nih.gov/pubmed/15834340

Ghinea, N., Lipworth, W., & Kerridge, I. (2015). Evidence, regulation and 'rational' prescribing: The case of gabapentin for neuropathic pain. *Journal of Evaluation in Clinical Practice, 21*(1), 28–33. http://dx.doi.org/10.1111/jep.12223

Gwilym, S. E., Filippini, N., Douaud, G., Carr, A. J., & Tracey, I. (2010). Thalamic atrophy associated with painful osteoarthritis of the hip is reversible after arthroplasty: A longitudinal voxel-based morphometric study. *Arthritis and Rheumatism, 62*(10), 2930–2940. http://dx.doi.org/10.1002/art.27585

Hansen, H., Manchikanti, L., Simopoulos, T. T., Christo, P. J., Gupta, S., Smith, H. S., et al. (2012). A systematic evaluation of the therapeutic effectiveness of sacroiliac joint interventions. *Pain Physician, 15*(3), E247–E278. Retrieved from http://www.ncbi.nlm.nih.gov/pubmed/22622913

Heddini, U., Bohm-Starke, N., Gronbladh, A., Nyberg, F., Nilsson, K. W., & Johannesson, U. (2014). Serotonin receptor gene (5HT-2A) polymorphism is associated with provoked vestibulodynia and comorbid symptoms of pain. *The Journal of Sexual Medicine, 11*(12), 3064–3071. http://dx.doi.org/10.1111/jsm.12685

Hu, L., Cai, M. M., Xiao, P., Luo, F., & Iannetti, G. D. (2014). Human brain responses to concomitant stimulation of Adelta and C nociceptors. *Journal of Neuroscience, 34*(34), 11439–11451. http://dx.doi.org/10.1523/jneurosci.1355-14.2014

Inoue, M., Hojo, T., Nakajima, M., Kitakoji, H., & Itoi, M. (2009). Comparison of the effectiveness of acupuncture treatment and local anaesthetic injection for low back pain: A randomised controlled clinical trial. *Acupunctutre Medicine, 27*(4), 174–177. http://dx.doi.org/10.1136/aim.2009.001164

Kim, H. W., Uh, D. K., Yoon, S. Y., Roh, D. H., Kwon, Y. B., Han, H. J., et al. (2008). Low-frequency electroacupuncture suppresses carrageenan-induced paw inflammation in mice via sympathetic post-ganglionic neurons, while high-frequency EA suppression is mediated by the sympathoadrenal medullary axis. *Brain Research Bulletin, 75*(5), 698–705. http://dx.doi.org/10.1016/j.brainresbull.2007.11.015

Kim, S. K., Park, J. H., Bae, S. J., Kim, J. H., Hwang, B. G., Min, B. I., et al. (2005). Effects of electroacupuncture on cold allodynia in a rat model of neuropathic pain: Mediation by spinal adrenergic and serotonergic receptors. *Experimental Neurology, 195*(2), 430–436. http://dx.doi.org/10.1016/j.expneurol.2005.06.018

Kmietowicz, Z. (2015). Guidance matches osteoarthritis patients to NSAIDs according to risk of side effects. *British Medical Journal, 350*, h1501. http://dx.doi.org/10.1136/bmj.h1501

Kongtharvonskul, J., Anothaisintawee, T., McEvoy, M., Attia, J., Woratanarat, P., & Thakkinstian, A. (2015). Efficacy and safety of glucosamine, diacerein, and NSAIDs in osteoarthritis knee: A systematic review and network meta-analysis. *European Journal Medicine Research, 20*(1), 24. http://dx.doi.org/10.1186/s40001-015-0115-7

Lawrence, R. C., Felson, D. T., Helmick, C. G., Arnold, L. M., Choi, H., Deyo, R. A., et al. (2008). Estimates of the prevalence of arthritis and other rheumatic conditions in the United States. Part II. *Arthritis and Rheumatism, 58*(1), 26–35. http://dx.doi.org/10.1002/art.23176

Lee, J. H., Jang, K. J., Lee, Y. T., Choi, Y. H., & Choi, B. T. (2006). Electroacupuncture inhibits inflammatory edema and hyperalgesia through regulation of cyclooxygenase synthesis in both peripheral and central nociceptive sites. *American Journal of Chinese Medicine, 34*(6), 981–988. http://dx.doi.org/10.1142/s0192415x06004454

Lee, M. S., Shin, B. C., & Ernst, E. (2008). Acupuncture for rheumatoid arthritis: A systematic review. *Rheumatology (Oxford), 47*(12), 1747–1753. http://dx.doi.org/10.1093/rheumatology/ken330

LeResche, L. (2005). International Association for the Study of Pain. 11th World Congress on Pain. August 21–26, 2005, Sydney, Australia. *Journal of Orofacial Pain, 19*(4), 345–346. Retrieved from http://www.ncbi.nlm.nih.gov/pubmed/16279487

Linde, K., Allais, G., Brinkhaus, B., Manheimer, E., Vickers, A., & White, A. R. (2009). Acupuncture for migraine prophylaxis. *Cochrane Database Systematic Reviews* (1), CD001218. http://dx.doi.org/10.1002/14651858.cd001218.pub2

Liu, G. P., Xue, F. S., Sun, C., & Li, R. P. (2015). Electroacupuncture for pain treatment after total knee arthroplasty. *Acupuncture Medicine, 33*(5), 433. http://dx.doi.org/10.1136/acupmed-2015-010859

Liu, L., Skinner, M., McDonough, S., Mabire, L., & Baxter, G. D. (2015). Acupuncture for low back pain: An overview of systematic reviews. *Evidence Based Complementry Alternative Medicine, 2015*, 328196. http://dx.doi.org/10.1155/2015/328196

Manheimer, E., Cheng, K., Linde, K., Lao, L., Yoo, J., Wieland, S., et al. (2010). Acupuncture for peripheral joint osteoarthritis. *Cochrane Database of Systematic Reviews* (1), CD001977. http://dx.doi.org/10.1002/14651858.cd001977.pub2

Mannion, A. F., Balague, F., Pellise, F., & Cedraschi, C. (2007). Pain measurement in patients with low back pain. *Nature Clinical Practice Rheumatology, 3*(11), 610–618. http://dx.doi.org/10.1038/ncprheum0646

Mansour, A. R., Baliki, M. N., Huang, L., Torbey, S., Herrmann, K. M., Schnitzer, T. J., et al. (2013). Brain white matter structural properties predict transition to chronic pain. *Pain, 154*(10), 2160–2168. http://dx.doi.org/10.1016/j.pain.2013.06.044

Molsberger, A. F., Schneider, T., Gotthardt, H., & Drabik, A. (2010). German Randomized Acupuncture Trial for chronic shoulder pain (GRASP) - a pragmatic, controlled, patient-blinded, multi-centre trial in an outpatient care environment. *Pain, 151*(1), 146–154. http://dx.doi.org/10.1016/j.pain.2010.06.036

National Academies. (2011). *Relieving pain in America: A blueprint for transforming prevention, care, education, and research.* Washington, DC: National Academies Press.

Nekovarova, T., Yamamotova, A., Vales, K., Stuchlik, A., Fricova, J., & Rokyta, R. (2014). Common mechanisms of pain and depression: are antidepressants also analgesics? *Front Behavioral Neuroscience, 8*, 99. http://dx.doi.org/10.3389/fnbeh.2014.00099

[NIH], N. I. o. H. (1997). Acupuncture. *NIH Consens Statement, 15*(5), 1–34.

NIH. (2014). *National Institute of Health Pathways to Prevention Workshop: The Role of Opioids in the Treatment of Chronic Pain.* Retrieved from https://prevention.nih.gov/docs/programs/p2p/ODPPainPanelStatementFinal_10-02-14.pdf

Nuckols, T. K., Anderson, L., Popescu, I., Diamant, A. L., Doyle, B., Di Capua, P., et al. (2014). Opioid prescribing: A systematic review and critical appraisal of guidelines for chronic pain. *Annals Internal Medicine, 160*(1), 38–47. http://dx.doi.org/10.7326/0003-4819-160-1-201401070-00732

Pachman, D. R., Barton, D. L., Watson, J. C., & Loprinzi, C. L. (2011). Chemotherapy-induced peripheral neuropathy: Prevention and treatment. *Clinical Pharmacology and Therapeutics, 90*(3), 377–387. http://dx.doi.org/10.1038/clpt.2011.115

Plank, S., & Goodard, J. (2009). The effectiveness of acupuncture for chronic daily headache: An outcomes study. *Military Medicine, 174*(12), 1276–1281. Retrieved from http://www.ncbi.nlm.nih.gov/pubmed/20055068

Plaster, R., Vieira, W. B., Alencar, F. A., Nakano, E. Y., & Liebano, R. E. (2014). Immediate effects of electroacupuncture and manual acupuncture on pain, mobility and muscle strength in patients with knee osteoarthritis: A randomised controlled trial. *Acupuncture in Medicine, 32*(3), 236–241. http://dx.doi.org/10.1136/acupmed-2013-010489

Qi, Z., & Kelley, E. (2014). The WHO Traditional Medicine Strategy 2014–2023: A perspective. *Science, 346*(6216), S5–S6. (Retrieved from <Go to ISI>://WOS:000346536500004)

Rittner, H. L., Brack, A., Machelska, H., Mousa, S. A., Bauer, M., Schafer, M., et al. (2001). Opioid peptide-expressing leukocytes: Identification, recruitment, and simultaneously increasing inhibition of inflammatory pain. *Anesthesiology, 95*(2), 500–508. Retrieved from http://www.ncbi.nlm.nih.gov/pubmed/11506126

Rosenow, D. E. (2002). Does neural blockade and other neurosurgical modalities offer a durable pain relief for spinal disorders? *Best Practice and Research Clinical Rheumatology, 16*(1), 155–164. http://dx.doi.org/10.1053/berh.2002.0206

Sekido, R., Ishimaru, K., & Sakita, M. (2003). Differences of electroacupuncture-induced analgesic effect in normal and inflammatory conditions in rats. *The American Journal of Chinese Medicine, 31*(6), 955–965. http://dx.doi.org/10.1142/s0192415x03001491

Silva, J. R., Silva, M. L., & Prado, W. A. (2011). Analgesia induced by 2- or 100-Hz electroacupuncture in the rat tail-flick test depends on the activation of different descending pain inhibitory mechanisms. *The Journal of Pain, 12*(1), 51–60. http://dx.doi.org/10.1016/j.jpain.2010.04.008

Song, Z., Meyerson, B. A., & Linderoth, B. (2011). Spinal 5-HT receptors that contribute to the pain-relieving effects of spinal cord stimulation in a rat model of neuropathy. *Pain, 152*(7), 1666–1673. http://dx.doi.org/10.1016/j.pain.2011.03.012

Strine, T. W., & Hootman, J. M. (2007). US national prevalence and correlates of low back and neck pain among adults. *Arthritis and Rheumatism, 57*(4), 656–665. http://dx.doi.org/10.1002/art.22684

Su, T. F., Zhang, L. H., Peng, M., Wu, C. H., Pan, W., Tian, B., et al. (2011). Cannabinoid CB2 receptors contribute to upregulation of beta-endorphin in inflamed skin tissues by electroacupuncture. *Molecular Pain, 7*(1), 98. http://dx.doi.org/10.1186/1744-8069-7-98

Taguchi, R., Taguchi, T., & Kitakoji, H. (2010). Involvement of peripheral opioid receptors in electroacupuncture analgesia for carrageenan-induced hyperalgesia. *Brain Research, 1355*, 97–103. http://dx.doi.org/10.1016/j.brainres.2010.08.014

Trigkilidas, D. (2010). Acupuncture therapy for chronic lower back pain: A systematic review. *The Annals of the Royal College Surgeons England, 92*(7), 595–598. http://dx.doi.org/10.1308/003588410x12699663904196

Tzeng, C. Y., Chang, S. L., Wu, C. C., Chang, C. L., Chen, W. G., Tong, K. M., et al. (2015). Single-blinded, randomised preliminary study evaluating the effects of 2 Hz electroacupuncture for postoperative pain in patients with total knee arthroplasty. *Acupuncture in Medicine, 33*(4), 284–288. http://dx.doi.org/10.1136/acupmed-2014-010722

Ussai, S., Miceli, L., Pisa, F. E., Bednarova, R., Giordano, A., Della Rocca, G., et al. (2015). Impact of potential inappropriate NSAIDs use in chronic pain. *Drug Design, Development and Therapy, 9*, 2073–2077. http://dx.doi.org/10.2147/dddt.s80686

Xue, F. S., Sun, C., Li, R. P., & Liu, G. P. (2015). Acupuncture for Pain Relief After Total Knee Arthroplasty: A Call for Clarification. *Regional Anesthesia and Pain Medicine, 40*(5), 640–641. http://dx.doi.org/10.1097/aap.0000000000000276

Yang, Y., Que, Q., Ye, X., & Zheng, G. H. (2015). Verum versus sham manual acupuncture for migraine: A systematic review of randomised controlled trials. *Acupuncture in Medicine, 34*(2), 76–83. http://dx.doi.org/10.1136/acupmed-2015-010903

Zhang, H., Sun, J., Wang, C., Yu, C., Wang, W., Zhang, M., et al. (2016). Randomised controlled trial of contralateral manual acupuncture for the relief of chronic shoulder pain. *Acupuncture in Medicine, 34*(3), 164–170. http://dx.doi.org/10.1136/acupmed-2015-010947

Zhang, R., Lao, L., Ren, K., & Berman, B. M. (2014). Mechanisms of acupuncture-electroacupuncture on persistent pain. *Anesthesiology, 120*(2), 482–503. http://dx.doi.org/10.1097/aln.0000000000000101

Zhang, Y., Zhang, R. X., Zhang, M., Shen, X. Y., Li, A., Xin, J., et al. (2012). Electroacupuncture inhibition of hyperalgesia in an inflammatory pain rat model: Involvement of distinct spinal serotonin and norepinephrine receptor subtypes. *British Journal of Anaesthesia, 109*(2), 245–252. http://dx.doi.org/10.1093/bja/aes136

Zhao, H. J., Tan, J. Y., Wang, T., & Jin, L. (2015). Auricular therapy for chronic pain management in adults: A synthesis of evidence. *Complementary Therapies in Clinical Practice, 21*(2), 68–78. http://dx.doi.org/10.1016/j.ctcp.2015.03.006

Zhao, L., Liu, J., Zhang, F., Dong, X., Peng, Y., Qin, W., et al. (2014). Effects of long-term acupuncture treatment on resting-state brain activity in migraine patients: A randomized controlled trial on active acupoints and inactive acupoints. *PLoS One, 9*(6), e99538. http://dx.doi.org/10.1371/journal.pone.0099538

CHAPTER 8

Anesthesia Involvement in Palliative Care

Amanda C. Faircloth

ABSTRACT

Palliative care teams require multidisciplinary support. While this is an emerging area in anesthesia practice, there are many avenues for certified registered nurse anesthetists (CRNAs) to share their unrivaled clinical knowledge. CRNAs may become involved with or consult on palliative sedation, medical management, interventional pain management, terminal wean/extubation, and organ donation. Additionally, CRNAs need to understand the unique needs of this patient population so that they can appropriately care for palliative care patients presenting to the operating room for palliative surgery. More research is needed to further explore CRNA involvement in palliative care. However, CRNAs have a specialized knowledge of pharmacology and physiology that perfectly complements the multidisciplinary palliative care team.

Death is the wish of some, the relief of many, and the end of all.
—Lucius Annaeus Seneca (4 BCE–65)

INTRODUCTION

Palliative care is a consultative discipline in the United States. It comprises an interdisciplinary team led by a palliative care physician. Palliative care experts address the physical, psychological, social, and spiritual aspects of life

http://dx.doi.org/10.1891/0739-6686.35.135

(Aslakson & Pronovost, 2011). While certified registered nurse anesthetists (CRNAs) may not routinely have exposure to palliative care patients, there is room to expand anesthesia's contribution to this medical specialty.

Background

Palliative care involves "aggressive symptom management, supported decision-making, and end-of-life care" (American Nurses Association, 2016, p. 4). The goal is to achieve the best quality of life for patients and their families (Pan, Morrison, Ness, Fugh-Berman, & Leipzia, 2000). The first step of palliative care is to outline realistic goals of care that encompass the patient and his or her family's wishes. Patient suffering (in the form of emotional distress) can begin with disease diagnosis (Ok, Meyers, & Evans, 2005). Early palliative care consultations can address this initial suffering, provide symptom management, and prognostic awareness (Strand, Kamdar, & Carey, 2013). The goal is to have a plan in place before the disease progresses.

Palliative care is not curative; the intent is to provide relief from symptoms (Kuziemsky, Jahnke, & Lau, 2006) and palliative care may be offered in conjunction with other medical treatments (Billings & Pantilat, 2001; Morrison & Meier, 2004). This leads to an overlap between palliative and curative models as these disciplines are synergistically linked (Figure 8.1).

Palliative care comprises three elements: goal setting, symptom management, and disease-directed therapy (Swetz & Kamal, 2012); see Figure 8.2. Goal

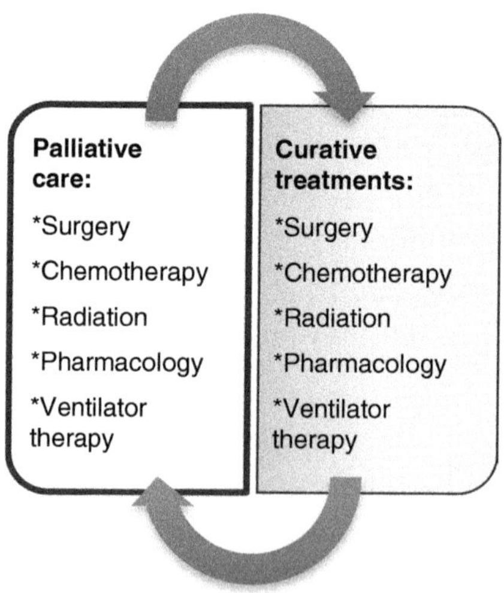

FIGURE 8.1 Overlap between palliative care and curative treatments.

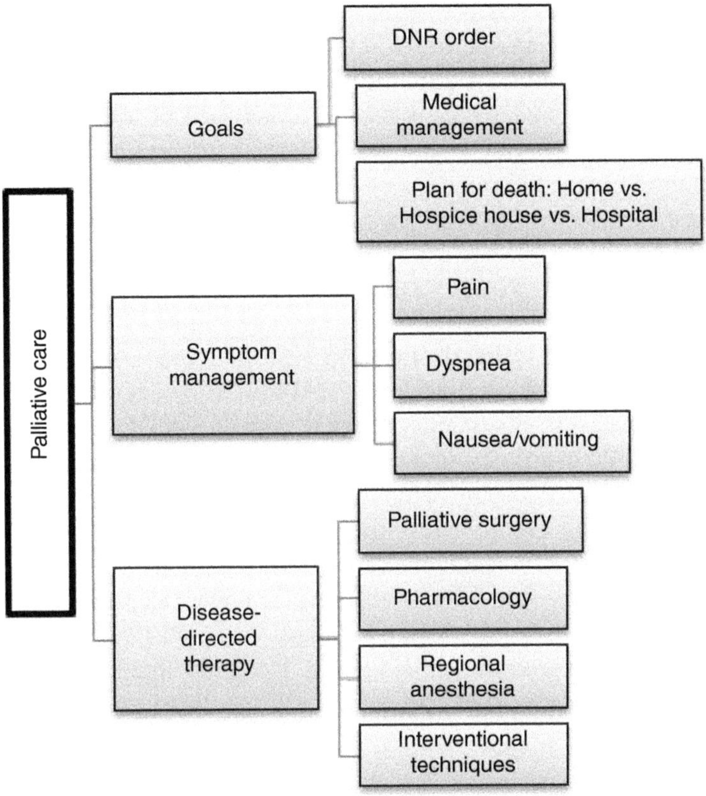

FIGURE 8.2 Components of palliative care.

setting is accomplished by initiating a clinical plan early in the disease process. During this period there are candid discussions about do-not-resuscitate (DNR) orders, medical management, and to ascertain where the patient would feel most comfortable during their remaining time. Symptom management and disease-directed therapy are addressed later in the chapter.

History of Hospice and Palliative Care

In 1879, the Sisters of Charity opened Our Lady's Hospice in Dublin (Desai, Kim, Fall, & Wang, 2007). Almost a century later, Dame Cicely Saunders founded St. Christopher's Hospice, in London in 1967, which provided the first research and teaching hospice (Stoddard, 1992). Hospice treats terminally ill patients with months left to live while palliative care provides services for the entire disease process, from diagnosis to death.

Palliative care emerged as a medical discipline in the latter half of the twentieth century as physicians began to understand that opioids could treat pain in cancer patients without the patients becoming addicted (Seymour, Clark, & Winslow, 2005). Pain management became a new area of study and this led to the development of modern hospice and palliative care services. The anesthesiologist, Dr. John Bonica, dedicated his career to understanding one's perception of pain and the methods available to adequately treat pain (Seymour et al., 2005). In 1947, Dr. Bonica established the first 24-hour pain service at Tacoma General Hospital (Seymour et al., 2005).

Palliative Care in the United States

The American Board of Medical Specialties (ABMS) recognizes palliative care as a medical subspecialty classified under internal medicine (ABMS, 2016). Currently, there are only 5,000 board-certified palliative care specialists in the United States (Quill & Abernethy, 2013). The demand for palliative care physicians outweighs the supply. This opens the door for other medical disciplines, such as intensive care unit (ICU) physicians, palliative care nurse practitioners (NPs), or anesthesia personnel to assume some care of this unique patient population. In an ideal setting, every hospital would house a palliative care unit (PCU); however, that is not the current reality in the United States. Hospitals should institute a triage system to engage palliative care specialists when necessary (Quill & Abernethy, 2013).

Intensive Care Unit

Not all palliative care patients are treated in PCUs as many patients receive care in the ICU. Similarly, during their stay some ICU patients may transition from a curative model to a palliative one (Truog et al., 2001).

One-third of patients with metastatic cancer die in the ICU and one-fifth of Americans die using ICU services (Angus et al., 2004). The goal of ICU care is to save lives; however, in many patients death becomes an inevitable outcome (Danis et al., 1999).

Multidisciplinary Team

Palliative care is a consultative discipline traditionally led by palliative care physicians (Billings & Pantilat, 2001). Palliative care requires multidisciplinary support including buy-in from medical institutions and hospital leadership (Danis et al., 1999). Health care providers involved in palliative care include, but are not limited to: anesthesia personnel, chaplains, psychiatrists, internal medicine physicians, palliative care NPs, palliative care nurses, social workers, psychosocial and psychiatric advanced practice nurses, and hospital administrators

(Lynch, 2003; Norton et al., 2007). Himelstein (2005) adds that pediatric palliative care teams also need specifically trained pediatric specialists including child psychologists or psychiatrists, child life therapists, art or music therapists, occupational therapists, physical therapists, and speech therapists.

Clinical staff should be appropriately trained to address end-of-life issues. Caring for patients whom you know will die can be mentally, spiritually, physically, and emotionally taxing on health care providers. Often health care providers are not adequately equipped and trained to address end-of-life care. This is especially apparent when caring for dying children as insufficient training can led to clinician burnout (Contro, Larson, Scofield, Sourkes, & Cohen, 2004). Providers may experience feelings of sadness, discouragement, and helplessness, and if not acknowledged, these feelings will affect patient care (ANA, 2010).

ECONOMICS OF PALLIATIVE CARE

There are 90 million Americans living with a serious or life-threatening illness (Strand et al., 2013) and 10 million cases of cancer are diagnosed worldwide each year (Brennan, Carr, & Cousins, 2007). Treating palliative care patients in a PCU leads to a decrease in ICU resource utilization, thereby saving hospitals, the government, and third-party payers money (Aslakson & Pronovost, 2011). Norton et al. (2007) report that proactive palliative care consultation, led by palliative care NPs, decreases medical ICU length of stays (8.06 vs. 16.28 days, $p = .0001$).

Housing terminal patients in a PCU yields a 66% decrease in hospital expenditures ($p < .0001$) and patient death costs are 59% lower when a patient dies in the PCU (Smith et al., 2003). Additionally, there is an average cost saving of $4,908 per admission for patients who die in the hospital under the care of a palliative care team (Strand et al., 2013).

PATIENT POPULATION

The old man smiled, 'I shall not die of a cold, my son. I shall die of having lived.'
—Willa Cather, *Death Comes for the Archbishop*

While anyone, regardless of age, gender, race, and ethnicity can become a candidate for palliative care, there are two distinct groups that require specific attention: geriatric and pediatric populations. Both of these vulnerable patient populations have unique palliative care characteristics.

Geriatric Population

Chronic pain affects 50% of the older population (Imani & Safari, 2011) and older adults may be less likely to receive appropriate pain management because untrained clinicians are worried about adverse side effects (Mercadante, Ferrera, Villari, & Casuccio, 2006). Not providing appropriate pain medications to the geriatric population could be construed as elder abuse and not addressing adequate pain relief could equate to negligence (Brennan et al., 2007).

In a study of 100 patients at the La Maddalena Cancer Center (Palermo, Italy) it was reported that opioid response and side effect profiles did not differ between patients less than 65 years of age versus patients over 65 years of age (Mercadante et al., 2006). Mercadante et al. (2006) concluded that elderly patients deserve the same individualization of opioid titration as their younger counterparts.

Pediatric Population

Pediatric palliative care is "about helping children and families to live to their fullest while facing complex medical conditions" (Himelstein, 2006, p. 163). In 2016 alone, 10,380 children under 15 years of age will be diagnosed with cancer and of those 1,250 are expected to die (American Cancer Society, 2016).

Death is often considered more acceptable in an adult versus a child, and this emotional strain can take its toll on families and health care providers alike. It is imperative that palliative care specialists working with pediatric patients be trained specifically in pediatrics. Children may not be able to voice their concerns and clinicians need to be trained to look at nonverbal signs of pain and distress (Himelstein, 2006). Also, health care providers should be aware that children grieve (Himelstein, Hilden, Boldt, & Weissman, 2004). Studies show that children as young as 3 years of age grasp the concept of death and by ages 8 to 9 they have a personal sense of mortality (Himelstein, 2006).

APPLICATION OF PALLIATIVE CARE

The good physician treats the disease; the great physician treats the patient who has the disease.

—Sir William Osler (1849–1919)

Disease Involvement

Palliative care covers a plethora of disease processes, which may or may not be malignant. Traditionally, palliative care services cover patients with a terminal disease such as metastatic cancer. However, palliative care may also include patients who have a chronic illness, but are not actively dying (Morrison & Meier, 2004). For adults this includes: end-stage congestive heart failure, chronic lung disease, pulmonary hypertension, progressive neurological disorders (e.g., Alzheimer's disease, Parkinson's disease, dementia, multiple sclerosis), drug-resistant tuberculosis (TB), end-stage renal disease, diabetes mellitus, HIV, and AIDS (Connor & Bermedo, 2014; Strand et al., 2013).

For children, palliative care conditions may include: cancer, congenital heart disease, HIV/AIDS, cystic fibrosis, severe gastrointestinal disorders, epidermolysis bullosa, renal failure (in patients who are not a candidate for transplant), muscular dystrophy, chromosomal abnormalities, cirrhosis of the liver, meningitis, neonatal conditions, and hypoxic/anoxic brain injuries (Connor & Bermedo, 2014; Himelstein, 2006).

Symptom Management

Patient symptom suffering exists in many forms including pain, dyspnea, delirium, nausea, vomiting, hopelessness, remorse, anxiety, and loneliness (Lynch, 2003). Symptom palliation for patient suffering is gaining traction in cancer treatment (Mercadante et al., 2006) and a large component of palliative care treatment is symptom management.

Pain

Pain is one of the most undertreated symptoms in palliative care and this undertreatment leads to both physical and psychological adverse effects (Brennan et al., 2007; Joshi & Chambers, 2010). Many patients will die with treatable pain because the perception of pain is subjective (Truog et al., 2001). Ten to fifty percent of palliative care patients report significant pain 1 week before death (Quill, Lo, & Brock, 1997) and some even experience "crescendo" pain as they near death (Fine, 2003).

Pain is described as both a sensory and emotional experience (Fine, 2005). Assessing pain in the dying may be difficult as some patients lose their ability to verbally communicate. When evaluating pain, CRNAs need to include physiological parameters such as hemodynamics, level of consciousness, breathing, and so forth in their assessment. The WHO analgesic ladder for adult cancer pain states that health care providers should start with nonopioids, then progress to mild opioids, and finally strong opioids until the patient is pain-free (WHO, 2016). The WHO recommends only a two-step ladder for children with cancer. The first step involves using paracetamol and ibuprofen for mild pain, and then if pain persists, introducing an opioid, preferably morphine, as the second step (WHO, 2012).

TREATMENT OPTIONS

There is only one ultimate and effectual preventative for the maladies to which flesh is heir, and that is death.

—Harvey Cushing, American neurosurgeon (1869–1939)

Treating palliative care patients requires a delicate balance of weighing all risks versus their benefit. While the overarching goal is to treat symptoms and alleviate suffering, clinicians must ensure that the treatments provided are appropriate for the patient's clinical condition and will not expedite death. Often concurrent treatments are required and patients' needs should be addressed daily as their ability to tolérate certain procedures, or their wishes regarding treatments, may change overnight.

Pharmacologic Options

Multimodal, co-analgesia pain management is the most effective way to manage pain in terminally ill patients. Anti-inflammatories, antidepressants, anticonvulsants, and corticosteroids in addition to opioids all are beneficial in treating pain in this patient population (Ferrell et al., 2008).

Some of the most commonly used sedative medications in palliative care include: haloperidol, midazolam, phenobarbital, ketamine, and chlorpromazine. Currently, propofol is being used when all other modalities have failed (McWilliams, Keeley, & Waterhouse, 2010).

Complementary and Alternative Medicine

As patients approach death they may experience pain, nausea, and dyspnea, and complementary and alternative medicine (CAM) is a useful adjunct in this patient population (Pan et al., 2000). CAM therapies are available in 39% of U.S. hospitals that have palliative care programs (Johnston et al., 2008). Modalities with successful use in palliative care include acupuncture, acupressure, transcutaneous electrical nerve stimulation, hypnosis, imagery, psychotherapy, music therapy, and aromatherapy massage (Pan et al., 2000).

Chemotherapy and Radiation

Palliative chemotherapy and palliative radiation provide symptom management and help patients with advance cancer maintain some semblance of normalcy in their lives (Desai et al., 2007). Bone pain is the most common source of pain in patients with metastatic prostate cancer and external beam radiation therapy is 90% effective at decreasing bone pain in this patient population (Ok et al., 2005).

Invasive Procedures

Palliative Surgery

CRNAs will encounter palliative care patients in the operating room (OR) as more and more high-risk, terminal patients are seeking surgical treatment for their symptoms. Palliative surgery is noncurative surgery intended to improve a patient's quality of life. The primary indications for palliative surgery are pain and uncontrolled bleeding (Desai et al., 2007). Surgical palliation should be considered a treatment option available to patients along with other palliative treatments such as pharmacology, chemotherapy, and radiation. Surgical procedures include: resection of gastric tumors (i.e., tumor debulking), cordotomy, dorsal rhizotomy, myelotomy, and deep brain stimulation (Desai et al., 2007).

Palliative surgery can improve quality of life through symptom control. In a year-long review of palliative surgery at City of Hope National Cancer Center 12.5% of all procedures performed that year were palliative in nature (Krouse et al., 2001). Krouse et al. (2001) report that the primary cancers for which palliative surgical procedures were employed include: lung, colorectal, breast, and prostate and that overall surgical morbidity is 21.3% (p = .004).

Palliative procedures may also be performed in the interventional radiology (IR) suite or at the bedside in a PCU or ICU. CRNAs may also provide sedation for symptom control interventions such as a paracentesis or thoracentesis (Mercadante, Villari, & Ferrera, 2003).

PALLIATIVE SEDATION

A controversial and yet germane area of palliative care is palliative sedation. CRNAs may be consulted to provide palliative sedation or to advise palliative care teams about the medications used in palliative sedation. The National Ethics Committee (NEC, 2007) defines palliative sedation as, "the administration of nonopioid drugs to sedate a terminally ill patient to unconsciousness as an intervention of last resort to treat severe, refractory pain or other clinical symptoms that have not been relieved by aggressive, symptom-specific palliation" (p. 484). With palliative sedation, patients are sedated to unconsciousness; death usually occurs in days (Quill et al., 1997).

There is much debate in the literature regarding the nomenclature surrounding "palliative" sedation and the term is often interchangeably used with "terminal" sedation. Other references include total sedation, controlled sedation, and deep sedation (Figure 8.3). However, regardless of the name used, the desired effect with this form of sedation is to relieve patient suffering (Bruce, Hendrix, & Gentry, 2006). For the remainder of this chapter, palliative sedation will be used to provide consistence and to remind the reader that while the end result is death (a terminal state), the intent and goal of palliative sedation is to provide *palliative* care.

Indications

Terminally ill patients may experience intolerable suffering at the end of life and palliative sedation is used to palliate symptoms. Sedation can treat physical,

Palliative sedation

- Terminal sedation
- Total sedation
- Controlled sedation
- Deep sedation

FIGURE 8.3 Nomenclature for palliative sedation.

spiritual, and psychological symptoms (McWilliams et al., 2010). Palliative sedation provides a conduit to alleviate refractory symptoms (Cowan & Walsh, 2001). It does not shorten survival as the median time to death after starting palliative sedation is one to two days (Cowan & Walsh, 2001; Lynch, 2003; Mercadante et al., 2003).

Palliative sedation is implemented when a symptom is truly refractory. Indications include agitation, restlessness, pain, confusion, respiratory distress, dyspnea, general malaise, nausea, and myoclonus (Lundström, Zachrisson, & Fürst, 2005; Mercadante et al., 2011; Schuman-Oliver, Brendel, Forstein, & Price, 2008). Dyspnea and delirium are the two most common reasons why palliative sedation is administered (Caraceni et al., 2012).

Medications

Midazolam is the preferred medication for palliative sedation (DeGraeff & Dean, 2007; Mercadante & Giarratano, 2012). Other medications frequently used include benzodiazepines (lorazepam), phenothiazine (chlorpromazine or methotrimeprazine), haloperidol, barbiturates (phenobarbital), and propofol (Davis, 2009).

A Dutch 4-year retrospective analysis of 157 palliative care patients revealed that 43% of patients received palliative sedation using midazolam and propofol (Rietjens et al., 2008).

Propofol also serves as an adjunct to decrease opioid consumption (Anghelescu, Hamilton, Faughnan, Johnson, & Baker, 2012). Propofol has also been successfully used for end-of-life sedation in children.

Another option to consider before instituting palliative sedation is to attempt "respite sedation" or palliative sedation for a predetermined time frame (usually 24–48 hours). Respite sedation provides patients with a reprieve from their symptoms and helps them to regain psychological strength to make sound end-of-life decisions (Schuman-Oliver et al., 2008).

ANESTHESIA INVOLVEMENT IN PALLIATIVE CARE

To die, to sleep-
To sleep, perchance to dream – ay, there's the rub,
For in this sleep of death what dreams may come . . .
—William Shakespeare, *Hamlet*

There are limited studies in the literature assessing anesthesia's involvement in palliative care. This is a unique area where CRNAs have the opportunity to make a difference, especially with regard to pain management. CRNAs are ideal candidates to serve on a multidisciplinary team because they have a solid understanding of pharmacology, drug titration, and experience dealing with critically ill patients in stressful situations (Fine, 2005). As palliative care centers grow, there will be more opportunity for collaborative, interdisciplinary work between anesthesia and palliative care teams. CRNAs should be prepared to provide consultation regarding pain management including pharmacologic and regional anesthesia recommendations.

Breakthrough Pain

A "pain crisis" or "breakthrough pain" requires immediate intervention. The Memorial Sloan Kettering Cancer Center Pain and Palliative Care service estimate they are called for a pain crisis 20–30 times/month (Moryl, Coyle, & Foley, 2008). Breakthrough pain is a very real issue in cancer patients and needs to be immediately addressed. Out of 66 palliative care patients, 624 episodes of breakthrough pain were reported, with intravenous (IV) morphine and transmucosal fentanyl decreasing pain in both groups within 15 minutes ($p < .001$) (Mercadante, Villari, Ferrera, Mangione, & Casuccio, 2010).

Anesthesia Drugs

Opioids

Opioids are used in palliative care to treat pain and control dyspnea (Mercadante & Giarratano, 2012) with morphine being the opioid of choice (Truog et al., 2001). Palliative care patients often need a combination of two to three opioids to obtain effective analgesia with tolerable side effects (Moryl et al., 2008). Providers should be sensitive to choosing a route of opioid administration (oral, rectal, transdermal, buccal, transmucosal, subcutaneous, IV, epidural, or intrathecal) that is appropriate for each patient's clinical situation as not every patient will have IV access (Moryl et al., 2008).

Ketamine

Ketamine is considered a front-line treatment for neuropathic pain including cancer pain, central pain, and postherpetic neuralgia phantom pain (Ben-Ari,

Lewis, & Davidson, 2007; Fitzgibbon & Viola, 2005). Low-dose ketamine is an effective co-analgesic medication (Fine, 2003; Moryl et al., 2008) and intrathecal ketamine has successfully been used in palliative care (Ben-Ari et al., 2007).

A benefit of ketamine is that it does not affect respiration and can be administered via many routes including: IV, subcutaneous, intranasal, intrathecal, epidural, rectal, and transdermal (Prommer, 2012). However, one should consider giving an opiate or a benzodiazepine to minimize ketamine's adverse effects (Soto et al., 2012).

Propofol

Moyle (1995) provided the first case report of propofol use in palliative care patients. Since then propofol has sporadically been used in palliative care. Low-dose propofol is helpful for decreasing anxiety and opioid requirements (Mercadante, DeConno, & Ripamonti, 1995).

Propofol also has valuable antiemetic properties. In a Swedish study of 35 palliative care patients, 13 patients received propofol for refractory nausea and 22 patients received propofol for unendurable suffering (Lundström et al., 2005). Propofol was shown to be a successful sedative and antiemetic in this patient population.

Propofol requires aseptic technique during administration, including a designated line, and the remaining, unused drug must be discarded within a specified time frame. CRNAs need to educate nurses about the unique considerations of this medication. Additionally, propofol does not have intrinsic analgesic properties; therefore providers should continue concurrent opioid use.

Dexmedetomidine

Dexmedetomidine has yet to gain traction in palliative care. Dexmedetomidine has key features that would make it an appropriate choice in the PCU: (a) it is compatible with other medications, (b) it has different routes of administration, and (c) it has an opioid-sparing effect. However, in spite of its potential for palliative sedation, it still has yet to become part of routine practice (Prommer, 2011).

Currently, only two studies have examined dexmedetomidine in the palliative care setting. Roberts, Wozencraft, Coyne, and Smith (2011) used dexmedetomidine (0.2 mcg/kg/hr) to control intractable cancer pain in a patient who had failed treatment with high-dose systemic opioids, ketamine, lidocaine, and intrathecal drug delivery. After initiation of dexmedetomidine the patient's pain became more tolerable, and the need for hydromorphone decreased. The Centro de Suporte Terapêutico Oncológico (Rio de Janeiro, Brazil) reported that dexmedetomidine was a useful adjunct for pain, anxiety, and restlessness in patients with metastatic cancer; however, they did not appreciate any opioid-sparing effects (Soares, Naylor, Martins, & Peixoto, 2002).

The Virginia Commonwealth University Massey Cancer Center has a protocol for dexmedetomidine use in the PCUs as bridge therapy (an adjunct for refractory pain); however, the potential for hypotension, bradycardia, and high cost have confined it to a secondary adjunct medication, as opposed to a primary drug (Coyne, Wozencraft, Roberts, Bobb, & Smith, 2010).

Substance Abuse

CRNAs should be acutely aware of a patient's medical history, especially a past medical history of substance abuse when involved in palliative care. Patients receiving methadone for substance abuse may not get an analgesic effect from their daily methadone dose and will need an increase in their medication dosing (Selwyn, 2005). Anesthetists and palliative care physicians should contact an addictionologist if they have specific questions about medications to give a patient with a history of substance abuse.

Pediatrics

CRNAs need to be meticulous and make sure their pain assessment and subsequent administration of medications to pediatric patients is age-appropriate. Often the oral or sublingual route is preferred in children to avoid IV access, which may not be available (Himelstein, 2006).

Pain Management Techniques

Neuraxial

When opioid therapy fails, palliative care physicians will consult anesthesia for pain management recommendations. Neuraxial techniques and nerve blocks are shown in the literature to be effective adjuncts to pharmacologic pain management in both adult and pediatric palliative care patients. For neuraxial techniques, intrathecal infusions are recommended with straight local anesthetics (LA) or a combination of LA and opioids. A benefit of intrathecal catheters is that patients can go home with them, providing pain therapy in a more comfortable, familiar setting.

A St. Jude's Children Hospital study reported that 12 out of 13 palliative pediatric patients had improved pain control with continuous blocks (epidural and/or peripheral nerve blocks; Anghelescu, Faughnan, Baker, Yang, & Kane, 2010). Of note, there should be a candid discussion with patients and their family members regarding the potential side effects of regional anesthesia. Side effects such as motor blockade or the potential loss of bladder function may cause more distress (especially in pediatric patients) than the pain relief provided (Collins, Grier, Kinney, & Berde, 1995). Another consideration is to discuss where the patient wants to die as some families may not want to deal with the apparatus associated with a regional technique (such as an indwelling catheter) at home (Rork, Berde, & Goldstein, 2013).

An intrathecal drug not commonly used by CRNAs, but that is becoming part of palliative care is ziconotide, a synthetic peptide that acts as a selective N-type voltage-gated calcium channel blocker. Ziconotide is indicated for patients with neuropathic or refractory pain not adequately treated by opioids. Staats et al. (2004) report that ziconotide provided moderate to complete pain relief in 53% of patients with cancer or AIDS ($p < .001$).

Celiac Plexus Blocks

Five–ten percent of advanced cancer patients will not achieve adequate pain relief from opioids and will require further interventions (Joshi & Chambers, 2010). Neurolytic celiac plexus blocks (CPB) have been shown to provide 90% pain relief for up to 3 months (Joshi & Chambers, 2010). In a study of 22 pancreatic cancer patients, CPB significantly decreased pain ($p < .0005$), opioid requirements ($p < .0005$), and nausea ($p < .005$; Mercadante, Catala, Arcuri, & Casuccio, 2003). Side effects of a CPB include postural hypotension and diarrhea, which can occur secondary to the sympathetic blockade of the abdominal viscera.

Anesthesia pain specialists may also consider a celiac plexus neurolysis as a permanent option to treat abdominal or pancreatic cancer pain. Neurolysis is a nerve destructive procedure that uses alcohol or phenol to provide pain relief for several months. Side effects of this block include: orthostatic hypotension and diarrhea (both resulting from the sympathectomy), alcohol intoxication, seizures, pneumothorax, incontinence, nerve damage, and paralysis (Erdek, King, & Ellsworth, 2013).

Other Regional Blocks

Superior hypogastric plexus blocks are becoming more popular to treat refractory pain from pelvic malignancies. This block does not obliterate cancer pain, but will help decrease opioid consumption (Mercadante, Fulfarro, & Casuccio, 2002).

Other palliative care blocks provided by anesthesia pain specialists include: superior hypogastric plexus, ganglion impar, stellate ganglion blocks, brachial plexus, suprascapular, paravertebral, lumbar plexus, psoas compartment, obturator, and femoral/sciatic nerve blocks (Joshi & Chambers, 2010).

Surgical Cases in the Operating Room

Palliative Surgery

Terminally ill patients may present to the OR for palliative surgery. It is important for CRNAs to have a thorough and extensive discussion with the patient, the patient's surrogate, and the surgical team regarding anesthetic and surgical goals. This discussion should provide clarification as to whether surgical intervention or medical symptom management is the best option to treat the offending symptoms (Mercadante & Giarratano, 2012).

DNR orders are a controversial topic among anesthesia providers. CRNAs may also face an Allow Natural Death statement. CRNAs should always discuss DNR orders with the patient or their proxy prior to surgery so that they can have a better understanding of the patient's level of comprehension surrounding the topic of resuscitation.

Some hospitals have a policy to routinely suspend DNR orders prior to surgery; however, this becomes a sensitive issue when dealing with hospice or palliative care patients presenting for surgery. Not all hospice patients have DNR orders, and likewise, just because a DNR order exists, it is not clear if the order should be blindly followed when presenting to the OR. Scott and Garvin (2012) recommend that health care providers treat each DNR order individually versus following a universal hospital protocol.

The American Association of Nurse Anesthetists in their Reconsideration of Advance Directives: Practice Guidelines (2015) policy recommend that a discussion about "reconsidering advance directives" occur during the informed consent process.

CRNAs can also impact palliative care through advocacy work (Callahan, Breakwell, & Suhayda, 2011). CRNAs may encounter terminally ill patients presenting for surgery who may not be aware of available palliative care options. This provides the opportunity for CRNAs to refer appropriate patients to palliative care teams.

Organ Harvesting

CRNAs may be called upon to harvest organs immediately after life support is withdrawn on a terminal patient. The University of Pittsburgh Medical Center developed the "Pittsburgh Protocol," which details the procedure for procuring an organ after a "controlled" death in the OR, ICU, or PCU (VanNorman, 2003). According to the protocol, teams must wait 2 minutes after the "irreversible" circulatory arrest to harvest the organs. VanNorman (2003) recommends that anesthesia providers who are involved with non-heart-beating cadaver organ donation have specific palliative care training. CRNAs may not always have the opportunity to be part of these end-of-life discussions or treatment plans and therefore must be emotionally and mentally prepared to harvest organs in the OR if necessary.

Surgical Cases Outside the Operating Room

Tracheostomy

In addition to supporting palliative patients in the OR, CRNAs need to be prepared to care for them outside the OR as well—whether in the ICU or PCU. CRNAs may be called upon to administer anesthesia for patients undergoing tracheostomies outside of the OR. Increasing numbers of amyotrophic lateral sclerosis (ALS) patients in PCUs are having beside tracheostomies (Chan & Devaiah, 2009).

Interventional Radiology

CRNAs may also encounter palliative patients in IR. Studies have shown that nerve blocks and radiofrequency ablations performed in IR can alleviate pain in patients with terminal cancer (Mercadante & Giarratano, 2012). These techniques, along with procedures such as permanent line placements, dural punctures, bone marrow biopsies, and transjugular intrahepatic portosystemic shunt (TIPS), may be performed in IR.

Electroconvulsive Therapy

Palliative care patients may present for electroconvulsive therapy (ECT) to treat severe depression, late-stage dementia, or psychosis (Rasmussen & Richardson, 2011). Rasmussen and Richardson (2011) argue that in some cases, ECT can be considered compassionate, depending on the clinical presentation.

Terminal Extubation and Weaning

A final area where CRNAs may interact with palliative care patients is in the ICU with terminal extubation. Terminal extubation involves removing an endotracheal tube (ETT) after a bolus of sedatives or analgesics to allow the patient to be free from an "unnatural" tube (Truog et al., 2001). A terminal wean involves gradually decreasing ventilator settings over several days, which can lead to hypoxemia and hypercarbia (Truog et al., 2001). Both practices are legal; however, neither should occur without an extensive interdisciplinary discussion with the family or patient surrogate.

ETHICS

Nothing hinders one act from having two effects, only one of which is intended, while the other is beside the intention.

—Thomas Aquinas (*Summa Theologica*)

Modern medicine affords us the ability to prolong life; however, is that always the right thing to do? This is a question that palliative care patients, families, and their health care teams must ask themselves. Every patient is unique and they have differing medical presentations, belief systems, customs, cultural traditions, and ethical principles, which influence their opinion regarding end-of-life options.

The tenets of medical philosophy are curative, which is a contrast to the palliative care philosophy, which does not seek to prolong life, but rather to improve whatever quality of life remains (Morrison & Meier, 2004). Patient-directed, life-ending options exist in palliative care. It is legal for a patient to voluntarily stop eating or drinking (Rady & Verheijde, 2010). It is also legal for a patient to request continuous sedation or to ask for life-sustaining therapies to be withdrawn or withheld (Rady & Verheijde, 2010). There is no moral or legal difference between withholding and withdrawing care; both are equally acceptable (Rady & Verheijde, 2010; Wellesley & Jenkins, 2009).

Euthanasia and Physician Assisted Suicide

Euthanasia, or intentionally killing an individual who is ill or injured to prevent further suffering, is illegal in the United States. Voluntary euthanasia, whereby the patient has requested death, is only legal worldwide in the Netherlands and Belgium. Physician-assisted suicide (PAS), whereby a physician assists a patient in committing suicide whether through knowledge about lethal dosages of drugs or actually providing those lethal doses, is recognized internationally in Switzerland. Two U.S. Supreme Court rulings, *Vacco v. Quill* (1997) and *Washington v. Glucksberg* (1997), returned the issue of PAS back to individual state legislature. While the Supreme Court does not support PAS, it does support sedation to avoid severe physical suffering in the dying. Currently, the Death with Dignity Act supports PAS and PAS is legal in Oregon, Washington, Montana, and Vermont.

Palliative sedation is ethically different from euthanasia or PAS (NEC, 2007). The American Medical Association in their 2008 *Sedation to Unconsciousness in End-of-Life Care* position acknowledge that palliative sedation is a rare intervention or last resort used to treat refractory pain and clinical symptoms.

Double Effect Doctrine

Palliative sedation is a morally and ethically weighted domain. In a European study of 17 countries, ICU physicians believe that the doses they ordered for terminal patients resulted in the death of 77% of those patients (Sprung et al., 2008). There is a fine line between relieving pain to alleviate patient suffering and hastening death. Pain and suffering are not synonymous, nor are they inherently distinct (Truog et al., 2001).

There are specific considerations to keep in mind with palliative sedation. Instituting palliative sedation may hasten one's death; however, by not providing this option patients may experience insufferable pain at the end of their life. The Doctrine of Double Effect (DDE) is used to morally and ethically justify palliative sedation. The DDE helps to assess the intended versus unintended consequence

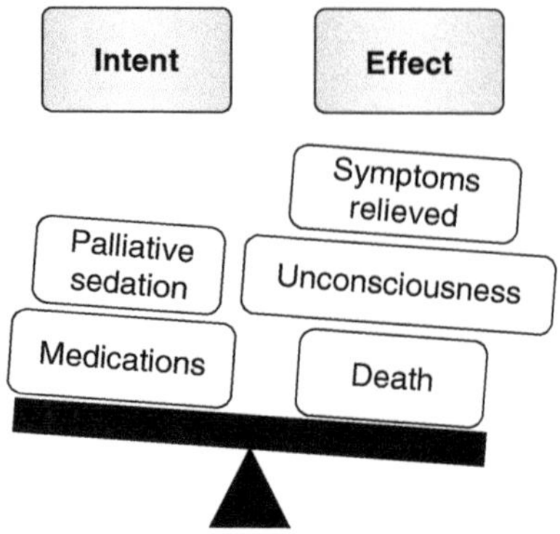

FIGURE 8.4 The Doctrine of Double Effect in palliative care.

of an action (Schuman-Oliver et al., 2008). The doctrine is rooted in Roman Catholic theology and stems from facing two choices, when neither choice is desirable (Bruce et al., 2006). The doctrine postulates that an act is conducted to achieve a good effect, and while bad effect consequences are foreseen, they are not intended. In the case of palliative sedation, the good effect is alleviating patient suffering; the bad effect, patient death (Figure 8.4).

While palliative sedation is considered an intervention of last resort, CRNAs should be prepared to administer medications for palliative sedation or to advise palliative care staff about palliative sedation pharmacologic options. As PCUs increase in numbers, CRNAs may have the opportunity for multidisciplinary work. This opens the door for research studies, clinical trials, and the chance for CRNAs to share their unique knowledge of multimodal medication use with the palliative care teams.

FUTURE RESEARCH

No one can confidently say that he will still be living tomorrow.

—Euripides (480–406 BCE)

Hospice and palliative medicine is now recognized as a medical subspecialty for anesthesiologists (ABMS, 2016). Ideally this certification will extend to CRNAs in the future. Callahan et al. (2011) recommend that palliative care content be included in nurse anesthesia education and likewise that CRNAs look at ways to integrate palliative care into their scope of practice. These recommendations are based on student registered nurse anesthetist (SRNA) participation in a National Institutes of Health R-25 grant supported course on interdisciplinary palliative care. Dickinson (2007) reports that 99% of medical and nursing schools offer some form of education on death and dying and 90% of students have participated in these learning opportunities. The burden now falls on nurse anesthesia faculty to consider incorporating palliative care education into nurse anesthesia curriculum.

CONCLUSION

Because I could not stop for Death –
He kindly stopped for me –
The carriage held but just Ourselves –
And Immortality.
—Emily Dickinson (1830–1886)

Unfortunately there is no panacea for palliative care patients. This is a distinct patient population comprising many different backgrounds, ages, comorbidities, and disease processes. CRNAs need to be aware of treatment options available to terminally ill patients. These patients should be continuously evaluated and reassessed as treatment plans, DNR decisions, and other aspects of their care may change day to day. Knowledge of palliative care will empower nurse anesthetists to provide tailored, compassionate care to these patients. Finally, as a profession, CRNAs are charged with the opportunity to use their unique skill set of understanding the symbiotic relationship between critical illness, pharmacology, and pain management and apply this knowledge to palliative care patients and teams.

REFERENCES

American Association of Nurse Anesthestists. (2015). *Reconsideration of advanced directives*. Retrieved from http://www.aana.com/resources2/professionalpractice/Pages/Reconsideration-of-Advance-Directives.aspx

American Board of Medical Specialties. (2016). *Specialty and subspecialty certifications*. Retrieved from http://www.abms.org/member-boards/contact-an-abms-member-board/american-board-of-psychiatry

American Cancer Society. (2016, January). *What are the key statistics for childhood cancer?* Retrieved from http://www.cancer.org/cancer/cancerinchildren/detailedguide/cancer-in-children-key-statistics

American Medical Association. (2016, June). *Opinion 5.6 - Sedation to unconsciousness in end-of-life care*. Retrieved from https://download.ama-assn.org/resources/doc/code-medical-ethics/code-2016-ch5.pdf

American Nurses Association Board of Directors. (2016). *Nurses' roles and responsibilities in providing care and support at the end of life*. Retrieved from http://www.nursingworld.org/MainMenuCategories/EthicsStandards/Ethics-Position-Statements/EndofLife-PositionStatement.pdf

Anghelescu, D. L., Faughnan, L. G., Baker, J. N., Yang, J., & Kane, J. R. (2010). Use of epidural and peripheral nerve blocks at end of life in children and young adults with cancer: The collaboration between a pain service and a palliative care service. *Paediatric Anaesthesia*, *20*(12), 1070–1077. http://dx.doi.org/10.1111/j.1460-9592.2010.03449.x

Anghelescu, D., Hamilton, H., Faughnan, L., Johnson, L. M., & Baker, J. (2012). Pediatric palliative sedation therapy with propofol: Recommendations based on experience in children with terminal cancer. *Journal of Palliative Medicine, 15*(10), 1082–1090. http://dx.doi.org/10.1089/jpm.2011.0500

Angus, D., Barnato, A., Linde-Zwirble, W., Weissfeld, L., Watson, R. S., Rickert, T., et al. (2004). Use of intensive care at the end of life in the United States: An epidemiologic study. *Critical Care Medicine, 32*(3), 638–643. http://dx.doi.org/10.1097/01.ccm.0000114816.62331.08

Aslakson, R., & Pronovost, P. (2011). Health care quality in end-of-life care: Promoting palliative care in the intensive care unit. *Anesthesiology Clinics, 29*(2011), 111–122. http://dx.doi.org/10.1016/j.anclin.2010.11.001

Ben-Ari, A., Lewis, M., & Davidson, E. (2007). Chronic administration of ketamine for analgesia. *Journal of Pain & Palliative Care Pharmacotherapy, 21*(1), 7–14. http://dx.doi.org/10.1300/j354v21n01_04

Billings, J. A., & Pantilat, S. (2001). Survey of palliative care programs in united states teaching hospitals. *Journal of Palliative Medicine, 4*(3), 309–314.

Brennan, F., Carr, D., & Cousins, M. (2007). Pain management: A fundamental human right. *Pain Medicine, 105*(1), 205–221. http://dx.doi.org/10.1213/01.ane.0000268145.52345.55

Bruce, S. D., Hendrix, C. C., & Gentry, J. H. (2006). Palliative sedation in end-of-life care. *Journal of Hospice and Palliative Nursing, 8*(6), 320–327.

Callahan, M. F., Breakwell, S., & Suhayda, R. (2011). Knowledge of palliative and end of-life care by student registered nurse anesthetists. *American Association of Nurse Anesthetists Journal, 79*(4), S15–S20.

Caraceni, A., Zecca, E., Martini, C., Gorni, G., Campa, T., Brunelli, C., et al. (2012). Palliative sedation at the end of life at a tertiary cancer center. *Support Care Cancer, 20*, 1299–1307. http://dx.doi.org/10.1007/s00520-011-1217-6

Chan, T., & Devaiah, A. K. (2009). Tracheostomy in palliative care. *Otolaryngologic Clinics of North America, 42*, 133–141. http://dx.doi.org/10.1016/j.otc.2008.09.002

Collins, J. J., Grier, H., Kinney, H. C., & Berde, C. B. (1995). Control of severe pain in children with terminal malignancy. *The Journal of Pediatrics, 126*(4), 653–657. http://dx.doi.org/10.1016/s0022-3476(95)70370-5

Connor, S., & Bermedo, M. C. S. (Ed.). (2014). *Global atlas of palliative care at the end of life.* Worldwide Palliative Care Alliance, London: World Health Organization. Retrieved from http://www.who.int/nmh/Global_Atlas_of_Palliative_Care.pdf

Contro, N., Larson, J., Scofield, S., Sourkes, B., & Cohen, H. (2004). Hospital staff and family perspectives regarding quality of pediatric palliative care. *Pediatrics, 114*(5), 1248–1252. doi: 10.1542/peds.2003-0857-L

Cowan, J. D., & Walsh, D. (2001). Terminal sedation in palliative medicine- definition and review of the literature. *Support Care Cancer, 9*, 403–407. http://dx.doi.org/10.1007/s005200100235

Coyne, P. J., Wozencraft, C. P., Roberts, S. B., Bobb, B., & Smith, T. J. (2010). Dexmedetomidine: Exploring its potential role and dosing guideline for its use in intractable pain in the palliative care setting. *Journal of Pain & Palliative Care Pharmacotherapy, 24*(4), 384–386. http://dx.doi.org/10.3109/15360288.2010.518227

Danis, M., Federman, D., Fins, J., Fox, E., Kastenbaum, B., Lanken, P., et al. (1999). Incorporating palliative care into critical care education: Principles, challenges, and opportunities. *Critical Care Medicine, 27*(9), 2005–2013.

Davis, M. P. (2009). Does palliative sedation always relieve symptoms? *Journal of Palliative Medicine, 12*(10), 875–877. http://dx.doi.org/10.1089/jpm.2009.0148

DeGraeff, A., & Dean, M. (2007). Palliative sedation therapy in the last weeks of life: A literature review and recommendations for standards. *Journal of Palliative Medicine, 10*(1), 67–85. http://dx.doi.org/10.1089/jpm.2006.0139

Desai, M., Kim, A., Fall, P., & Wang, D. (2007). Optimizing quality of life through palliative care. *The Journal of the American Osteopathic Association, 107*(12), ES9–ES14.

Dickinson, G. E. (2007). End-of-life and palliative care issues in medical and nursing schools in the United States. *Death Studies, 31*, 713–726. http://dx.doi.org/10.1080/07481180701490602

Erdek, M. A., King, L. M., & Ellsworth, S. G. (2013). Pain management and palliative care in pancreatic cancer. *Current Problems in Cancer, 37*, 266–272.

Ferrell, B., Levy, M., & Paice, J. (2008). Managing pain from advanced cancer in the palliative care setting. *Clinical Journal of Oncology Nursing, 12*(4), 575–581. http://dx.doi.org/10.1188/08.cjon.575-581

Fine, P. G. (2003). Ketamine: From anesthesia to palliative care. *Quarterly newsletter of the American academy of hospice and palliative medicine, 3*(3), 1–6.

Fine, P. G. (2005). The evolving and important role of anesthesiology in palliative care. *Anesthesia & Analgesia, 100*, 183–188. http://dx.doi.org/10.1213/01.ane.0000141061.74294.de

Fitzgibbon, E. J., & Viola, R. (2005). Parenteral ketamine as an analgesic adjuvant for severe pain: Development and retrospective audit of a protocol for a palliative care unit. *Journal of Palliative Medicine, 8*(1), 49–57.

Himelstein, B. (2005). Palliative care in pediatrics. *Anesthesiology Clinics of North America, 23*(2005), 837–856. http://dx.doi.org/10.1016/j.atc.2005.07.005

Himelstein, B. (2006). Palliative care of infants, children, adolescents, and their families. *Journal of Palliative Medicine, 9*(1), 163–181.

Himelstein, B., Hilden, J., Boldt, A., & Weissman, D. (2004). Pediatric palliative care. *New England Journal of Medicine, 350*, 1752–1762.

Imani, F., & Safari, S. (2011). "Pain relief is an essential human right," we should be concerned about it. *Anesthesiology and Pain Medicine, 1*(2), 55–57. http://dx.doi.org/10.5812/kowsar.22287523.2306

Johnston, D., Nagel, K., Friedman, D., Meza, J., Hurwitz, C., & Friebert, S. (2008). Availability and use of palliative care and end-of-life services for pediatric oncology patients. *Journal of Clinical Oncology, 26*(28), 4646–4650. http://dx.doi.org/10.1200/jco.2008.16.1562

Joshi, M., & Chambers, W. A. (2010). Pain relief in palliative care: A focus on interventional pain management. *Expert Review of Neurotherapeutics, 10*(5), 747–756.

Krouse, R., Nelson, R., Farrell, B., Grube, B., Juarez, G., Wagman, L., & Chu, D. (2001). Surgical palliation at a cancer center. *Archives of Surgery, 136*(7), 773–778. http://dx.doi.org/10.1001/archsurg.136.7.773

Kuziemsky, C., Jahnke, J., & Lau, F. (2006). The e-hospice—beyond traditional boundaries of palliative care. *Telematics and Informatics, 23*(2006), 117–133. http://dx.doi.org/10.1016/j.tele.2005.05.003

Lundström, S., Zachrisson, U., & Fürst, C. J. (2005). When nothing helps: Propofol as sedative and antiemetic in palliative cancer care. *Journal of Pain and Symptom Management, 30*(6), 570–577. http://dx.doi.org/10.1016/j.jpainsymman.2005.05.017

Lynch, M. (2003). Palliative sedation. *Clinical Journal of Oncology Nursing, 7*(6), 653–667.

McWilliams, K., Keeley, P., & Waterhouse, E. (2010). Propofol for terminal sedation in palliative care: A systematic review. *Journal of Palliative Medicine, 13*(1), 73–76.

Mercadante, S., Catala, E., Arcuri, E., & Casuccio, A. (2003). Celiac plexus block for pancreatic cancer pain: Factors influencing pain, symptoms and quality of life. *Journal of Pain and Symptom Management, 26*(6), 1140–1147.

Mercadante, S., DeConno, F., & Ripamonti, C. (1995). Propofol in terminal care. *Journal of Pain and Symptom Management, 10*(8), 639–642.

Mercadante, S., Ferrera, P., Villari, P., & Casuccio, A. (2006). Opioid escalation in patients with cancer pain: The effect of age. *Journal of Pain and Symptom Management, 32*(5), 413–419. http://dx.doi.org/10.1016/j.jpainsymman.2006.05.015

Mercadante, S., Fulfaro, F., & Casuccio, A. (2002). Pain mechanisms involved and outcome in advanced cancer patients with possible indications for celiac plexus block and superior hypogastric plexus block. *Tumori*, *88*, 243–245.

Mercadante, S., & Giarratano, A. (2012). The anesthesiologist and end-of-life care. *Current Opinion in Anesthesiology*, *25*, 371–375. http://dx.doi.org/10.1097/aco.0b013e3283530e7d

Mercadante, S., Porzio, G., Valle, A., Fusco, F., Aielli, F., & Costanzo, V. (2011). Palliative sedation in patients with advanced cancer followed at home: A systematic review. *Journal of Pain and Symptom Management*, *41*(4), 754–760. http://dx.doi.org/10.1016/j.jpainsymman.2010.07.013

Mercadante, S., Villari, P., & Ferrera, P. (2003). A model of acute symptom control unit: Pain relief and palliative care unit of La Maddalena cancer center. *Support Care Cancer*, *11*, 114–119. http://dx.doi.org/10.1016/j.jpainsymman.2007.04.018

Mercadante, S., Villari, P., Ferrera, P., Mangione, S., & Casuccio, A. (2010). The use of opioids for breakthrough pain in acute palliative care unit by using doses proportional to opioid basal regimen. *Clinical Journal of Pain*, *26*(4), 306–309.

Morrison, S., & Meier, D. (2004). Palliative care. *The New England Journal of Medicine*, *350*(25), 2582–2590.

Moryl, N., Coyle, N., & Foley, K. M. (2008). Managing an acute pain crisis in a patient with advanced cancer. *The Journal of the American Medical Association*, *299*(12), 1457–1467. http://dx.doi.org/10.1001/jama.299.12.1457

Moyle, J. (1995). The use of propofol in palliative medicine. *Journal of Pain and Symptom Management*, *10*(8), 643–646.

National Ethics Committee. (2007). The ethics of palliative sedation as a therapy of last resort. *American Journal of Hospice & Palliative Medicine*, *23*(6), 483–491. http://dx.doi.org/10.1177/1049909106294883

Norton, S., Hogan, L., Holloway, R., Temkin-Greener, H., Buckley, M., & Quill, T. (2007). Proactive palliative care in the medical intensive care unit: Effects on length of stay for selected high-risk patients. *Crit Care Med*, *35*(6), 1530–1534.

Ok, J., Meyers, F., & Evans, C. (2005). Medical and surgical palliative care of patients with urological malignancies. *The Journal of Urology*, *174*, 1177–1182.

Pan, C., Morrison, S., Ness, J., Fugh-Berman, A., & Leipzig, R. (2000). Complementary and alternative medicine in the management of pain, dyspnea, and nausea and vomiting near the end of life: A systematic review. *Journal of Pain and Symptom Management*, *20*(5), 374–387.

Prommer, E. (2011). Dexmedetomidine: Does it have potential in palliative medicine? *American Journal of Hospice & Palliative Medicine*, *28*(4), 276–283. http://dx.doi.org/10.1177/1049909110389804

Quill, T., & Abernethy, A. (2013). Generalist plus specialist palliative care—creating a more sustainable model. *The New England Journal of Medicine*, 368(13), 1173–1175.

Quill, T., Lo, B., & Brock, D. (1997). Palliative options of last resort: A comparison of voluntarily stopping eating and drinking, terminal sedation, physician-assisted suicide, and voluntary active euthanasia. *The Journal of the American Medical Association*, *278*(23), 2099–2104.

Rady, M. Y., & Verheijde, J. L. (2010). Continuous deep sedation until death: Palliation or physician-assisted death? *American Journal of Hospice & Palliative Medicine*, *27*(3), 205–214. http://dx.doi.org/10.1177/1049909109348868

Rasmussen, K. G., & Richardson, J. W. (2011). Electroconvulsive therapy in palliative care. *American Journal of Hospice & Palliative Medicine*, *28*(5), 375–377. http://dx.doi.org/10.1177/1049909110390203

Rietjens, J., van Zuylen, L., van Veluw, H., van der Wijk, L., van der Heide, A., & van der Rijt, C. C. (2008). Palliative sedation in a specialized unit for acute palliative care in a cancer hospital: comparing patients dying with and without palliative sedation. *Journal of Pain and Symptom Management*, *36*(3), 228–234. http://dx.doi.org/10.1016/j.jpainsymman.2007.10.014

Roberts, S., Wozencraft, C. P., Coyne, P. J., & Smith, T. J. (2011). Dexmedetomidine as an adjuvant analgesic for intractable cancer pain. *Journal of Palliative Medicine, 14*(3), 371–373. http://dx.doi.org/10.1089/jpm.2010.0235

Rork, J. F., Berde, C. B., & Goldstein, R. D. (2013). Regional anesthesia approaches to pain management in pediatric palliative care: A review of current knowledge. *Journal of Pain and Symptom Management, 46*(6), 859–873.

Schuman-Olivier, Z., Brendel, D. H., Forstein, M., & Price, B. H. (2008). The use of palliative sedation for existential distress: A psychiatric perspective. *Harvard Review of Psychiatry, 16*(6), 339–351. http://dx.doi.org/10.1080/10673220802576917

Scott, T. H., & Gavrin, J. R. (2012). Palliative surgery in the do-not-resuscitate patient: Ethics and practical suggestions for management. *Anesthesiology Clinics, 30*, 1–12. http://dx.doi.org/10.1016/j.anclin.2012.02.001

Selwyn, P. A. (2005). Palliative care for patient with human immunodeficiency virus/acquired immune deficiency syndrome. *Journal of Palliative Medicine, 8*(6), 1248–1268.

Seymour, J., Clark, D., & Winslow, M. (2005). Pain and palliative care: The emergence of new specialties. *Journal of Pain and Symptom Management, 29*(1), 2–13.

Smith, T., Coyne, P., Cassel, B., Penberthy, L., Hopson, A., & Hager, M. A. (2003). A high volume specialist palliative care unit and team may reduce in-hospital end of-life care costs. *Journal of Palliative Medicine, 6*(5), 699–705.

Soares, L. G., Naylor, C., Martins, M., & Piexoto. (2002). Dexmedetomidine: A new option for intractable distress in the dying. *Journal of Pain and Symptom Management, 24*(1), 6–8. http://dx.doi.org/10.1016/s0885-3924(02)00423-2

Soto, E., Stewart, D. R., Mannes, A. J., Ruppert, S. L., Baker, K., Zlott, D., et al. (2012). Oral ketamine in the palliative care setting: A review of the literature and case report of a patient with neurofibromatosis type 1 and glomus tumor-associated complex regional pain syndrome. *American Journal of Palliative Care, 29*(4), 308–317. http://dx.doi.org/10.1177/1049909111416345

Sprung, C. L., Ledoux, D., Bulow, H. H., Lippert, A., Wennberg, E., Baras, M., et al. (2008). Reliving suffering or intentionally hastening death: Where do you draw the line? *Critical Care Medicine, 36*(1), 8–13. http://dx.doi.org/10.1097/01.ccm.0000295304.99946.58

Staats, P. S., Yearwood, T., Charapata, S. G., Presley, R. W., Wallace, M. S., Byas-Smith, M., et al. (2004). Intrathecal ziconotide in the treatment of refractory pain in patients with cancer or AIDS. *The Journal of the American Medical Association, 291*(1), 63–70. http://dx.doi.org/10.1001/jama.291.1.63

Stoddard, S. (1992). *Hospice movement: A better way of caring for the dying*. New York, NY: Vintage Books.

Strand, J., Kamdar, M., & Carey, E. (2013). Top 10 things palliative care clinicians wished everyone knew about palliative care. *Mayo Clinic Proceedings, 88*(8), 859–865. http://dx.doi.org/10.1088/1475-7516/2013/05/020

Swetz, K. M., & Kamal, A. H. (2012). Palliative care. *Annals of Internal Medicine, 156*(3), ITC2-ITC16. http://dx.doi.org/10.7326/0003-4819-156-3-201202070-01002

Truog, R. D., Cist, A. F., Brackett, S. E., Burns, J. P., Curley, M. A., Danis, M., et al. (2001). Recommendations for end-of-life care in the intensive care unit: The ethics committee of the society of critical care medicine. *Critical Care Medicine, 29*(12), 2332–2348.

Vacco v Quill. (1997). 521 US 793. *NH Rev Stat Ann Section.*

VanNorman, G. A. (2003). Another matter of life and death: What every anesthesiologist should know about the ethical, legal, and policy implications of the non-heart beating cadaver organ donor. *Anesthesiology, 98*, 763–773.

Washington v Glucksberg. (1997). 521 US 702.

Wellesley, H., & Jenkins, I. A. (2009). Withholding and withdrawing life-sustaining treatment in children. *Pediatric Anesthesia, 19*, 972–978. http://dx.doi.org/10.1111/j.1460-9592.2009.03027.x

World Health Organization. (2012). *WHO guidelines on the pharmacological treatment of persisting pain in children with medical illnesses.* Retrieved from http://apps.who.int/iris/bitstream/10665/44540/1/9789241548120_Guidelines.pdf

World Health Organization. (2016). *WHO's cancer pain ladder for adults.* Retrieved from http://www.who.int/cancer/palliative/painladder/en/

CHAPTER 9

Treatment and Prevention of Spinal-Induced Hypotension in the Cesarean Section Patient

What Does the Evidence Say?

Joseph E. Pellegrini

ABSTRACT

Most anesthesia providers prefer to do a subarachnoid block (SAB) for cesarean section because of its rapid onset and reliability to provide adequate anesthesia. However an effect of the SAB is that it causes a spinal-induced hypotension (SIH) in up to 85% of the population. There have been multiple studies that assessed fluid administration, vasopressor administration, maternal positioning, or serotonin blockers given prophylactically to attenuate the SIH response. Despite these multiple studies, the method to prevent and treat SIH remains varied from one anesthesia practice to another. The purpose of this chapter is to review the evidence on the various methods used to prevent and treat SIH.

INTRODUCTION

The anesthesia technique of choice for cesarean section delivery is spinal anesthesia or a subarachnoid block (SAB) because of its reliable sensory and motor

http://dx.doi.org/10.1891/0739-6686.35.159

blockade, fast onset, and reduced risk of local anesthesia toxicity (Shibli & Russell, 2000). While these benefits are well known, spinal anesthesia is also associated with a fairly significant side effect profile. Foremost among these side effects is hypotension. In fact, hypotension has been reported to occur in up to 85% of cesarean section patients following SAB placement (Riley, Cohen, Rubenstien, & Flanagan, 1995). The reason this incidence is so high is because patients undergoing a cesarean section require a high sensory level (T-4) for surgical anesthesia, are less responsive to in vivo vasopressors and more prone to aortocaval compression (AAC). All of these factors then culminate in a sympathetic blockade that results in profound peripheral vasodilation and an increased venous capacitance that can be refractory to vasopressor agents. This condition is called spinal-induced hypotension (SIH). Those sequelae associated with SIH in the cesarean section patient include possible placental hypoperfusion, fetal hypoxia, acidosis, fetal neurological injury, and maternal nausea and vomiting (Cyna, Andrew, Emmett, Middleton, & Simmons, 2006). While there are multiple strategies proposed to prevent and treat SIH in the cesarean section patient, the most commonly used techniques include: maternal pelvic tilting, administration of crystalloid and colloid solutions, administration of vasopressor agents, maternal positioning during SAB placement, use of lower extremity compression devices, and the use of 5-HT3 antagonists administered as a prophylactic agent (Cyna et al., 2006; Gao, Zheng, Han, Wang, & Zheng, 2015). While this is not a complete list of measures, these are the most commonly used methods in clinical practice. The purpose of this review is to focus on the evidence for these commonly used strategies in an effort to better inform the practitioner and to facilitate recommendations to clinical practice.

UTERINE DISPLACEMENT

In late pregnancy it has been long believed that assumption of the supine position induces a hypotensive response in some parturients. This syndrome was first described in 1953 by Howard, Goodson, and Mengert where they noted near "shock-like" conditions in 10% of the late term parturients they placed in a supine position for several minutes. They postulated that these symptoms were secondary to occlusion of the inferior vena cava (IVC) from the weight of the gravid uterus and recommended that all late term pregnancy patients should avoid supine positioning. Additional research by Scott and Kerr (1963) noted that supine positioning of a late term parturient resulted in a 20% to 50% reduction in the cardiac output (CO) as compared to when they are maintained in a lateral position. Later research discovered that this fall in CO was not only due to compression on the IVC but also from abdominal aorta compression

(Lees, Schott, Kerr, & Taylor, 1967). This dual compression phenomenon is now termed aortocaval compression, and some of the clinical manifestations that are attributed to AAC include maternal nausea, vomiting, weakness and pallor, and fetal bradycardia, acidosis, and hypoxia (Goodlin, 1971; Kinsella & Lohmann, 1994).

It was soon discovered that a 15- to 20-degree wedge placed under the parturients pelvis facilitated a left uterine displacement (LUD), which helped alleviate AAC and improved CO (Crawford, Burton, & Davies, 1972). Multiple studies have shown the clinical and radiographic benefits from positioning the patient away from the supine to a more lateral position (Bieniarz et al., 1968; Dhekne, Barron, & Koch, 1987). Some of these benefits include reductions in hypotension and improvement in neonatal umbilical pH levels and Apgar scores (Bamber & Dresner, 2003; Buley, Downing, Brock-Utne, & Cuerden, 1977; Downing, Coleman, Mohemedy, Jeal, & Mohemedy, 1974; Kundra et al., 2012; Kohler, Sorensen, & Helbo-Hansen, 2002; Rees, Thurlow, Gardner, Scrutton, & Kinsella, 2002). This technique of placing a 15- to 20-degree pelvic wedge or "hip roll" was quickly adopted as the standard of care. Recently some studies have indicated that a greater benefit might be derived from placement of a right lumbar wedge as compared to a right pelvic wedge. The first study to compare the differences in SIH incidence between pelvic and lumbar wedge placement was done by Zhou, Shao, Zeng, Song, and Yang in 2008. They randomized 60 parturients scheduled for an elective cesarean section under combined spinal–epidural (CSE) into either the pelvic and lumbar wedge groups. They reported a higher incidence of SIH in the pelvic wedge group (77%) as compared to the lumbar wedge group (47%) but no differences in neonatal outcomes. Based on this they concluded that added benefits could be derived by lumbar versus pelvic wedge placement.

Another study to investigate this phenomenon was done by Calvache, Munoz, and Baron (2011) in which they analyzed the incidences of hypotension, vasopressor requirements, and nausea in 80 SAB cesarean section patients. One group was randomized to receive modified supine position (defined as placement of a 20-degree lumbar wedge), whereas the other group was placed in a supine position without LUD. They reported no significant differences in SIH between the supine group (50%) and lumbar wedge group (42%), but did note significant increased vasopressor requirements, nausea, and vomiting in the supine group, thereby showing some benefit in LUD.

Providing LUD at the recommended 15- to 20-degree tilt can be challenging in some parturients secondary to the changing body habitus of the cesarean section patient. The prevalence of obesity in pregnancy is increasing in the United States and with obesity comes an increase in the risk for hypotension, especially

SIH, following SAB placement for a cesarean delivery (Harvey, Hodgson, & Kinsella, 2013). There are studies that indicate that up to 20% of all women of normalized weight (body mass index [BMI] < 30 kg/m^2) fail to achieve a 15-degree LUD lateral tilt when conventional tilting techniques are used. The failure rate is even higher in women who are obese or morbidly obese. It has been reported that approximately 33% of women with a BMI 35 kg/m^2 or greater fail to achieve a 15-degree tilt when conventional tilting techniques are used, and these women may require a tilt as high as 30 degrees to achieve adequate LUD. The cause of this failure to achieve LUD is speculated to be secondary to the variability of adipose tissue in the obese patient (Harvey et al., 2013). While most practitioners would argue that providing a 30-degree tilt may be unachievable in many clinical practices based on surgeon needs and the patient's ability to tolerate such an extreme tilt, almost all will agree that providing at least a 15-degree tilt is the standard of care. Some of the recognized methods that can be used in conjunction with a 15-degree wedge device to ensure adequate tilt is maintained can include doing a manual displacement of the uterus until delivery of the neonate, providing a tilt to the operative table or using a device such as the inflatable wedge device (Cyna et al., 2006; Grewal & Suir, 2009). This inflatable device has the ability to offer a range of degrees of tilt and can be used solely or in concert with a conventional wedge device.

In conclusion, to help prevent SIH symptoms in patients presenting for a cesarean section under SAB the overall body of evidence indicates that placing a 15-degree (or greater) wedge under the lower lumbar region facilitates LUD and should be considered as the standard of care. In the obese patient it may be difficult to achieve a 15-degree tilt using a standardized wedge device and alternative methods to facilitate LUD may be required.

CRYSTALLOID LOADING

Another standard of care technique often employed to prevent SIH has been to administer a fluid bolus of crystalloid solution prior to administration of spinal anesthesia for a cesarean section. This was based on research performed in the latter 1960s, which showed efficacy in preventing SIH when patients are "preloaded" with a crystalloid solution. A bolus dose of 15 to 20 ml/kg was the recommended bolus dose of crystalloid given 14 to 20 minutes before SAB injection for many years. However, in the early 1990s many obstetrical anesthesia practitioners questioned the value of the crystalloid preload (Rout, Rocke, Levin, Gouws, & Reddy, 1993). Some practitioners hypothesized that it might be more beneficial to administer the solution as a co-load, given at the time of the SAB injection (Dyer et al., 2004; Mojica, Melendez, & Bautista, 2002). Therefore the purpose of this section is to review the utility of crystalloid preloading and coloading as it relates to prevention of SIH.

Crystalloid Preloading

The first study to determine the effect of prophylactic fluid administration on hypotension following placement of an SAB for cesarean section was done by Wollman and Marx in 1968. They showed a significant reduction in SIH symptoms when parturients were administered a fluid preload of 20 ml/kg of D5LR given 14 to 20 minutes before injection of an SAB for cesarean section. This original study was small (14 patients in the experimental group and 10 in the control group) and only included 11 patients in active labor. Of these only 14 underwent a cesarean section (9 hydrated; 5 nonhydrated). However, despite these small numbers they reported a remarkable zero percent incidence of SIH in the hydrated group and an 80% incidence in the nonhydrated group. Subsequent studies also supported these findings and as a result preloading became the standard of care to prevent SIH in most anesthesia practices (Clark, Cotton, & Lee, 1976; Marx, Cosmi, & Wollman, 1969). It needs to be noted that this earlier research used dextrose containing solutions as their preload, which was in conflict with what many practitioners were using in their clinical practices. Research performed in the early 1980s reported that administration of a dextrose containing solution to a late term pregnant patient could result in maternal hyperglycemia and neonatal hypoglycemia and jaundice (Kenepp et al., 1982). Based on this, many practitioners began using nonglucose containing solutions such as lactated Ringer's (LR) or 0.9% NaCl solution for preloading prior to an SAB and they quickly noted that it was less effective in preventing SIH than when a dextrose containing solution was used. The first study to analyze the value of volume preloading with a crystalloid solution was done by Rout et al. in 1993 where they performed a two-stage open sequential study in which they allocated 140 cesarean section patients into one of two groups. One group was allocated to receive standardized preloading with 20 ml/kg of crystalloid solution over 15 to 20 minutes prior to spinal anesthesia placement whereas the other group was only administered intravenous (IV) crystalloid at a keep-vein-open rate. These researchers did report that the incidence of hypotension was 16% higher in those who did not receive a preloading bolus of crystalloid but no differences were noted in the duration of hypotension, ephedrine requirements, nor neonatal outcomes. The authors concluded that preloading with a crystalloid solution such as LR was not effective in preventing SIH and the subsequent symptoms and recommended that the mandate requiring a fixed preload volume of crystalloid solution prior to SAB placement be abandoned, especially when the cesarean section is considered urgent. Subsequent studies were also performed and reported similar results, and also recommended that the mandatory fluid preloading before SAB injection in the cesarean section patient be abandoned (Jackson, Reid, & Thorburn, 1995; Oh et al., 2014). Subsequent research identified that crystalloids do not remain in the intravascular space and distribute rapidly into the extracellular space; therefore the timing of infusion may be the key to prevent SIH (Oh et al., 2014; Ueyama, Yan-Ling, Tanigami, Mashimo, & Yoshiya, 1999). Based on this, the attention was turned toward the timing of when to administer the crystalloid solution.

Timing of Crystalloid Infusion

One of the first to analyze the effect the timing of the prophylactic crystalloid bolus on the incidence and severity of SIH was Mojica, Melendez, and Bautista (2002) in which they randomized general surgery patients receiving an SAB into three groups. One group was randomized to receive no preload (placebo) group, another was randomized to receive the traditional preload of 20 ml/kg administered 20 minutes before SAB injection, and a third group was assigned to receive 20 ml/kg initiated at the time of the SAB injection (co-load). These investigators reported the incidence of SIH was significantly reduced in the co-load group and no differences were found between the placebo and preload groups. All co-load fluids were administered rapidly (over 6–10 minutes) and no differences in demographics, surgeries, and SAB or adjunct medications were noted between the groups. However, it should be noted that this study was done on a nonobstetrical population and it was unknown if a similar effect could be demonstrated in an obstetrical population receiving an SAB for cesarean section.

The first investigator to analyze the effect of a co-load of crystalloid solution on the incidence and severity of SIH in groups of cesarean section patients given an SAB was done by Dyer et al. (2004). They randomized 50 women to receive either a preload of 20 ml/kg crystalloid given over 20 minutes prior to SAB injection or an equivalent volume administered rapidly as a co-load and noted a lower incidence of hypotension and vasopressor requirements at 7, 8, and 9 minutes after SAB injection in the co-load group (Dyer et al., 2004). Although the only differences in Mean Arterial Pressure were noted at 7, 8, and 9 minutes after SAB placement, this is significant in that the greatest impact on maternal hemodynamics occurs 5 to 10 minutes following injection of the spinal anesthetic (Williamson et al., 2009). Based on this, they concluded that 20 ml/kg of crystalloid solution administered as a rapidly infused co-load was superior to conventional preloading techniques in preventing hypotension.

The use of a co-load was further validated in a recent randomized controlled study in which patients were co-loaded or preloaded with 15 ml/kg in an effort to reduce SIH from an SAB at cesarean section. These investigators reported that those in the co-load group had a significantly lower incidence of SIH (53.3% vs. 83.3%), decreased ephedrine requirements (7.5 mg vs. 15 mg) and a lower incidence of nausea (27% vs. 60%) as compared to the preload group (Oh et al., 2014). However, there have been studies that have shown no differences between crystalloid preloading and co-loading. In fact, a 2009 meta-analysis that included a subgroup analysis of crystalloid co-loading and preloading found no differences between the groups (Banerjee, Stocche, Angle, & Halpern, 2009). These authors concluded that in patients undergoing elective cesarean section under SAB the timing of fluid loading does not have an impact on the incidence of SIH. This review had several limitations in that it was a subgroup analysis on only five small studies, which the authors combined into one analysis. As a result, an effect size for each bolus volume could not be established, calling into question the generalizability of the results. However, overall it appears that the body of evidence suggests a benefit of co-loading over preloading and should remain the preferable practice for SIH prophylaxis as it relates to fluid loading.

COLLOID ADMINISTRATION

The premise behind prophylactic administration of any IV solution is to increase the blood volume in an effort to decrease the incidence of SIH. While this has been shown to be ineffective when crystalloids are used as a preloading solution, it is less clear if colloids would be ineffective if administered as a preload. Multiple studies that include the use of 5% albumin, 6% hydroxyethyl starch (HES), and gelatin have been done to determine if they prevent SIH and report that preloading with a colloidal solution is highly effective in preventing SIH as compared to crystalloid preloading (Dahlgren, Granath, Wessel, & Irestedt, 2006; French, White, Howell, & Popat, 1999; Riley et al., 1995; Siddick, Aouad, Kai, Sfeir, & Barska, 2000; Teoh & Sia, 2009). This was further validated by a recent Cochrane collaboration analysis (Cyna et al., 2006) and a meta-analysis (Li, Zhang, Tan, & Xu, 2013) in which they also concluded that prophylactic administration of colloids is significantly more effective than crystalloid preloading in preventing SIH. However it should be noted that most studies used a synthetic colloid solution such as HES and not serum albumin. Recently the use of synthetic colloid solutions have fallen into some disfavor secondary to the reports that the use of HES was associated with acute kidney injury and decreased survivability in critically ill patients with sepsis (Perner, Haase, & Guterormsen, 2012). Based on these findings, the use of synthetic colloids remains limited in practice, especially in the critically ill population, and most practitioners opt to use serum albumin as their standard colloid solution. Although limited, there have been studies that have used serum albumin and one of the first studies to evaluate serum albumin preloading was done by Malthru et al. in 1980. A total of 85 patients receiving an SAB for cesarean delivery were included. The patients were randomly assigned into four groups; group 1 (n = 21) received D5LR (15 ml/kg); group 2 (n = 20) D5LR plus ephedrine 25 mg IM (intramuscular); group 3 (n = 24) received 5% albumin in D5LR (15 ml/kg); and group 4 (n = 22) received 5% albumin in D5LR (15 ml/kg) plus 25 mg IM ephedrine. These investigators reported that subjects in the 5% albumin groups had significantly lower incidence of SIH and higher Apgar scores as compared to crystalloid only (with and without ephedrine). Based on this, they concluded the prophylactic administration of 5% albumin in D5LR solution is an effective method to prevent SIH.

Clearly colloids are effective if given as a preloading solution but some investigators speculated if similar results could be obtained if administered as a co-load solution. The reason that this query was first raised was because it was noted that some cesarean sections were being delayed because practitioners were often waiting until the colloid solution was fully administered before performing the SAB. One of the first studies to determine the effect administering a colloid as a co-load solution was done by Carvalho, Mercier, Riley, Brummel, and Cohen (2009). In this study they randomized 46 parturients to receive either a preload or a co-load of 500 ml of 6% HES solution. No differences in maternal hemodynamics or neonatal outcomes were reported. Therefore the investigators concluded that both methods were equally effective in preventing SIH symptoms in cesarean section patients receiving an SAB. At approximately the same time, a similar study was done by Teoh and Sia (2009) in which they randomized 40 parturients scheduled for cesarean section under SAB to receive either 15 ml/kg of HES solution as a preload or as a co-load. Maternal heart rate (HR), blood pressure (BP), CO, and stroke volume (SV) measurements were obtained with a noninvasive ultrasonic CO monitor. They reported that maternal CO was significantly higher in the preload group but not sustained throughout the entire procedure and no differences in overall outcomes were noted between the groups. Based on these and similar results, it can be concluded that administration of colloidal solution either as a preload or co-load is effective in preventing SIH.

VASOPRESSORS

There has been a long-standing debate as to what is the most appropriate vasopressor to use to prevent and treat SIH in parturients receiving an SAB for cesarean section. Based on some early studies the choice of vasopressors in obstetrics was largely limited to ephedrine because of its predominantly beta-adrenergic agonist effects, which were shown to preserve uterine blood flow (UBF) while increasing maternal BP (James, Greiss, & Kemp, 1970). The models used in these early studies were pregnant, paralyzed ewes and these findings were then extrapolated to a human population.

In 1965, Greiss and Crandell reported that when pregnant sheep were administered a spinal anesthetic, profound hypotension ensued with a resultant drop in UBF. To treat the hypotension the investigators administered doses of norepinephrine, phenylephrine, or angiotensin. They noted that all of these antihypertensives were able to increase the BP but also resulted in a profound decrease in UBF with an increase in fetal acidosis. Based on these results they concluded that vasopressors should only be used as a last resort to treat hypotension and therapy should first consist of fluid bolus and positioning. Shortly after these experiments, Shnider, Lorimier, Holl, Chapler, and Morishima (1968) also induced hypotension in pregnant ewes and showed that when ephedrine was used to treat SIH, maternal BP was maintained without a subsequent increase in fetal acidosis. However, these experiments did not measure UBF and were not a good reflection of clinical conditions; therefore further investigations were warranted. A more definitive study was done by James, Griess, and Kemp (1970), which showed that ephedrine was superior to phenylephrine in maintaining UBF when used to treat SIH. Additional research by Ralston, Shnider, and deLorimier (1974) compared the alpha- and beta-adrenergic effects of ephedrine and found that ephedrine was effective in preventing and treating SIH without impacting UBF. Based on these studies the American College of Obstetrics and Gynecology made ephedrine the vasopressor of choice to treat and prevent SIH (Chestnut & Gibbs, 1991).

Ephedrine

Ephedrine was noted to have a beneficial effect on UBF secondary to its mixed alpha and beta pharmacology. It was not until 1976 that a study was performed to determine if the prophylactic administration of ephedrine would be effective in preventing SIH in patients undergoing a cesarean section under SAB. A prospective randomized study was performed by Gutsche (1976) in which he assigned 17 patients to receive either 50 mg ephedrine IM (8 patients) or placebo (9 patients) approximately 5 to 23 minutes prior to SAB placement. Gutsche noted that those assigned to receive the ephedrine had significantly lower incidences of SIH and nausea and vomiting and proposed that 50 mg ephedrine IM was a viable treatment to prevent SIH. One of the first studies to investigate the effectiveness of administration of a prophylactic dose of IV ephedrine was done by King and Rosen (1998) in which they looked at the differences between prophylactic infusions, boluses or placebo and noted no differences between the groups as it related to SIH prevention. However, this was only one study and only included 10 patients per group; therefore the sample size may not be substantial enough to show significance. Since that time there have been multiple studies that also reported that ephedrine prophylaxis is beneficial in preventing SIH, and it quickly became a standardized SIH prophylactic regimen (Kang, Aboluliesh, & Cartis, 1982; Mahajan, Anand, & Gombar, 2009; Ngan Kee et al., 2008). However, while these studies did support the use of ephedrine as a treatment and prophylactic regimen, some questioned the overall effect it had on the fetus.

Phenylephrine

It was not until the late 1980s that phenylephrine was reexamined as a viable option to treat SIH and its overall effect on the fetus and neonate questioned. As noted earlier the use of alpha-agonists such as phenylephrine to treat SIH was discouraged based on some early animal studies that reported that direct alpha stimulation resulted in decreased UBF, with a resultant decreasing placental perfusion. In 1988, Ramanthan and Grant conducted a study in which they assessed hemodynamic changes and neonatal acid–base status in 127 elective cesarean sections done under epidural analgesia. All patients were divided to receive placebo, ephedrine, or phenylephrine to treat SIH. These investigators reported that both the ephedrine and phenylephrine groups increased CO and reversed hypotension but in contrast to the earlier animal studies these researchers noted that those administered phenylephrine had a lower reported incidence of fetal acidosis and a faster resolution of hypotension. Based on these results they recommended that phenylephrine should be reconsidered a first-line treatment regimen for SIH. Despite this evidence, the practice of not using phenylephrine to treat SIH continued and it was not until 1991 when Moran, Perillo, LaPorta, Bader, and Datta reported similar results that supported the use of phenylephrine over ephedrine that phenylephrine began to be considered as a viable option to ephedrine. Following this, multiple studies were performed, which included the use of low-dose phenylephrine infusions or bolus doses to treat SIH and these studies also reported that phenylephrine was effective in treating and preventing SIH without causing subsequent maternal bradycardia and adverse fetal outcomes (Allen, George, White, Muir, & Habib, 2010; Doherty, Ohashi, Downey, & Cavalho, 2012; Dyer et al., 2009; Lee et al., 2015; Ngan Kee, Khaw, Ng, & Lee, 2004; Veeser et al., 2012). Eventually the American Society of Anesthesiologists (ASA) Task Force on Obstetric Anesthesia changed its position and came out with a 2007 consensus statement supporting the use of phenylephrine over ephedrine in the prevention and treatment of SIH (Hawkins et al., 2007). In addition to the consensus statement from the ASA, the Canadian and Belgian guidelines also came out with a recommendation that supported phenylephrine over ephedrine as the vasopressor of choice to treat and prevent SIH, in the absence of maternal bradycardia (Loubert, 2012; Van De Velde, 2013).

ONDANSETRON (5-HT3 ANTAGONISM)

Spinal anesthesia results in a diminished venous return secondary to blockade of sympathetic nerves. Patients receiving an SAB for a cesarean section require a high level of sensory and sympathetic blockade that results in vasodilation as well as an increased incidence of bradycardia from a relative parasympathetic dominance (Liu & McDonald, 2001; Salo, Woods, Anderson, & McAllen, 2007; Yamano, Ito, Kamato, & Miyata, 1995). The hypotension is largely due to the decreases in CO and systemic vascular resistance from the sympathectomy, whereas the bradycardia is primarily due to a mechanism called Bezold–Jarisch reflex (BJR). This BJR is caused from the reduced filling of the right atrium from the sympathectomy, which reduces outflow from intrinsic chronotropic stretch mechanoreceptors in the ventricular wall (Yamano et al., 1995). Animal studies have suggested that serotonin is an important factor in the induction of the BJR and blockade of this reflex may be beneficial in decreasing the severity of SIH. To test this hypothesis, studies have been performed to determine if the patients undergoing spinal anesthesia would have a decreased incidence of SIH, if they were prophylactically administered a serotonin antagonist such as ondansetron.

The first study to investigate the effect of prophylactic administration of the 5-HT3 antagonist ondansetron on SIH was done by Owczuk et al. (2008) in which they randomly administered to SAB patients either 8 mg IV ondansetron or placebo. It was noted that those patients in receipt of ondansetron had a significant reduction in both bradycardia and hypotension, as compared to placebo. Some of the criticisms regarding this study were that it used a higher dose of ondansetron (8 mg) than is typically administered in clinical practice (4 mg) and it did not include patients who received an SAB for a cesarean section. In 2012, a study was done by Sahoo, SenDasgupta, Goswami, and Hazra in which they administered 4 mg ondansetron or placebo approximately 5 minutes before SAB injection to 52 patients scheduled for an elective cesarean section. These investigators reported that those in the ondansetron group had a decreased incidence of SIH, a lower need for supplemental vasopressors, and a significantly lower incidence of nausea and vomiting, as compared to the placebo group. However, no differences in maternal HRs were noted between the groups. Overall, these findings were shown to be beneficial and they concluded that 4 mg of IV ondansetron given 5 minutes before SAB placement is an effective method to prevent SIH symptoms, possibly due to blockade of the BJR reflex. Other studies have also reported that prophylactic ondansetron is effective in preventing SIH (Rashad & Farmawy, 2013; Wang et al., 2014). In fact, in a recent meta-analysis by Gao et al. (2015) in which they analyzed 10 clinical trials (863 patients) they reported that overall the incidence of SIH, nausea and vomiting and the need for rescue vasopressors were reduced when ondansetron is administered approximately

5 minutes prior to SAB injection, as compared to placebo. In addition, this meta-analysis also reported that prophylactic ondansetron was effective in preventing bradycardia, thereby supporting the result that the BJR may be instrumental in SIH.

There has been at least one well-designed clinical trial that reports that prophylactic administration of ondansetron has little effect on SIH incidence and adverse events. Ortiz-Gomez et al. (2014) reported no differences in SIH and vasopressor requirements in groups of patients given 2, 4, or 8 mg ondansetron, or placebo administered 5 minutes before spinal anesthesia. All patients in this study were given a calculated dose of bupivacaine (bupivacaine [mg] = height [cm] × 0.06) plus 20 micrograms (mcg) fentanyl. The total dose of bupivacaine was noted to be similar to that provided in other studies but the dose of fentanyl did exceed the doses used in many clinical practices. Most practitioners limit their intrathecal fentanyl to 10 mcg and administration of a larger fentanyl dose may have attenuated a possible central action of ondansetron on SIH symptoms. The previous studies cited did not include an opioid; therefore it is difficult to determine if the co-administration of an opioid is an instrumental factor in blocking the beneficial effects from ondansetron in the SAB patient. In general, this preceding study did not have much of an impact on the overall body of evidence that does report that prophylactic ondansetron can alleviate the hypotension, bradycardia, nausea and vomiting caused by SIH as well as reduce vasopressor requirements in patients receiving an SAB for cesarean delivery (Gao et al., 2015). Further studies need to be performed to determine if these effects are attenuated by co-administration of an opioid with the SAB.

POSITIONING AT TIME OF SAB

An area that is often associated with hypotension following the placement of an SAB in the cesarean section patient is the parturient's position during and immediately after the subarachnoid injection. The most common local anesthetic agent used to produce an SAB in the cesarean section population is hyperbaric bupivacaine. Most CRNAs and anesthesiologists have adopted the sitting position for induction of neuraxial anesthesia because it allows for rapid and reliable identification of the parturient's midline, especially in the morbidly obese patient (Wong, Nathan, & Brown, 2009). In 1995, Inglis, Daniel, and McGrady reported that ephedrine requirements following SAB injection were significantly lower if the injection was performed while the parturient was in a sitting position as compared to a lateral position. These authors hypothesized that the sitting position delayed a cephalic spread of the local anesthetic by gravitational effects thereby resulting in a lower level of sympathectomy overall. A subsequent study by

Coppejans, Hendrickx, Goossens, and Vercauteren in 1998 was done that randomized effects of sitting versus lateral injection on SIH in groups receiving low-dose bupivacaine–sufentanil CSE for elective cesarean section. They reported that less incidence of SIH in the sitting (18%) as compared to the lateral (40%) group. However, this study was done using a CSE technique and lower doses of bupivacaine than traditionally used in clinical practice thereby questioning the generalizability of the results. A recent study by Obasuyi, Fyneface-Ogan, and Mato (2013) evaluated the effect of the lateral and sitting positions during SAB injection of hyperbaric bupivacaine for cesarean section. A total of 100 patients were randomized to receive a dose of 10 to 12 mg (based on maternal height) while positioned in a lateral or sitting position. Following injection all the parturients were immediately placed in a modified supine position with LUD. In this study they reported the incidence of hypotension was significantly lower in the lateral group (34%) as compared to the sitting group (56%) for up to 30 minutes following SAB injection. Based on this they concluded that the lateral position during SAB injection provided a more stable BP for an extended period following SAB injection. Similar results were also reported in earlier studies that showed a lower incidence of SIH when the SAB was performed with the parturient in the lateral versus the sitting position (Russell, Popat, Richards, & Burry, 2002; Yun, Marx, & Santos, 1998). Based on the conflicting results and because of the lack of homogeneity between the studies no definitive recommendation regarding sitting versus lateral during SAB injection as it relates to SIH prevention can be made and further investigations will be required.

LOWER LIMB COMPRESSION

A major mechanism that precipitates hypotension following an SAB is the redistribution of blood from the central to the peripheral compartment due to sympathetic vasodilation. There have been several different techniques and mechanisms described in the literature to suppress this redistribution and augment the venous return. These included studies that analyzed the use of inflatable splints (Gouldie, Winter, & Ferguson, 1988), leg elevation (Rout, Rocke & Gouws, 1993), combination therapy using Esmarch dressings and leg elevation (Christensen, Trautnera, Stokela, & Nielsen, 1986), and thromboembolic deterrant (TED) stockings (Sood, Cooper, Michel, Wee, & Pickering, 1996). Overall the findings supported the use of compression and leg elevation using these interventions. This is supported in the Cochrane review by Cyna et al. (2006) in which they pooled the results from seven clinical trials and showed lower limb compression is effective in preventing SIH as compared to control.

One of the most commonly used devices in the operative suite on the cesarean section patient is the sequential compression device (SCD). This device contains a pump that applies pressure sequentially using a milking motion over the lower extremities to avoid deep vein thrombosis. It has also been hypothesized that use of SCDs can result in less SIH in cesarean section patients who have been given an SAB. Pressure is sequentially applied and released in a milking motion over the lower extremity and it is hypothesized that it would also decrease overall SIH. The first study to test this hypothesis was done by Sujata, Arora, Panigrahi, and Hanjorra (2012) in which they randomized 100 SAB patients scheduled for an elective cesarean delivery. One group was randomly selected to receive the SCD intervention whereas the other received no treatment. These investigators reported the overall incidence of SIH was only 25.5% in the SCD group as compared to 60% incidence in the control group.

DISCUSSION AND RESEARCH RECOMMENDATIONS/IMPLICATIONS

The most frequently used method to prevent SIH is the use of a lateral "hip" roll placed under the right hip. When the evidence was reviewed it indicated that a left lateral tilt of at least 20 to 30 degrees by placement of a lower lumbar hip roll is most effective in preventing SIH. Most often many practitioners will use a one-liter IV bag to facilitate LUD and this may not provide the LUD required to prevent SIH, and often they will place it under the hip as opposed to the lower lumbar region. The evidence clearly showed that at least 15 degrees of displacement must be provided by a wedge placed under the right lower lumbar region to provide reduction of SIH risk, and more displacement may be required in the obese patient. Another technique that is often used in combination with uterine displacement is lower limb compression provided by either passive or mechanical means. Studies have shown that using passive compression methods such as TEDs or Esmarch dressings to the lower extremities along with SCDs is most effective in preventing SIH when LUD is provided.

The controversy over preloading versus co-loading of a crystalloid solution prior to an SAB remains despite the evidence that indicates that crystalloid preloading does little to prevent SIH. The evidence clearly indicates that if a crystalloid solution is used to facilitate an expanded intravascular volume it should be administered at the time of the SAB injection using a rapid infusion technique to produce optimal results, and administration of a colloid as a preload or a co-load is most effective in preventing SIH. Administration of colloid volumes as small as 500 ml have been shown to be effective in preventing SIH, which is advantageous in a parturient who is fluid restricted such as a severe preeclamptic patient. Caution must be exercised if a synthetic colloid solution is used, especially if the patient has renal compromise or sepsis. An alternative to synthetic colloids is serum albumin, which can be administered as a 5% solution to most patients. Prior to administering albumin to patients the risks should be weighed against the benefits. Very limited research is available as to the detriment of using synthetic colloids in the parturient population and the withdrawal of synthetics from the hospital inventory is based on data from the critically ill septic patient; therefore more research is needed in this area as well.

Vasopressors will remain a mainstay in preventing and treating SIH. The evidence and recommendations from both anesthesia and obstetrics disciplines state that phenylephrine should be considered the first-line choice to treat and prevent SIH whereas ephedrine can be considered when the hypotension is also accompanied by bradycardia. Another class of medications that has shown some promise in helping attenuate SIH effects are the 5-HT3 antagonists. However, only small studies have been performed thus far using these agents and further research is required to determine if they are truly effective in decreasing SIH incidence and severity. The effect of positioning during placement of an SAB and its effect on SIH remains a controversial topic. Most practitioners report that they prefer placing the SAB with the parturient in the sitting position and the evidence is mixed regarding the value of sitting versus lateral positioning during SAB injection. To provide a more definitive answer a large, sufficiently powered, prospective study will need to be done.

Finally, the evidence overwhelmingly supports the use of lower limb extremity compression devices or techniques that should be used during the entire perioperative period, including during SAB injection. This includes the current recommended SCDs most commonly used for deep venous thrombosis (DVT) prophylaxis in all surgical patients.

CONCLUSIONS

SIH remains a significant problem in obstetrical anesthesia and there have been multiple studies and techniques evaluated to reduce the incidence and severity in the cesarean section population receiving an SAB. Whatever the preventive or treatment regimen used by the anesthesia provider, the most effective method to prevent and treat SIH is constant monitoring by the anesthesia professional and immediate treatment of any adverse effects during the performance of an anesthetic for cesarean section, which includes monitoring of not only the mother but the fetus as well.

REFERENCES

Allen, T. K., George, R. B., White, W. D., Muir, H. A., & Habib, A. S. (2010). A double-blind, placebo controlled trial of four fixed rate infusion regimens of phenylephrine for hemodynamic support during spinal anesthesia for cesarean delivery. *Anesthesia and Analgesia, 111*, 1221–1229.

Buley, R. J. R., Downing, J. W., Brock-Utne, J. G., & Cuerden, C. (1977). Right versus left lateral tilt for caesarean section. *British Journal of Anaesthesia, 49*(10), 1009–1015.

Bamber, J. H., & Dresner, M. (2003). Aortocaval compression n pregnancy: The effect of changing the degree and direction of lateral tilt on maternal cardiac output. *Anesthesia and Analgesia, 97*(1), 256–258.

Banerjee, A., Stocche, R. M., Angle, P., & Halpern, S. H. (2009). Pre-load or coload for spinal anesthesia for elective cesarean delivery: A meta-analysis. *Canadian Journal of Anesthesia, 57*(1), 24–31.

Bieniarz, J., Crottogini, J. J., Curuchet, E., Romero-Salinas, G., Yoshida, T., Poseiro, J. J., et al. (1968). Aortocaval compression by the uterus in late human pregnancy II. An arteriographic study. *American Journal of Obstetrics and Gynecology, 100*(2), 203–217.

Calvache, J. A., Munoz, M. F., & Baron, F. J. (2011). Hemodynamic effects of a right lumbar-pelvic wedge during spinal anesthesia for cesarean section. *International Journal of Obstetric Anesthesia, 18*(3), 307–311.

Carvalho, B., Mercier, F. J., Riley, E. T., Brummel, C., & Cohen, S. E. (2009). Hetastarch co-loading is as effective as pre-loading for the prevention of hypotension following spinal anesthesia for cesarean delivery. *International Journal of Obstetric Anesthesia, 18*(2), 150–155.

Chestnut, D. H., & Gibbs, C. P. (1991). Obstetric Anesthesia. In S. G, Gabbe, J. R, Niebyl & J. L, Simpson (Eds.), *Obstetrics normal and problem pregnancies* (2nd ed, p. 504). New York, NY: Churchill Livingstone.

Christensen, K. S., Trautnera, S., Stokela, M., & Nielsen, J. F. (1986). Inflatable splints: Do they cause tissue ischemia? *Injury, 17*(3), 167–170.

Clark, S. L., Cotton, D. B., & Lee, W. (1989). Central hemodynamic assessment of normal term pregnancy. *American Journal of Obstetrics and Gynecology, 161*, 1439–1442.

Crawford, J. S., Burton, M., & Davies, P. (1972). Time and lateral tilt at caesarean section. *British Journal of Anaesthesia, 44*, 477–484

Cyna, A. M., Andrew, M., Emmett, R. S., Middleton, P., & Simmons, S. W. (2006). Techniques for preventing hypotension during spinal anaesthesia for caesarean section. *Cochrane Database Systematic Review*, (4), CD002251.

Dahlgren, G., Granath, F., Wessel, H., & Irestedt, L. (2006). Prediction of hypotension during spinal anesthesia for cesarean section and its relation to the effect of crystalloid or colloid pre-load. *International Journal of Obstetric Anesthesia, 16*, 128–134.

Dhekne, R. D., Barron, B. J., & Koch, E. R. (1987). Radionuclide venography in pregnancy. *Journal of Nuclear Medicine, 28*, 1290–1293.

Doherty, A., Ohashi, Y., Downey, K., & Cavalho, J. C. (2012). Phenylephrine versus bolus regimens during delivery under spinal anesthesia: A double-blind randomized clinical trial to assess hemodynamic changes. *Anesthesia and Analgesia, 115*, 1343–1350.

Downing, J. W., Coleman, A. J., Mohemedy, M. C., Jeal, D. E., & Mohemedy, Y. H. (1974). Lateral table tilt for cesarean section. *Anaesthesia, 29*(6), 696–703.

Dyer, R. A., Farina, Z., Joubert, I. A., DuToit, P., Meyer, M., Torr, G., et al. (2004). Crystalloid preload versus rapid crystalloid administration after induction of spinal anesthesia (coload) for elective cesarean section. *Anaesthesia and Intensive Care, 32*(3), 351–357.

Dyer, R. A., Reed, A. R., Van Dyk, D., Arache, M. J., Hodges, O., Lombard, C. J., et al. (2009). Hemodynamic effects of ephedrine, phenylephrine, and the coadministration of pheynylpherine with oxytocin during spinal anesthesia for elective cesarean delivery. *Anesthesiology, 111*(4), 763–765.

French, G. W., White, J. B., Howell, S. J., & Popat, M. (1999). Comparison of pentastarch and hartmann's solution for volume pre-loading in spinal anaesthesia for elective caesarean section. *British Journal of Anaesthesia, 83*, 475–477.

Gao, L., Zheng, G., Han, J., Wang, Y., & Zheng, J. (2015). Effects of prophylactic ondansetron on spinal anesthesia-induced hypotension: A meta-analysis. *International Journal of Obstetric Anesthesia, 24*(4), 335–343.

Goodlin, R. C. (1971). Aortocaval compression during caesarean section. A cause of newborn depression. Obstetrics and Gynecology, 37(5), 702–705.

Goudie, T. A., Winter, A. W., & Ferguson, D. L. M. (1988). Lower limb compression using inflatable splints to prevent hypotension during spinal anesthesia. Acta Anaesthesiologica Scandinavica, 32, 541–544.

Greiss, F. C., & Crandell, D. L. (1965). Therapy for hypotension induced by spinal anesthesia during pregnancy. *Journal of the American Medical Association, 191*(10), 793–796.

Grewal, B. S., & Suir, I. (2009). Measured angle of tilt achieved by an inflatable balloon wedge: Is visual assessment a valid predictor? *International Journal of Obstetric Anesthesia, 18*(Suppl.), S40.

Gutsche, B. B. (1976). Prophylactic ephedrine preceding spinal analgesia for cesarean section. *Anesthesiology, 45*(4), 462–465.

Harvey, N. L., Hodgson, R. L., & Kinsella, S. M. (2013). Does body mass index influence the degree of pelvic tilt produced by a Crawford wedge. *International Journal of Obstetric Anesthesia, 22*(2), 129–132.

Hawkins, J. L., Arens, J. F., Bucklin, B. A., Connis, R. T., Dailey, P. A., Gambling, D. R., et al. (2007). Practice guidelines for obstetric anesthesia; An updated report by the American Society of Anesthesiologists Task Force on Obstetric Anesthesia and Analgesia. *Anesthesiology, 106*(4), 843–863.

Howard, B. K., Goodson, J. H., & Mengert, W. F. (1953). Supine hypotensive syndrome in late pregnancy. *Obstetrics & Gynecology, 1*(4), 371–377.

Inglis, A., Daniel, M., & McGrady, E. (1995). Maternal position during induction of spinal anaesthesia for caesarean section. A comparison of right lateral and sitting positions. *Anaesthesia, 50*(4), 363–365.

Jackson, R., Reid, J. A., & Thorburn, J. (1995). Volume pre-loading is not essential to prevent spinal induced hypotension at caesarean section. *British Journal of Anaesthesia, 75*(3), 262–265.

James, F. M., Greiss, F. C., & Kemp, R. A. (1970). An evaluation of vasopressor therapy for maternal hypotension during spinal anesthesia. *Anesthesiology, 33*(1), 25–34.

Kang, Y. G., Abouleish, E., & Cartis, S. (1982). Prophylactic intravenous ephedrine infusion during spinal anesthesia for cesarean section. *Anesthesia and Analgesia, 61*(10), 839–842.

Kenepp, N. B., Kumar, S., Shelly, W. C., Stanley, C. A., Gabbe, S. G., & Gutsche, B. B. (1982). Fetal and neonatal hazards of maternal hydration with 5% dextrose before caesarean section. *Lancet, 1*(8282), 1150–1152.

King, S. W., & Rosen, M. A. (1998). Prophylactic ephedrine and hypotension associated with spinal anesthesia for cesarean delivery. *International Journal of Obstetric Anesthesia, 7*(1), 18–22.

Kinsella, S. M., & Lohmann, G. (1994). Supine hypotensive syndrome. *Obstetrics & Gynecology, 83*(5), 774–778.

Kohler, F., Sorensen, F., & Helbo-Hansen, H. S. (2002). Effect of delayed supine positioning after induction of spinal anesthesia for caesarean section. *Acta Anaesthesiologica Scandinavica, 46*(4), 441–446.

Kundra. P, Velraj, J., Amirthalingam, U., Habeebullah, S., Yuvaraj, K., Elangovan, S., et al. (2012). Effect of positioning from supine and left lateral positions to left lateral tilt on maternal blood flow velocities and waveforms in full-term parturients. *Anaesthesia, 67*, 889–893.

Lee, H.-M., Kim, S.-H., Hwang, B.-Y., Yoo, B.-W., Koh, W.-U., Jang, D.-M., et al. (2016). The effects of prophylactic bolus phenylephrine on hypotension during low-dose spinal anesthesia for cesarean section. *International Journal of Obstetric Anesthesia, 25*, 17–22.

Lees, M. M., Schott, D. B., Kerr, M. G., & Taylor, S. H. (1967). The circulatory effects of recumbent postural change in late pregnancy. *Clinical Science, 32*(3), 453–465.

Li, L., Zhang, Y., Tan, Y., & Xu, S. (2013). Colloid or crystalloid solution on maternal and neonatal hemodynamics for cesarean section: A meta-analysis of randomized controlled trials. *Journal of Obstetrics and Gynaecology Research, 39*(5), 932–941.

Liu, S. S., & McDonald, S. B. (2001). Current issues in spinal anesthesia. *Anesthesiology, 94*(5), 888–906.

Loubert, C. (2012). Fluid and vasopressor management for cesarean delivery under spinal anesthesia: continuing professional development. *Canadian Journal of Anaesthesia, 59*(6), 604–619.

Mahajan, L., Anand, L. K., & Gombar, K. K. (2009). A randomized double-blind comparison of ephedrine, phenylephrine and mephentermine infusions to maintain blood pressure during spinal anaesthesia for cesarean delivery: The effects on fetal acid-base status and haemodynamic control. *Journal of Anaesthesiology Clinical Pharmacology, 25*(4), 427–432.

Malthru, M., Rao, T. L. K., Kartha, R. K., Radha, K., Shanmugham, M., & Jacobs, H. K. (1980). Intravenous albumin administration for prevention of spinal hypotension during cesarean section. *Anesthesia and Analgesia, 59*(9), 655–658.

Marx, G. F., Cosmi, E. V., & Wollman, S. B. (1969). Biochemical status and clinical condition of mother and infant at cesarean section. *Anesthesia and Analgesia, 48*(6), 986–993.

Mojica, J. L., Melendez, H. J., & Bautista, L. E. (2002). The timing of intravenous crystalloid administration and incidence of cardiovascular side effects during spinal anesthesia: The results from a randomized controlled trial. *Anesthesia and Analgesia, 94*(2), 432–437

Moran, D. H., Perillo, M., LaPorta, R. F., Bader, A. M., & Datta, S. (1991). Phenylephrine in the prevention of hypotension following spinal anesthesia for cesarean delivery. *Journal of Clinical Anesthesia, 3*(4), 301–305.

Ngan Kee, W. D., Khaw, K. S., Ng, F. F., & Lee, B. B. (2004). Prophylactic phenylephrine infusion for preventing hypotension during spinal anesthesia for cesarean delivery. *Anesthesia and Analgesia, 98*(3), 815–821.

Ngan Kee, W. D., Lee, A., Khaw, K. S., Ng, F. F., Karmakar, M. K., & Gin, T. (2008). A randomized double-blind comparison of phenylephrine and ephedrine infusion combinations to maintain blood pressure during spinal anesthesia for cesarean delivery the effects on fetal acid-base status and hemodynamic control. *Anesthesia and Analgesia, 107*(4), 1295–1302.

Obasuyi, B. I., Fyneface-Ogan, S., & Mato, C. N. (2013). A comparison of the haemodynamic effects of lateral and sitting positions during induction of spinal anesthesia for caesarean delivery. *International Journal of Obstetric Anesthesia, 22*(2), 124–128.

Oh, A.-Y., Huan, J.-W., Song, I.-A., Kim, M.-H., Ryu, J.-H., Park, H.-P., et al. (2014). Influence of the timing of administration of crystalloid on maternal hypotension during spinal anesthesia for cesarean delivery: Pre-load versus coload. *BMC Anesthesiology, 14*(36), 1–5.

Ortiz-Gomez, J. R., Palaciao-Abizanda, F. J., Morrillas-Ramirez, F., Fornet-Ruiz, A., Lorenzo-Jimenez, A., & Bermejo-Albares, M. L. (2014). The effect of intravenous ondansetron on maternal haemodynamics during elective caesarean delivery under spinal anesthesia: A double-blind, randomized, placebo-controlled trial. *International Journal of Obstetric Anesthesia, 23*(2), 138–143.

Owczuk, R., Wenski, W., Polak-Krzeminska, P., Twardowski, P., Arszulowicz, R., Dylczyk-Sommer, A., et al. (2008). Ondansetron given intravenously attenuates arterial blood pressure drop due to spinal anesthesia: A double-blind, placebo-controlled study. *Regional Anesthesia and Pain Medicine, 33*(4), 332–339.

Perner, A., Haase, N., Guterormsen, A. B., Britto, M. T., Hornung, R., Cassedy, A., et al. (2012). Hydroxyethyl starch 130/0.4.2 versus Ringer's acetate in severe sepsis. *New England Journal of Medicine, 367*(124), 124–134.

Ralston, D. H., Shnider, S. M., & deLorimier, A. A. (1974). Effects of equipotent ephedrine, metaraminol, mephentermine, and methoxamine on uterine blood flow in the pregnant ewe. *Anesthesiology, 40*(4), 354–370.

Ramanthan, S., & Grant, G. J. (1988). Vasopressor therapy for hypotension due to epidural anesthesia for cesarean section. Acta Anaesthesiologica Scandinavica, 32(7), 559–565.

Rashad, M. M., & Farmawy, M. S. (2013). Effects of intravenous ondansetron and granisetron on hemodynamic changes and motor and sensory blockade induced by spinal anesthesia in parturients undergoing a cesarean section. *Egyptian Journal of Anaesthesia, 29*(4), 369–374.

Rees, S. G. O., Thurlow, J. A., Gardner, I. C. D., Scrutton, M. J. L., & Kinsella, S. M. (2002). Maternal cardiovascular consequences of positioning after spinal anesthesia for Cesarean section: Left 15 degree table tilt vs. left lateral. *Anaesthesia, 57*(1), 15–20.

Riley, E. T., Cohen, S. E., Rubenstien, A. J., & Flanagan, B. (1995). Prevention of hypotension after spinal anesthesia for cesarean section: Six percent hetastarch versus lactated ringer's solution. *Anesthesia and Analgesia, 81*(4), 838–842.

Rout, C. C., Rocke, D. A., & Gouws, E. (1993). Leg elevation and wrapping in the prevention of spinal hypotension following spinal anesthesia in elective caesarean section. *Anaesthesia, 48*(4), 304–308.

Rout, C. C., Rocke, D. A., Levin, J., Gouws, E., & Reddy, D. (1993). A reevaluation of the role of crystalloid pre-load in the prevention of hypotension associated with spinal anesthesia for elective cesarean section. *Anesthesiology, 79*(2), 262–269.

Russell, R., Popat, M., Richards, E., & Burry, J. (2002). Combined spinal epidural anaesthesia for caesarean section: A randomized comparison of oxford, lateral and sitting positions. *International Journal of Obstetric Anesthesia, 11*(3), 190–195.

Sahoo, T., SenDasgupta, C., Goswami, A., & Hazra, A. (2012). Reduction in spinal-induced hypotension with ondansetron in parturients undergoing caesarean section: A double-blind randomized, placebo-controlled study. *International Journal of Obstetric Anesthesia, 2,* 24–28.

Salo, L. M., Woods, R. L., Anderson, C. R., & McAllen, R. M. (2007). Nonuniformity in the von Bezold-Jarisch reflex. *American Journal of Physiology Regulatory, Integrative and Comparative Physiology, 293*(2), 714–720.

Scott, D. B., & Kerr, M. G. (1963). Inferior vena caval pressure in late pregnancy. *British Journal of Obstetrics and Gynaecology, 70*(6), 1044–1049.

Shibli, K. U., & Russell, I. F. (2000). A survey of anaesthetic techniques used for caesarean section in the UK in 1997. *International Journal of Obstetric Anesthesia, 9*(3), 160–167.

Shnider, S. M., Lorimier, A. A., Holl, J. W., Chapler, F. K., & Morishima, H. O. (1968). Vasopressors in obstetrics. I. Correction of fetal acidosis with ephedrine during spinal hypotension. *American Journal of Obstetrics & Gynecology, 102*(7), 911–919.

Siddick, S. M., Aouad, M. T., Kai, G. E., Sfeir, M. M., & Baraka, A. S. (2000). Hydroxyethylstarch 10% is superior to ringer's solution for pre-loading before spinal anesthesia for cesarean section. *Canadian Journal of Anesthesia, 47*(7), 616–621.

Sood, P. K., Cooper, P. J., Michel, M. Z., Wee, M. Y., & Pickering, R. M. (1996). Thromboembolic deterrent stockings fail to prevent hypotension associated with spinal anaesthesia for elective caesarean section. *International Journal of Obstetric Anesthesia, 5*(3), 172–175.

Sujata, N., Arora, D., Panigrahi, B. P., & Hanjorra, V. M. (2012). A sequential compression mechanical pump to prevent hypotension during elective cesarean section under spinal anesthesia. *International Journal of Obstetric Anesthesia, 21*(2), 140–145.

Teoh, W. H. L., & Sia, A. T. H. (2009). Colloid pre-load versus coload for spinal anesthesia for cesarean delivery: The effects on maternal cardiac output. *Anesthesia and Analgesia, 108*(5), 1592–1598.

Ueyama, H., Yan-Ling, H., Tanigami, H., Mashimo, T., & Yoshiya, I. (1999). Effects of crystalloid and colloid pre-load on blood volume in the parturient undergoing spinal anesthesia for elective cesarean section. *Anesthesiology, 91*(6), 1571–1576.

Van De Velde, M. (2013). Belgian guidelines for safe regional anesthesia and obstetric anesthesia and analgesia. *Acta Anaesthesiolgica Belgica, 64*(3), 95–96.

Veeser, M., Hofmann, T., Roth, R., Klohr, S., Rossaint, R., & Heesen, M. (2012). Vasopressors for the management of hypotension after spinal anesthesia for elective caesarean section. Systematic review and cumulative meta-analysis. *Acta Anaesthesiolgica Scandinavica, 56*(7), 810–816.

Wang, Q., Zhuo, L., Shen, M. K., Yu, Y. Y., Yu, J. J., & Wang, M. (2014). Ondansetron pre-loading with crystalloid infusion reduces maternal hypotension during cesarean section. *American Journal of Perinatology, 31*(10), 913–921.

Williamson, W., Burks, D., Pipkin, J., Burkard, J. F., Osborne, L. A., & Pellegrini, J. E. (2009). Effect of timing of fluid bolus on reduction of spinal-induced hypotension in patients undergoing elective cesarean section. *American Association of Nurse Anesthetists Journal*, 77(2), 130–136.

Wollman, S. B., & Marx, G. F. (1968). Acute hydration for prevention of hypotension of spinal anesthesia in parturients. *Anesthesiology, 29*(2), 374–380.

Wong, C. A., Nathan, N., & Brown, D. L. (2009). Spinal, epidural and caudal anesthesia: Anatomy, physiology and technique. In D. H. Chestnut, L. S. Polley, L. C. Tsen, & C. A. Wong (Eds.), *Obstetric anesthesia, principles and practice* (4th ed., pp. 223–245). Philadelphia, PA: Mosby.

Yamano, M., Ito, H., Kamato, T., & Miyata, K. (1995). Characteristics of inhibitory effects of serotonin (5-HT) 3 – receptor antagonists, YM060 and YM114 (KAE-393), on the von Bezold-Jarisch reflex induced by 2-Methyl-5HT, veratridine and electrical stimulation of vagus nerves in rats. *Japan Journal of Pharmacology, 69*(4), 351–356.

Yun, E. S., Marx, G. F., & Santos, A. C. (1998). The effects of maternal position during induction of combined spinal-epidural anesthesia for cesarean delivery. *Anesthesia and Analgesia, 87*(4), 614–618.

Zhou, Z. Q., Shao, Q., Zeng, Q., Song, J., & Yang, J. J. (2008). Lumbar wedge versus pelvic wedge in preventing hypotension following combined spinal epidural anaesthesia for caesarean delivery. *Anesthesia & Intensive Care, 36*(6), 835–839.

CHAPTER 10

Forced-Air Warmers and Surgical Site Infections in Patients Undergoing Knee or Hip Arthroplasty

Paul N. Austin

ABSTRACT

The majority of the evidence indicates preventing inadvertent perioperative hypothermia reduces the incidence of many perioperative complications. Among the results of inadvertent perioperative hypothermia are increased bleeding, myocardial events, impaired wound healing, and diminished renal function. Most researchers agree there is an increased incidence of surgical site infections in patients who experience inadvertent perioperative hypothermia.

Forced-air warming is effective in preventing inadvertent perioperative hypothermia. Paradoxically, forced-air warmers have been implicated in causing surgical site infections in patients undergoing total knee or hip arthroplasty. The results of investigations suggest these devices harbor pathogens and cause unwanted airflow disturbances. However, no significant increases in bacterial counts were found when forced-air warmers were used according to the manufacturer's directions. The results of one study suggested the incidence of surgical

http://dx.doi.org/10.1891/0739-6686.35.179

site infections in patients undergoing total joint arthroplasty was increased when using a forced-air warmer. However these researchers did not control for other factors affecting the incidence of surgical site infections in these patients.

Current evidence does not support forced-air warmers causing surgical site infections in patients undergoing total knee or hip arthroplasty. Clinicians must use and maintain these devices as per the manufacturer's directions. They may consider using alternative warming methods. Well-conducted studies are needed to help determine the role of forced-air warmers in causing infections in these patients.

INTRODUCTION

Many agree inadvertent perioperative hypothermia leads to complications including surgical site infections (Schmied, Kurz, Sessler, Kozek, & Reiter, 1996; Scott & Buckland, 2006). Forced-air warmers are often used perioperatively to prevent inadvertent perioperative hypothermia. The use of these devices is described in various clinical practice guidelines (Association of periOperative Registered Nurses [AORN], 2016; Hooper et al., 2010; National Collaborating Centre for Nursing and Supportive Care [NCC-NSC], 2008). Some have questioned the role of forced-air warmers in causing surgical site infections, particularly in patients undergoing total joint arthroplasty (Augustine, 2014). Discussions in trade journals of this alleged problem and resulting lawsuits have caused concern (Gapinski, 2015). This review examines inadvertent perioperative hypothermia, the role of forced-air warmers in preventing inadvertent perioperative hypothermia, and the role of forced-air warmers in surgical site infections in patients undergoing total knee or hip arthroplasty.

INADVERTENT PERIOPERATIVE HYPOTHERMIA

Definition and Incidence

Hypothermia is often defined as a body temperature less than or equal to 36°C (96.8°F; Hooper et al., 2010). The overall incidence of inadvertent perioperative hypothermia is hard to determine. The incidence of inadvertent perioperative hypothermia in patients undergoing total hip or knee arthroplasty has been reported to be approximately 27% (Leijtens, Koëter, Kremers &, Koëter, 2013). A group from China examined data from 830 patients who received general anesthesia for a variety of surgical procedures randomly selected from 24 hospitals in Beijing and found an overall incidence of inadvertent perioperative hypothermia of 39.9% with only 10.7% of patients receiving intraoperative warming (Yi et al., 2015). In addition, approximately 30% of over 3,000 operating nurse survey respondents indicated prevention of inadvertent perioperative hypothermia was a high priority (Steelman, Graling, & Perkhounkova, 2013).

Complications Resulting From Inadvertent Perioperative Hypothermia

Serious complications may result from inadvertent perioperative hypothermia. Most agree the complications due to inadvertent perioperative hypothermia include increased bleeding (Schmied, Kurz, Sessler, Kozek, & Reiter, 1996) and an increased risk of myocardial ischemia (Frank et al., 1997). Inadvertent perioperative hypothermia may also lead to an increased incidence of surgical site infections (Scott & Buckland, 2006).

Inadvertent Perioperative Hypothermia and Surgical Site Infection

Results of investigations suggest inadvertent perioperative hypothermia leads to a greater risk of surgical site infection. Authors of a systematic review of 26 randomized clinical studies reported hypothermic subjects had an increased risk of developing a surgical site infection (Scott & Buckland, 2006). For example, the authors of a randomized controlled trial included in that systematic review found an increased risk of surgical site infections when the patient experienced inadvertent perioperative hypothermia: In that study, 19% of subjects undergoing colorectal surgery who suffered inadvertent perioperative hypothermia had a surgical site infection compared with 6% of normothermic subjects (Kurz, Sessler, & Lenhardt, 1996). Authors of another randomized controlled trial included in that review reported that for subjects undergoing surgeries with minimal risk of infection (breast, hernia, varicose vein) who were actively warmed preoperatively, 14% of non-prewarmed subjects developed a surgical site infection compared with 5% of prewarmed subjects (p = .001; Melling, Ali, Scott, & Leaper, 2001).

Some investigators reported inadvertent perioperative hypothermia was not associated with surgical site infection. The results of a descriptive study involving over 1,000 subjects suggested there was no relationship between inadvertent perioperative hypothermia and surgical site infections (Melton et al., 2013). The results of a retrospective review of data from 79 patients undergoing colorectal surgery indicated body temperatures less than 36°C (96.8°F) may be protective in preventing surgical site infections; however, the difference in surgical site infections between the group experiencing perioperative hypothermia and the normothermic did not reach statistical significance (p = .062; Geiger et al., 2012). However, inferring causality is difficult as the study was retrospective. A retrospective study of pediatric spinal surgery subjects also indicated hypothermia was protective against surgical site infections

(Linam et al., 2009). The authors of the AORN clinical practice guideline for preventing inadvertent perioperative hypothermia (2016) named inconsistent methods of temperature monitoring as a possible cause of the disagreement between studies. In addition, some investigators used body temperature <35°C (95°F) rather than <36°C (96.8°F) as the definition of inadvertent perioperative hypothermia (AORN, 2016). The AORN (2016) recommends monitoring temperature at core or "near-core" sites in patients at risk for inadvertent perioperative hypothermia.

Clinical practice guidelines call for maintaining normothermia as a method of preventing surgical site infections despite the conflicting evidence. These include guidelines from the AORN (2016), the American Society of PeriAnesthesia Nurses (Hooper et al., 2010), and the Association for Professionals in Infection Control and Epidemiology (APIC, 2010). The Institute for Healthcare Improvement (2012) suggests preventing hypothermia for patients undergoing colorectal surgery. In addition, the NCC-NSC (2008) in the United Kingdom also calls for preventing surgical site infections by maintaining normothermia.

THE ROLE OF FORCED-AIR WARMERS IN PREVENTING INADVERTENT PERIOPERATIVE HYPOTHERMIA

Forced-air warming for perioperative patients was introduced into practice in the United States over 20 years ago (Augustine, 1991). The majority of the evidence supported using forced-air warmers to prevent inadvertent perioperative hypothermia (AORN, 2016). A brief review of this evidence is as follows.

Evidence Supporting the Use of Forced-Air Warmers to Prevent Inadvertent Perioperative Hypothermia

The evidence supporting using forced-air warmers to prevent inadvertent perioperative hypothermia includes a 2009 systematic review of 14 randomized controlled trials. The authors concluded forced-air warmers as well as carbon-fiber blankets prevent inadvertent perioperative hypothermia (Galvao, Marck, Sawada, & Clark, 2009). Four subsequently published studies examining subjects who underwent total knee arthroplasty (Kim et al., 2009; Trentman, Weinmeister, Hentz, Laney, & Simula, 2009), shoulder arthroscopy (Yoo, Park, Yi, Kwon, & Rhee, 2009), and laparoscopic abdominal surgery (Pu et al., 2014) also supported the efficacy of forced-air warmers. Authors of a 2011 evidence synthesis also found forced-air warming is effective in preventing inadvertent perioperative hypothermia (Moola & Lockwood, 2011).

Alternatives to Forced-Air Warmers

Others have shown alternatives to the forced-air warmer may be as or more effective in preventing inadvertent perioperative hypothermia. Some have suggested resistive heating blanket (Tanaka et al., 2013), using a passive insulation system (Rathinam, Annam, Steyn, & Raghuraman, 2009), and an electric heating blanket (Ng, Lai, & Ho, 2006) are as effective as forced-air warmers. Resistive polymer heating blankets have also been found to be as effective as forced-air warmers (Brandt et al., 2010; Kimberger et al., 2008). Other devices may be even more effective than forced-air warmers. These include circulating water garments (Galvao, Liang, & Clark, 2010), direct heat conduction thermal pads (Calcaterra et al., 2009), and circulating water garments combined with a water mattress (Hasegawa, Negishi, Nakagawa, & Ozaki, 2012). One of the greatest barriers to using these devices is the cost for facilities currently using forced-air warmers, difficulty in using with certain surgical procedures, and user inconvenience.

Recommendations From Clinical Practice Guidelines

Authors of many clinical practice guidelines found the evidence supports the use of forced-air warmers as per the manufacturer's directions. These groups include the AORN (2016), Society of PeriAnesthesia Nurses (Hooper et al., 2010), and the National Collaborating Centre for Nursing and Supportive Care (2008). However, there has recently been a concern that using forced-air warmers for patients undergoing total joint arthroplasty is linked to surgical site infections (Augustine, 2014).

TOTAL KNEE AND HIP ARTHROPLASTY INFECTIONS AND FORCED-AIR WARMERS

Over 700,000 total knee and 300,000 total hip arthroplasties are performed annually in the United States (National Center for Health Statistics, 2010). The incidence of surgical site infection following these surgeries is approximately 0.5% to 2.4%. Some factors have been proposed that increase the risk of surgical site infection after total knee and hip arthroplasty. These are classified as patient- (e.g., carrying *Staphylococcus aureus*, smoking, male gender, morbid obesity, diabetes, and rheumatoid arthritis) or procedure-specific (e.g., low volume surgeon). The risk factors may be modifiable (e.g., smoking) or nonmodifiable (e.g., male gender); see APIC (2010) and Zhu et al. (2015).

Infections of knee and hip prosthetic joints are often catastrophic. Treatment may involve removing the infected prosthesis and debridement of surrounding tissue. A new prosthesis is not implanted at that time resulting in additional pain and immobility. If the infection is eradicated, the patient has to undergo a third operation to implant a replacement prosthesis. The patient is at increased risk for morbidity and mortality from not only the infected prosthesis but also prolonged immobility and additional surgical procedures (APIC, 2010; Matar et al., 2010).

Biofilm plays an important role in prosthetic hip and knee infections (Song et al., 2013). Biofilm, microorganisms enclosed in a polysaccharide matrix produced by the organisms, adheres to solid surfaces of the body or to implanted prostheses. Biofilm has been shown to readily form on hip and knee prostheses. The biofilm makes is very difficult for antibiotics and the immune system to access and treat bacteria embedded in the biofilm. Bacteria traveling on microscopic particles in the air can seed the wound leading to prosthesis infection involving the formation of biofilm (Song et al., 2013). Proposed mechanisms of this seeding include deposition of harbored microorganisms and causing unwanted airflow disturbances (Augustine, 2014).

Evidence Addressing Forced-Air Warmers as a Cause of Surgical Site Infections

The relationship between forced-air warmers and surgical site infections has been reviewed by the author's group (Kellam, Dieckmann, & Austin, 2013) and others (ECRI Institute, 2013; Sikka & Prielipp, 2014; Wood, Moss, Keenan, Reed, & Leaper, 2014). Investigators used four methods examining the relationship between forced-air warmers and surgical site infections. These were culturing forced-air warmers to determine if they harbor pathogens and investigating if forced-air warmers cause unwanted airflow disturbances that impair the effect of operating room ventilation systems that promote the flow of filtered air toward the surgical field. Other methods included culturing areas near or on patients, manikins or volunteers in real or simulated settings, and examining the incidence of surgical site infections.

Most of the studies suffered from methodological concerns. Some may have been underpowered as none of the investigators described how they determined the sample size of forced-air warmers or subjects. None described maintaining and using the forced-air warmer according to the manufacturer's directions. There was also no random allocation or blinding.

Forced-Air Warmers Harboring Pathogens

Forced-air warmers may harbor bacteria (Table 10.1). Researchers used methods including swabbing the surface of the forced-air warmer, filters, and air path surfaces (Albrecht, Gauthier, & Leaper, 2009; Albrecht, Gauthier, Belani,

TABLE 10.1

Summary of Evidence From Sources Examining the Intake, Air Path, Output Hose, or the Air Emitting Directly From the Forced-Air Warmer Device for Bacteria or Particles

Evidence Source[a]	Number of Devices Examined Culture Locations	Findings	Comments[b]
Avidan et al. (1997)	10[c] Multiple locations	4/10 FAWs: growth from air from output hose 10/10: no growth from air from perforated FAW blanket Upstream side of filter evidence of colonization No growth when output hose fitted with filter[d]	Organisms included *Staphylococcus epidermis* FAWs from various ORs Fitting outlet hose with filter may prevent emission of bacteria from FAW
Baker, King, and Smith (2002)	1[e] Interior and exterior of FAW and inside of output hose	"Heavy growth" of bacteria from all sites	
Bernards, Harinck, Dijkshoorn, van der Reijden, and van den Broek (2004)	1[f] Exterior and internal FAW filters	Same strain of *Acinetobacter baumanii* causing outbreak, organism not cultured after removal of dust inside FAW	Part of investigation of *Acinetobacter baumanii* outbreak in a medical ICU
Albrecht, Gauthier, and Leaper (2009)	25 FAWs[g] from 5 hospitals Air from intake and output hoses, interior of intake and output hoses	8/25 FAW: lower filtration efficiencies 17 FAWs: bacteria cultured from inside of 71% of intake and 88% of output hoses 9 FAWs: 89% cultures positive from liquid from rinsing inside of output hose	Implied FAWs emitting internally generated contamination within the size range of free floating bacteria (<4 μm)

(*Continued*)

TABLE 10.1

Summary of Evidence From Sources Examining the Intake, Air Path, Output Hose, or the Air Emitting Directly From the Forced-Air Warmer Device for Bacteria or Particles (Continued)

Evidence Source[a]	Number of Devices Examined Culture Locations	Findings	Comments[b]
Albrecht, Gauthier, Belani, Litchy, and Leaper (2011)	5 new intake filters[f] 5 used intake filters[f] 52 FAWs[f]: internal air path surfaces, hose outlet particle counts	Newer filters: retention efficiency of 93.8% Used filters: had 61.3% efficiency 92.3% of FAWs had bacteria cultured from internal air path surfaces	Increased efficiency of new filters may be due to design change About 50% FAWs likely internally generating and emitting airborne contaminants
Reed, Kimberger, McGovern, and Albrecht (2013)	5 new intake filters 23 used intake filters 23 FAWs	Mean efficiency 63.8% Performed within specification 95% of FAWs generated significant levels of contamination >0.3 μm in size 70% of FAWs had hose-end airflows with higher contamination levels than in intake airflows 100% of FAWs: viable microorganisms swabbed from internal air path	Unknown if the FAWs were maintained as per manufacturer recommendations Coverlet not used when sampling outflow

Note. FAW = forced-air warmer; ICU = intensive care unit; OR = operating room.

[a]All studies were Level IV (C) quasi-experimental studies (Stetler et al., 1998). [b]No mention of sample size calculation or if FAWs were maintained according to manufacturer's directions. [c]9 Bair Huggers (Arizant Healthcare, Eden Prairie, MN), 1 Warm Touch (Mallinkrodt Medical, St Louis, MO). [d]DAR Hygroback filter (Covidien Respiratory and Monitoring Solutions, Boulder, CO) for breathing systems. [e]WarmAir (Cincinnati Sub-Zero, Cincinnati, OH). [f]Bair Hugger (Arizant Healthcare, Eden Prairie, MN). [g]Unknown FAW manufacturer.

Source: From Kellam, Dieckmann, and Austin (2013).

Litchy, & Leaper, 2011; Avidan et al., 1997; Baker, King, & Smith, 2002; Bernards, Harinck, Dijkshoorn, van der Reijden, & van den Broek, 2004; Reed, Kimberger, McGovern, & Albrecht, 2013). Other methods include counting hose outlet particles (Albrecht et al., 2011), examining bacterial emission from the forced-air warmer coverlet (Avidan et al., 1997), and determining if parts of the subject's body coming into contact with the forced-air warmer coverlet had increased bacterial counts (Huang, Shah, Vinodkumar, Hegarty, & Greatorex, 2003). Importantly, the results of the studies looking at bacterial counts when used as per the manufacturer's directions with the appropriate coverlet suggested that no bacteria emitted from the coverlet (Avidan et al., 1997) and bacterial counts on areas of the body in the path of air from the coverlet did not increase (Huang et al., 2003).

Forced-Air Warmers Causing Unwanted Airflow Disturbances

Total joint arthroplasties are often performed in operating rooms fitted with air handling systems that supply a constant laminar flow of filtered air flowing toward the surgical field. The flow may be vertical or horizontal. Laminar flow is thought to decrease the likelihood of particles such as dust, lint, or skin cells containing bacteria being deposited in the wound. However, some have questioned the value of laminar flow, given the high cost of these units and its marginal effectiveness when proper rates of operating room air exchange are maintained and antibiotic prophylaxis is administered (Kapadia et al., 2013).

Five groups of investigators (Belani, Albrecht, McGovern, Reed, & Nachtsheim, 2012; Dasari, Albrecht, & Harper, 2012; Legg, Cannon, & Hamer, 2012; Legg & Hamer, 2013; McGovern et al., 2011) determined that forced-air warmers disrupt laminar flow (Table 10.2) and the photos illustrating how forced-air warmers disrupt laminar flow are dramatic. The results of two other investigations suggested forced-air warmers did not produce unwanted disruptions in laminar flow (Sessler, Olmsted, & Kuelpmann, 2011; Sharp, Chesworth, & Fern, 2002). These studies contain serious limitations. All were performed in a simulated setting where all personnel were motionless. The scrubbed surgical team constantly moves in the path of the laminar airflow during actual operations. Additionally, laminar flow is disrupted by normal operating room traffic such as opening and closing the operating room door. These limitations, along with the questionable value of laminar flow in preventing surgical site infections in patients undergoing total joint arthroplasty (Kapadia et al., 2013), make it difficult to conclude the use of forced-air warmers increases surgical site infections due to causing unwanted airflow disturbances.

TABLE 10.2

Summary of Evidence Sources Examining Unwanted Airflow Disturbances in the Operating Room Due to the Forced-Air Warmer

Evidence Source[a]	Setting Subjects Intervention	Assessment of Airflow Disturbance	Findings	Comments[b]
Sharp, Chesworth, and Fern (2002)	Laminar flow ultra-clean-air-ventilated OR (Howorth enclosure) 12 different conditions ranging from empty OR to 4 different volunteers on OR table covered with FAW[c] blanket	Smoke test	No significant effect on OR airflow with FAW[b] unit on or off	
McGovern et al. (2011)	Laminar flow ultra-clean-air-ventilated OR (Howorth enclosure) Draped manikin simulating hip replacement (repeated once) and draped lumbar spinal procedure (not repeated) Upper or lower body FAW[d] coverlet or torso conductive fabric blanket[e]	Neutral-buoyancy detergent bubbles released near manikin head or near floor Area near surgical site observed	Air currents with FAW on were more toward the surgical site compared with conductive fabric	Single surgeon and anesthesia provider but no OR traffic
Sessler, Olmsted, and Kuelpmann (2011)	2 laminar flow ORs Volunteer draped patient Warmed manikins represented surgical team FAW[d] with upper body cover or underbody blanket	Smoke with visual tracer	FAW with upper body cover or underbody blanket: no impairment in laminar flow and unwanted airflow disturbances	No OR traffic

Legg, Cannon, and Hamer (2012)	Laminar flow ultra-clean-air-ventilated OR (Howorth enclosure) 1 draped volunteer simulating lower limb procedure Torso FAW[d] cover or torso conductive fabric blanket[e]	Particle counts (size 0.3, 0.5, 5 µm) 10 cm over surgical site	Particle counts increased with FAW compared with conductive fiber blanket (p = .0038 to .0087)	Wall extensions used to maximize airflow Surgeon present with hood and body exhaust system No other team member present
Dasari, Albrecht, and Harper (2012)	Laminar flow ultra-clean-air-ventilated OR (Howorth enclosure) Manikin draped for abdominal operation Lower body FAW[d], overbody conductive fiber blanket[e], underbody resistive blanket[f]	Air temperature measured 5 heights including floor, table, patient, ceiling at 5 locations including surgical site	Greater increase in temperature over surgical site with FAW (+2.73°C) higher compared with conductive fiber blanket (+2.73°C) or resistive blanket (+3.63°C)	Based on changes in air temperature at various locations, authors concluded FAW generates convection currents near surgical site and may produce unwanted airflow disturbances
Belani, Albrecht, McGovern, Reed, and Nachtsheim (2013)	Downward displacement ventilated OR Manikin draped for total knee replacement FAW[d] with torso cover, torso conductive fiber blanket[e], no warming device Experiment repeated once	Neutral-buoyancy detergent bubbles released under drape near head of manikin, sampled over surgical site	Increase in average bubble counts over surgical site with FAW (132.5) compared with conductive fiber blanket (0.48); $p < .003$	Motionless anesthesia provider at head of table No simulated OR team or traffic

(*Continued*)

TABLE 10.2

Summary of Evidence Sources Examining Unwanted Airflow Disturbances in the Operating Room Due to the Forced-Air Warmer (Continued)

Evidence Source[a]	Setting Subjects Intervention	Assessment of Airflow Disturbance	Findings	Comments[b]
Legg and Hamer (2013)	Laminar flow ultra-clean-air-ventilated OR (Howorth enclosure) Manikin draped for total knee replacement Torso FAW[d] cover or torso conductive fabric blanket[e]	Neutral-buoyancy helium soap bubbles	Air currents generated from increased temperature of the surgical side of the drape FAW: 174,000 particles/m^3 Conductive fiber blanket: 1,000 particles/m^3 Control: 2,000 particles/m^3	Scrubbed surgeon present

Note. FAW = forced-air warmer; OR = operating room.

[a]All studies were Level IV (C) quasi-experimental studies (Stetler et al., 1998). [b]No mention of sample size calculation or if FAWs were maintained according to manufacturer's directions. [c]Warm Touch (Mallinkrodt Medical, St Louis, MO). [d]Bair Hugger (Arizant Healthcare, Eden Prairie, MN). [e]Hot Dog (Augustine Temperature Management, Eden Prairie, MN). [f]Initherm (OTM1, Rotherham, UK).

Source: From Kellam, Dieckmann, and Austin (2013).

Comparing Bacterial Counts Near or on Patients or Volunteers in Real or Simulated Settings

Five groups of investigators examined bacterial counts near or on patients or volunteers when forced-air warmers were used in the operating room (Huang et al., 2003; Moretti et al., 2009; Sharp et al., 2002; Tumia & Ashcroft, 2002; Zink & Iaizzo, 1993; Table 10.3). One group found bacterial loads were increased at various locations near the operating room table when forced-air warming was used, but that increase was similar to or lower than the bacterial load detected when the patient was placed on the operating room table (Moretti et al., 2009). The others found no increase in bacterial loads near or on patients or volunteers when using a forced-air warmer (Huang et al., 2003; Moretti et al., 2009; Sharp et al., 2002; Tumia & Ashcroft, 2002; Zink & Iaizzo, 1993). The forced-air warmers were used with a coverlet as per the manufacturer's directions.

Incidence of Surgical Site Infections in Subjects Warmed With and Without the Use of a Forced-Air Warmer

The results of an adequately powered well-conducted interventional or observational study could help determine the role of forced-air warmers in causing surgical site infections. Unfortunately, investigators have not conducted such a study. Three groups of investigators sought to determine if the use of forced-air warmers increased the risk of surgical site infections (Huang et al., 2003; McGovern et al., 2011; Moretti et al., 2009; Table 10.4). Two groups found no increase in surgical site infections in subjects where forced-air warmers were used perioperatively. The first group of investigators included a small ($n = 16$) sample of vascular surgery patients who were followed up to 6 months postoperatively (Huang et al., 2003). The second group examined 30 subjects undergoing total hip arthroplasty (Moretti et al., 2009). The third group conducted an observational study that included a large ($n = 1,437$) sample of subjects undergoing total knee or hip arthroplasty. Three hundred seventy-one subjects were warmed using a conductive fiber blanket and the remainder with a forced-air warmer. They found subjects who were warmed using a forced-air warmer had a significantly greater risk of developing a deep wound infection (odds ratio, 3.8; $p = .024$). There were multiple methodological concerns including no records of incontinency, blood transfusion, or overall physical status. Surgical antibiotic prophylaxis was changed partway through the trial. There was no control for potentially confounding factors such as factors that may predispose total knee or hip patients to surgical site infections. Thus, history may have played a role in the results as the study was conducted over a two-year period (McGovern et al., 2011).

TABLE 10.3

Summary of Evidence Sources Examining Bacterial Counts Near or on Patients, Volunteers, or Manikins in an Operating Room When a Forced-Air Warmer Was Used in a Real or Simulated Setting

Evidence Source[a]	Setting Subjects Intervention	Site(s) Sampled	Findings	Comments[b]
Zink and Iaizzo (1993)	3 ORs 9 draped volunteer simulated patients Lower body FAW[c] blanket 2 study periods (2 hours FAW off, 2 hours FAW on)	Abdomen	No difference in total number of bacterial colonies between 2 study periods More coagulase negative colonies when FAW off ($p < .05$)	Presumed OR air handling met standards Volunteers had normal skin and not taking antibiotics Skin not prepped No surgical team/traffic in OR
Sharp, Chesworth, and Fern (2002)	Laminar flow ultra-clean-air-ventilated OR 12 different conditions ranging from empty OR to 4 different volunteers on OR table covered with FAW[d] blanket with unit on and off	30 cm from simulated operating site	No detectable airborne contamination at sample site with any condition	Pilot study found low levels of CFU/m^3 3 of 4 volunteers had psoriasis of varying degrees No surgical team or traffic in the OR
Tumia and Ashcroft (2002)	2 ultra-clean-air-ventilated ORs 2 collection periods with empty OR 4 collection periods with orthopedic cases FAW[e] cover (unknown location) applied to patient	Close to middle of OR, 1 m off floor	Nonsignificant increase in CFU with FAW on ($p = .48$) compared to when off	Unknown patient characteristics

Huang, Shah, Vinodkumar, Hegarty, and Greatorex (2003)	Unknown number of ORs 16 patients undergoing aortic surgery with prosthetic graft (mean 234 minutes, range 180–270 minutes) FAW[c] with upper body cover	6 sites including around the OR, near axilla, wound edge, FAW[c] filter and output hose at various times during case	Significant decrease in colony counts at sites around OR and near axilla FAW filter and wound edge sterile	No mention of air handling method used in the OR, presumed met standards
Moretti et al. (2009)	Unknown number of ORs 30 hip arthroplasty patients 20 of these had a FAW[c] cover placed (mean procedure time 90 minutes)	6 sites including around the OR, near axilla, wound edge, FAW[c] filter and output hose at various times during case	While bacterial loads increased at some but not all locations near the OR table with use of FAW, the increase was comparable to or lower than the load present at time of placement of patient on OR table	

Note. CFU, colony forming units; FAW, forced-air warmer; OR, operating room.

[a]All studies were Level IV (C) quasi-experimental studies (Stetler et al., 1998). [b]No mention of sample size calculation or if FAWs were maintained according to manufacturer's directions. [c]Bair Hugger (Arizant Healthcare Medical, Eden Prairie, MN). [d]Warm Touch (Mallinkrodt Medical, St Louis, MO). [e]Unknown FAW manufacturer.

Source: From Kellam, Dieckmann, and Austin (2013).

TABLE 10.4

Incidence of Infection in Patients Who Were Warmed Intraoperatively Using a Forced-Air Warmer

Evidence Source[a]	Subjects and Procedure Intervention	Findings and Comments[c]
Huang et al. (2003)	16, aortic surgery with graft Forced-air warmer[b] with upper body cover (mean 234 minutes)	No postoperative surgical site infections at 6 months postop
Moretti et al. (2009)	30, hip replacement 20 forced-air warmer[b] cover placed (mean 90 minutes), 10 no forced-air warmer	No postoperative surgical site infections, unknown follow-up period Unknown location of forced-air warmer cover
McGovern et al. (2011)	1,437, hip or knee replacement Forced-air warmer[b] 1,066 Conductive fiber blanket[d] 371	Increased risk for developing deep infections great for subjects warmed with forced-air warmer (odds ratio 3.8, $p = .024$) No impact of factors such as age, diabetes No records on blood transfusions, incontinency, and overall physical status

[a]All studies were Level IV (C) quasi-experimental studies (Stetler et al., 1998). [b]Bair Hugger (Arizant Healthcare, Eden Prairie, MN). [c]No mention of randomization, patient selection, sample size calculation, blinding. [d]Hot Dog (Augustine Temperature Management, Eden Prairie, MN).

Source: From Kellam, Dieckmann, and Austin (2013).

CONCLUSION

The evidence supporting maintaining normothermia to prevent surgical site infection is conflicting; however, most clinical practice guidelines support maintaining normothermia (AORN, 2016; Hooper et al., 2010). Maintaining normothermia is important for patients undergoing total joint arthroplasty (APIC, 2010). Avoiding hypothermia has benefits beyond preventing surgical site infections such as decreasing the risk of cardiovascular and coagulation problems (AORN, 2016). Forced-air warmers have been shown to be effective in preventing inadvertent perioperative hypothermia (Galvao et al., 2009; Moola & Lockwood, 2011).

The results suggest there is no conclusive evidence that the use of forced-air warmers increases the risk of surgical site infections (Kellam et al., 2013). A group reported finding insufficient evidence suggesting the use of forced-air warmers increases the risk of surgical site infections (ECRI Institute, 2013). Others concluded forced-air warmers should be carefully maintained including changing the intake filter at the recommended interval and cleaning the outside of the hose between uses. Although further research is needed to show if the use of forced-air warmers causes surgical site infection in patients undergoing total joint arthroplasty, clinicians should consider using other methods of warming patients undergoing these procedures (Sikka & Prielipp, 2014; Wood et al., 2014).

An adequately powered study aimed at determining if the use of a forced-air warmer increases the risk of a surgical site infection in patients undergoing total joint arthroplasty will need a large sample size because of the low overall risk of a surgical site infection in these patients. A well-conducted, adequately powered observational study may be an alternative to a randomized controlled trial. Potentially confounding factors will also have to be addressed. These include the factors known to increase (e.g., diabetes) or decrease (e.g., proper use of perioperative antibiotics) the risk of a surgical site infection (APIC, 2010).

Clinicians have to weigh the risks and benefits of using a forced-air warmer perioperatively, especially in patients undergoing total knee or hip arthroplasty. These include both medical and economic benefits. The forced-air warmer must be maintained and used according to the manufacturer's directions. Maintaining the filters and cleaning the forced-air warmer units must be done meticulously. Use of alternative warming methods may be considered. Clinicians must consider the risks and benefits of these alternative devices.

REFERENCES

Albrecht, M., Gauthier, R. L., Belani, K., Litchy, M., & Leaper, D. (2011). Forced-air warming blowers: An evaluation of filtration adequacy and airborne contamination emissions in the operating room. *American Journal of Infection Control, 39*(4), 321–328. http://dx.doi.org/10.1016/j.ajic.2010.06.011

Albrecht, M., Gauthier, R., & Leaper, D. (2009). Forced-air warming: A source of airborne contamination in the operating room? *Orthopedic Reviews, 1*(2), e28. http://dx.doi.org/10.4081/or.2009.e28

Association for Professionals in Infection Control and Epidemiology. (2010). *Guide to the elimination of orthpedic surgical site infections*. Retrieved from http://www.apic.org/Resource_/EliminationGuideForm/34e03612-d1e6-4214-a76b-e532c6fc3898/File/APIC-Ortho-Guide.pdf

Association of periOperative Registered Nurses. (2016). *AORN guidelines for perioperative practice*. Denver, CO: Author.

Augustine, S. (1991). The Bair Hugger Patient Warming System. *Journal of Post Anesthesia Nursing*, (1), 2–4.

Augustine, S. (2014). Another perspective on forced-air warming and the risk of surgical site infection. *Association of periOperative Registered Nurses Journal, 99*(3), 350–351. http://dx.doi.org/10.1016/j.aorn.2013.12.010

Avidan, M. S., Jones, N., Ing, R., Khoosal, M., Lundgren, C., & Morrell, D. F. (1997). Convection warmers–not just hot air. *Anaesthesia, 52*(11), 1073–1076.

Baker, N., King, D., & Smith, E. G. (2002). Infection control hazards of intraoperative forced air warming. *The Journal of Hospital Infection, 51*(2), 153–154.

Belani, K. G., Albrecht, M., McGovern, P. D., Reed, M., & Nachtsheim, C. (2012). Patient warming excess heat: The effects on orthopedic operating room ventilation performance. *Anesthesia andAnalgesia, 117*(2), 406–411. http://dx.doi.org/10.1213/ane.0b013e31825f81e2

Bernards, A. T., Harinck, H. I., Dijkshoorn, L., van der Reijden, T. J., & van den Broek, P. J. (2004). Persistent acinetobacter baumannii? Look inside your medical equipment. *Infection Control and Hospital Epidemiology: The Official Journal of the Society of Hospital Epidemiologists of America, 25*(11), 1002–1004. http://dx.doi.org/10.1086/502335

Brandt, S., Oguz, R., Huttner, H., Waglechner, G., Chiari, A., Greif, R., et al. (2010). Resistive-polymer versus forced-air warming: Comparable efficacy in orthopedic patients. *Anesthesia and Analgesia, 110*(3), 834–838. http://dx.doi.org/10.1213/ane.0b013e3181cb3f5f

Calcaterra, D., Ricci, M., Lombardi, P., Katariya, K., Panos, A., & Salerno, T. A. (2009). Reduction of postoperative hypothermia with a new warming device: A prospective randomized study in off-pump coronary artery surgery. *Journal of Cardiovascular Surgery, 50*(6), 813–817.

Dasari, K. B., Albrecht, M., & Harper, M. (2012). Effect of forced-air warming on the performance of operating theatre laminar flow ventilation. *Anaesthesia, 67*(3), 244–249. http://dx.doi.org/10.1111/j.1365-2044.2011.06983.x

ECRI Institute. (2013). Forced-air warming and surgical site infections. Our review finds insufficient evidence to support changes in current practice. *Health Devices, 42*(4), 122–125. Retrieved from http://www.fawfacts.com/_asset/4f12x7/Forced-Air_Warming_and_Surgical_Site_InfectionsHealth_Devices.pdf

Frank, S. M., Fleisher, L. A., Breslow, M. J., Higgins, M. S., Olson, K. F., Kelly, S., et al. (1997). Perioperative maintenance of normothermia reduces the incidence of morbid cardiac events. A randomized clinical trial. *Journal of the American Medical Association, 277*(14), 1127–1134.

Galvao, C. M., Liang, Y., & Clark, A. M. (2010). Effectiveness of cutaneous warming systems on temperature control: Meta-analysis. *Journal of Advanced Nursing, 66*(6), 1196–1206. http://dx.doi.org/10.1111/j.1365-2648.2010.05312.x

Galvao, C. M., Marck, P. B., Sawada, N. O., & Clark, A. M. (2009). A systematic review of the effectiveness of cutaneous warming systems to prevent hypothermia. *Journal of Clinical Nursing, 18*(5), 627–636. http://dx.doi.org/10.1111/j.1365-2702.2008.02668.x

Gapinski, K. (2015). What to make of these bair hugger lawsuits. *Outpatient Surgery Magazine*. Retrieved from https://www.outpatientsurgery.net/outpatient-surgery-news-and-trends/general-surgical-news-and-reports/what-to-make-of-these-bair-hugger-lawsuits--09-23-15

Geiger, T. M., Horst, S., Muldoon, R., Wise, P. E., Enrenfeld, J., Poulose, B., et al. (2012). Perioperative core body temperatures effect on outcome after colorectal resections. *American Surgeon, 78*(5), 607–612.

Hasegawa, K., Negishi, C., Nakagawa, F., & Ozaki, M. (2012). Core temperatures during major abdominal surgery in patients warmed with new circulating-water garment, forced-air warming, or carbon-fiber resistive-heating system. *Journal of Anesthesia, 26*(2), 168–173. http://dx.doi.org/10.1007/s00540-011-1306-1

Hooper, V. D., Chard, R., Clifford, T., Fetzer, S., Fossum, S., Godden, B., et al. (2010). ASPAN's evidence-based clinical practice guideline for the promotion of perioperative normothermia: second edition. *Journal of Perianesthesia Nursing, 25*(6), 346–365. http://dx.doi.org/10.1016/j.jopan.2010.10.006

Huang, J. K., Shah, E. F., Vinodkumar, N., Hegarty, M. A., & Greatorex, R. A. (2003). The Bair Hugger patient warming system in prolonged vascular surgery: An infection risk? *Critical Care (London, England), 7*(3), R13–R16. http://dx.doi.org/10.1186/cc1888

Institute for Healthcare Improvement. (2012). *How-to guide: Prevent surgical site infections.* Cambridge, MA: Author. Retrieved from http://www.ihi.org/resources/pages/tools/howtoguidepreventsurgicalsiteinfection.aspx

Kapadia, B. H., Pivec, R., Johnson, A. J., Issa, K., Naziri, Q., Daley, J. A., et al. (2013). Infection prevention methodologies for lower extremity total joint arthroplasty. *Expert Review of Medical Devices, 10*(2), 215–224. http://dx.doi.org/10.1586/erd.12.76

Kellam, M. D., Dieckmann, L. S., & Austin, P. N. (2013). Forced-air warming devices and the risk of surgical site infections. *Association of periOperative Registered Nurses Journal, 98*(4), 354–366; quiz 367–369. http://dx.doi.org/10.1016/j.aorn.2013.08.001

Kim, Y. S., Jeon, Y. S., Lee, J. A., Park, W. K., Koh, H. S., Joo, J. D., et al. (2009). Intra-operative warming with a forced-air warmer in preventing hypothermia after tourniquet deflation in elderly patients. *Journal of International Medical Research, 37*(5), 1457–1464.

Kimberger, O., Held, C., Stadelmann, K., Mayer, N., Hunkeler, C., Sessler, D. I., et al. (2008). Resistive polymer versus forced-air warming: Comparable heat transfer and core rewarming rates in volunteers. *Anesthesia and Analgesia, 107*(5), 1621–1626. http://dx.doi.org/10.1213/ane.0b013e3181845502

Kurz, A., Sessler, D. I., Lenhardt, R. (1996). Perioperative normothermia to reduce the incidence of surgical-wound infection and shorten hospitalization. Study of Wound Infection and Temperature Group. *New England Journal of Medicine, 334*(19), 1209–1215.

Legg, A. J., Cannon, T., & Hamer, A. J. (2012). Do forced air patient-warming devices disrupt unidirectional downward airflow? *The Journal of Bone and Joint Surgery (British volume), 94*(2), 254–256. http://dx.doi.org/10.1302/0301-620x.94b2.27562

Legg, A. J., & Hamer, A. J. (2013). Forced-air patient warming blankets disrupt unidirectional airflow. *The Bone and Joint Journal, 95-B*(3), 407–410. http://dx.doi.org/10.1302/0301-620x.95b3.29121

Leijtens, B., Koëter, M., Kremers, K., & Koëter, S. (2013). High incidence of postoperative hypothermia in total knee and total hip arthroplasty: A prospective observational study. *The Journal of Arthroplasty, 28*(6), 895–898. http://dx.doi.org/10.1016/j.arth.2012.10.006

Linam, W. M., Margolis, P. A., Staat, M. A., Britto, M. T., Hornung, R., Cassedy, A., et al. (2009). Risk factors associated with surgical site infection after pediatric posterior spinal fusion procedure. *Infection Control and Hospital Epidemiology, 30*(2), 109–116. http://dx.doi.org/10.1086/605323

Matar, W. Y., Jafari, S. M., Restrepo, C., Austin, M., Purtill, J. J., & Parvizi, J. (2010). Preventing infection in total joint arthroplasty. *Journal of Bone and Joint Surgery (American volume), 92*(Suppl. 2), 36–46. http://dx.doi.org/10.2106/jbjs.j.01046

McGovern, P. D., Albrecht, M., Belani, K. G., Nachtsheim, C., Partington, P. F., Carluke, I., et al. (2011). Forced-air warming and ultra-clean ventilation do not mix: An investigation of theatre ventilation, patient warming and joint replacement infection in orthopaedics. *The Journal of Bone and Joint Surgery (British volume), 93*(11), 1537–1544. http://dx.doi.org/10.1302/0301-620x.93b11.27124

Melling, A. C., Ali, B., Scott, E. M., & Leaper, D. J. (2001). Effects of preoperative warming on the incidence of wound infection after clean surgery: A randomised controlled trial. *The Lancet, 358*(9285), 876–880. http://dx.doi.org/10.1016/s0140-6736(01)06071-8

Melton, G. B., Vogel, J. D., Swenson, B. R., Remzi, F. H., Rothenberger, D. A., & Wick, E. C. (2013). Continuous intraoperative temperature measurement and surgical site infection risk: Analysis of anesthesia information system data in 1008 colorectal procedures. *Annals of Surgery, 258*(4), 606–612; discussion 612–603. http://dx.doi.org/10.1097/sla.0b013e3182a4ec0f

Moola, S., & Lockwood, C. (2011). Effectiveness of strategies for the management and/or prevention of hypothermia within the adult perioperative environment. *International Journal of Evidence-Based Healthcare (Wiley-Blackwell), 9*(4), 337–345. http://dx.doi.org/10.1111/j.1744-1609.2011.00227.x

Moretti, B., Larocca, A. M., Napoli, C., Martinelli, D., Paolillo, L., Cassano, M., et al. (2009). Active warming systems to maintain perioperative normothermia in hip replacement surgery: A therapeutic aid or a vector of infection? *The Journal of Hospital Infection, 73*(1), 58–63. http://dx.doi.org/10.1016/j.jhin.2009.06.006

National Center for Health Statistics. (2010). *Inpatient surgery*. Retrieved from http://www.cdc.gov/nchs/fastats/inpatient-surgery.htm

National Collaborating Centre for Nursing and Supportive Care. (2008). *The management of inadvertent perioperative hypothermia in adults*. (2008). Retrieved from https://www2.rcn.org.uk/__data/assets/pdf_file/0006/197358/003_282.pdf

Ng, V., Lai, A., & Ho, V. (2006). Comparison of forced-air warming and electric heating pad for maintenance of body temperature during total knee replacement. *Anaesthesia, 61*(11), 1100–1104. http://dx.doi.org/10.1111/j.1365-2044.2006.04816.x

Pu, Y., Cen, G., Sun, J., Gong, J., Zhang, Y., Zhang, M., et al. (2014). Warming with an underbody warming system reduces intraoperative hypothermia in patients undergoing laparoscopic gastrointestinal surgery: A randomized controlled study. *International Journal of Nursing Studies, 51*(2), 181–189. http://dx.doi.org/10.1016/j.ijnurstu.2013.05.013

Rathinam, S., Annam, V., Steyn, R., & Raghuraman, G. (2009). A randomised controlled trial comparing Mediwrap heat retention and forced air warming for maintaining normothermia in thoracic surgery. *Interactive Cardiovascular and Thoracic Surgery, 9*(1), 15–19. http://dx.doi.org/10.1510/icvts.2008.195347

Reed, M., Kimberger, O., McGovern, P. D., & Albrecht, M. C. (2013). Forced-air warming design: evaluation of intake filtration, internal microbial buildup, and airborne-contamination emissions. *American Association of Nurse Anesthetists Journal, 81*(4), 275–280.

Schmied, H., Kurz, A., Sessler, D. I., Kozek, S., & Reiter, A. (1996). Mild hypothermia increases blood loss and transfusion requirements during total hip arthroplasty. *The Lancet, 347*(8997), 289–292.

Scott, E. M., & Buckland, R. (2006). A systematic review of intraoperative warming to prevent postoperative complications. *Association of periOperative Registered Nurses Journal, 83*(5), 1090–1104; 1107–1013.

Sessler, D. I., Olmsted, R. N., & Kuelpmann, R. (2011). Forced-air warming does not worsen air quality in laminar flow operating rooms. *Anesthesia and Analgesia, 113*(6), 1416–1421. http://dx.doi.org/10.1213/ane.0b013e318230b3cc

Sharp, R. J., Chesworth, T., & Fern, E. D. (2002). Do warming blankets increase bacterial counts in the operating field in a laminar-flow theatre? *The Journal of Bone and Joint Surgery (British volume), 84*(4), 486–488.

Sikka, R. S., & Prielipp, R. C. (2014). Forced air warming devices in orthopaedics: A focused review of the literature. *Journal of Bone and Joint Surgery (American volume), 96*(24), e200. http://dx.doi.org/10.2106/jbjs.n.00054

Song, Z., Borgwardt, L., Hoiby, N., Wu, H., Sorensen, T. S., & Borgwardt, A. (2013). Prosthesis infections after orthopedic joint replacement: The possible role of bacterial biofilms. *Orthopedic Reviews, 5*(2), 65–71. http://dx.doi.org/10.4081/or.2013.e14

Steelman, V. M., Graling, P. R., & Perkhounkova, Y. (2013). Priority patient safety issues identified by perioperative nurses. *Association of periOperative Registered Nurses Journal, 97*(4), 402–418. http://dx.doi.org/10.1016/j.aorn.2012.06.016

Stetler, C. B., Morsi, D., Rucki, S., Broughton, S., Corrigan, B., Fitzgerald, J., et al. (1998). Utilization-focused integrative reviews in a nursing service. *Applied Nursing Research, 11*(4), 195–206.

Tanaka, N., Ohno, Y., Hori, M., Utada, M., Ito, K., & Suzuki, T. (2013). A randomised controlled trial of the resistive heating blanket versus the convective warming system for preventing hypothermia during major abdominal surgery. *Journal of Perioperative Practice,* 23(4), 82–86.

Trentman, T. L., Weinmeister, K. P., Hentz, J. G., Laney, M. B., & Simula, D. V. (2009). Randomized non-inferiority trial of the vitalHEAT temperature management system vs the bair hugger warmer during total knee arthroplasty. *Canadian Journal of Anaesthesia, 56*(12), 914–920. http://dx.doi.org/10.1007/s12630-009-9199-2

Tumia, N., & Ashcroft, G. P. (2002). Convection warmers–a possible source of contamination in laminar airflow operating theatres? *The Journal of Hospital Infection, 52*(3), 171–174.

Wood, A. M., Moss, C., Keenan, A., Reed, M. R., & Leaper, D. J. (2014). Infection control hazards associated with the use of forced-air warming in operating theatres. *Journal of Hospital Infection (American volume),* 88(3), 132–140. http://dx.doi.org/10.1016/j.jhin.2014.07.010

Yi, J., Xiang, Z., Deng, X., Fan, T., Fu, R., Geng, W., et al. (2015). Incidence of inadvertent intraoperative hypothermia and its risk factors in patients undergoing general anesthesia in beijing: A prospective regional survey. *PloS One, 10*(9), e0136136. http://dx.doi.org/10.1371/journal.pone.0136136

Yoo, H. S., Park, S. W., Yi, J. W., Kwon, M. I., & Rhee, Y. G. (2009). The effect of forced-air warming during arthroscopic shoulder surgery with general anesthesia. *Arthroscopy,* 25(5), 510–514. http://dx.doi.org/10.1016/j.arthro.2008.10.022

Zhu, Y., Zhang, F., Chen, W., Liu, S., Zhang, Q., & Zhang, Y. (2015). Risk factors for periprosthetic joint infection after total joint arthroplasty: A systematic review and meta-analysis. *Journal of Hospital Infection,* 89(2), 82–89. http://dx.doi.org/10.1016/j.jhin.2014.10.008

Zink, R. S., & Iaizzo, P. A. (1993). Convective war therapy does not increase the risk of wound contamination in the operating room. *Anesthesia and Analgesia,* 76(1), 50–53.

CHAPTER 11

The Neurotoxicity of General Anesthetic Drugs

Emphasis on the Extremes of Age

Chuck Biddle and Vincent Ford

ABSTRACT

A substantial body of research suggests that anesthetic exposure to patients who are very young or very old may impair cognitive, behavioral, and emotional development or recovery. In lower animal models of pre- and postnatal age, anesthetic exposure may impact inflammation, synaptogenesis, neuronal apoptosis, and glial cell development. To date, research in humans is inconclusive regarding the long-term cognitive and behavioral sequelae of general anesthesia in the young child. In older adults, postoperative cognitive dysfunction and cognitive delirium are identified as markers of anesthetic neurotoxicity. Existing neurological degenerative processes and other comorbidities in combination with the stress of surgery make evaluating the independent impact of anesthetic exposure difficult. Advances in research, imaging, and partnerships have enhanced the potential for understanding the impact of anesthetic exposure. In both populations, the resulting data and limitations faced in initial research efforts are catalysts for current prospective studies.

http://dx.doi.org/10.1891/0739-6686.35.201

INTRODUCTION

Anesthesia, allowing for painful interventions of all types to be performed, ranks among a conspicuous handful of interventions impacting the quality of life of citizens worldwide. It most certainly rivals antibiotic therapy, insulin, vaccination, and blood transfusion in terms of facilitating positive outcomes. With more than 250 million of Earth's citizens undergoing surgical procedures each year, the impact of anesthesia services is clearly substantial (Weiser et al., 2008).

Despite the use of agents creating the state of general anesthesia for over 165 years, the precise mechanism(s) of their action and their cellular toxicity remain unclear. However, a growing and robust body of literature reveals vexing concerns about the lasting neurocognitive effects of anesthetic drugs, especially those employed in creating a state of general anesthesia. Although moderating the experience of pain occurred from the earliest times of our historical record, we date the advent of creating a state of general anesthesia to the 1840s with the use of inhaled anesthetics.

The site of action of anesthetic drugs is the central nervous system (CNS), effects that have largely been viewed as brief, controllable, and devoid of long-term consequences. In this review we critique the extant literature regarding the acute and long-term CNS effects of drugs producing general anesthesia in what we term the "vulnerable" populations of the very young and the older patient.

NEUROTOXICITY IN THE PEDIATRIC PATIENT

Advances in the anesthetic care of the pediatric patient have evolved rapidly since the 1980s fueled by research, newer anesthetic agents, innovative technology, and provider specialization. Prior to the mid-1980s, avoiding anesthetic exposure to infants and young children, due to the risk of death resulting from hypotension, arrhythmia, or hypoxia, was not an uncommon practice (Wise-Faberowski, Quienonez, & Hammer, 2014). Today, an estimated 6 million children undergo surgical care each year in the United States alone (Shen et al., 2013). The prevalence of anesthesia administered to children has prompted very important questions regarding the short- and long-term effects of anesthesia from clinicians and parents alike.

Recent research reveals that drugs commonly used in the anesthetic care of children, alone or in combination, may cause significant and widespread neuroapoptotic degeneration of developing neurons in various mammalian species (Jevtovic-Todorovic, 2011). The majority of this research is based on animal models including rhesus monkeys, mice, and guinea pigs aimed to examine the anesthetic drug impact on neurological development and subsequent cognitive or behavioral impairment.

The Developing Brain

The developing mammalian brain differs from the adult brain in ways that provide a biological foundation for enhanced susceptibility to drug effects. In early mammalian CNS development, there is accelerated neuronal formation followed by rapid synaptogenesis; this proliferation is eventually reduced to establish behaviorally relevant connections between neurons (Hudson & Hemmings Jr., 2011). Gamma-amino butyric acid (GABA) receptor excitation is imperative for synaptogenesis. The GABA receptor, a ligand-gated ion channel, allows for the transportation of chloride into the neuron producing hyperpolarization of the cell and suppression of neuronal activity in adults. However, early in mammalian brain development, the gradient for chloride is reversed such that chloride permeability results in depolarization and neuronal excitation. N-methyl-D-aspartate (NMDA) receptors are primarily excitatory in nature, playing a role in memory formation and learning. Stimulation of ligand-gated NMDA receptors results in an influx of sodium and calcium and an efflux of potassium. The excitatory nature of NMDA receptors remain constant throughout the life span of the mammalian brain.

The mammalian brain undergoes a rapid growth spurt during the last trimester of gestation until the third year of life. This period of neurogenesis/synaptogenesis results in the production of superfluous neurons and neurons with erroneous connections that are eventually removed by apoptosis and synaptic regression (Aker, Block, & Biddle, 2015). Normally, apoptosis, or programmed cell death, is responsible for the elimination of 50% to 70% of neurons. Neurons are also removed during times of physiologic insult, withdrawal of neurotrophic factors, and after exposure to anesthesia.

Timing May Be Everything: Peak Periods of Synaptogenesis

As the effects of anesthetic drugs are CNS-based, their potential detrimental effect on impairing neuronal growth or promoting apoptosis best occurs during the peak of normal synaptogenic activity. Differences in CNS developmental timelines vary widely among species, making human extrapolation complicated and tenuous at best. For example, the murine critical period for exposure resulting in neurotoxicity, postnatal day 0 to 14, approximates the 20th week of gestation in humans. The rhesus monkey critical period for anesthetic neurodegeneration approximates the 26th week of gestation (Hudson & Hemmings Jr., 2011). The premature human fetus would appear to be at greatest risk for anesthetic neurotoxicity, but there is little evidence to support direct extrapolation from animal data, only biological plausibility.

Recognition of peak periods of synaptogenesis in the developing human brain aids in limiting anesthetic vulnerability and the potential for neurotoxicity.

There are significant regional differences in the timing for peak synaptogenesis. The earliest is in the primary sensorimotor cortex, occurring around birth. The parietal and temporal association cortex, important in language and spatial attention, peaks at around 9 months. The last region to peak is in the prefrontal cortex, which occurs at 2 to 3 years of age. The prefrontal cortex is key in executive function as well as integrative and modulatory brain function. Since peak synaptogenesis occurs between birth and 3 years of age, it may be appropriate to consider the vulnerable period for anesthetic-induced neurotoxicity to be during this time frame (Sun, 2010).

The Role of Inflammation

Neuroinflammation is a recognized mechanism of cognitive impairment. Proinflammatory cytokines, tumor necrosis factor (TNF)-a, and interleukin (IL)-6 are released by microglia during activation by stress, certain drugs, trauma, and infection, fueling brain inflammation and leading to cognitive impairment. Shen et al. (2013) exposed both 6- and 60-day-old mice to anesthesia regimens including sevoflurane and desflurane of varying duration. The effects of the anesthetic regimen were assessed by learning and memory tests, levels of proinflammatory cytokine IL-6 and TNA-a factor in brain tissue, and the amount of ionized calcium binding to select cells that are markers for microglial activation in the hippocampus. The researchers demonstrated that the anesthesia regimen of 3% sevoflurane for 2 hours daily for three consecutive days induced both cognitive impairment and neuroinflammation in younger but not adult mice. These results suggest that anesthesia-related cognitive impairment may depend on numerous factors including stage of neurological development, number and duration of exposures, degree of inflammatory response elicited, and type of anesthetic agent.

Progression of Studies in Nonhuman Primates to Human Trials

While neurotoxicity and neuronal apoptosis are demonstrable in laboratory models, the clinical significance in humans is unsettled. Nonhuman primates are genetically and physiologically the closest to human models. Paule et al. (2011) performed a randomized controlled trial of long-term cognitive development of rhesus monkeys exposed to ketamine during the early period of brain development. A continuous infusion of low-dose ketamine was administered to maintain a light plane of surgical anesthesia. The infusion was administered during postnatal day 5 or 6, a critical period of brain development. Significant, persistent cognitive impairment was observed in ketamine exposed monkeys compared to unexposed monkeys. The Operant Test Battery, designed to assess learning, motivation, color discrimination, and short-term memory was the assessment tool used. Other researchers reported that ketamine treated monkeys (postnatal day 5 or 6) demonstrate lower scores in all aspects of the Operant Test Battery, starting at 10 months of postnatal age and lasting beyond 3 years of age (Jevtovic-Todorovic, 2011).

Zou et al. (2011) conducted a study on rhesus monkeys to determine if prolonged exposure to combinations of nitrous oxide (N_2O) and isoflurane produced neurotoxicity using 16 rhesus monkeys (4 male, 12 female) on postnatal day 5 or 6. The animals were randomly assigned to four groups (Table 11.1) and exposed to 8 hours of the inhalational agents. A rabbit polyclonal antibody that detects human cleaved caspase-3, one of the key effectors of apoptosis, degeneration selective silver staining, and Fluoro-Jade C staining were utilized as markers to make neuronal damage visible and measurable. A computer-based image analysis system was employed to determine the number of damaged neural cells. It was determined that the effects of inhaled anesthetic exposure (N_2O or isoflurane) on the monkey brains were primarily contained within the cortical brain regions, especially the frontal cortex, temporal gyrus, and hippocampus. No significant neurotoxic effects were observed for those exposed to N_2O or isoflurane alone. However, neuronal damage was apparent when N_2O was combined with isoflurane as indicated by increased numbers of caspase-3-, silver-staining- and Fluoro-Jade C-positive cells in the frontal cortex, temporal gyrus and hippocampus.

Creeley et al. (2014) evaluated the impact of isoflurane on both neurons and oligodendrocytes administered to pregnant rhesus monkeys at 120 days gestational age, which approximates to mid-third trimester in humans. The experimental group was induced with propofol, exposed to isoflurane (end tidal 1.0%–1.5%) for five hours, and then discontinued. Three hours after cessation of isoflurane, the fetus was delivered by cesarean section and submitted for histopathological evaluation. The control group was induced with propofol and then received intravenous normal saline instead of general anesthesia. They were

TABLE 11.1

Zou et al. Study of Rhesus Monkeys and Inhaled Anesthetics

Group	Agent	Gender
1	Nitrous oxide (70%) alone	1 male/2 female
2	Isoflurane (1.0%) alone	3 female
3	70% Nitrous oxide + 1.0% isoflurane	1 male/4 female
4	Control—Air	2 male/3 female

then returned to their cage, with access to food and water, for the remainder of the experimental period. At 8 hours after time zero, the fetus was delivered by cesarean section and submitted for histopathological evaluation. Neuronal apoptosis was quantified by computerized brain mapping and staining, particularly with activated caspase-3, to track morphological changes and demarcate apoptotic neurons and glial cells. Results demonstrated neuroapoptosis most prominently in the cerebellum, caudate, putamen, amygdala, and many cerebrocortical regions. Compared to the control group, there was a 4.1 fold increase in the number of apoptotic profiles (neurons and oligodendrocytes) in the isoflurane exposed fetus. Oligodendrocyte apoptosis occurred throughout white and gray matter regions. These glial cells appear to be most vulnerable when they are early in their potential to myelinate axons.

Research regarding human exposure to anesthesia and resultant cognitive and behavioral impairment is conflicting. The majority of studies involving human subjects are retrospective, observational, case-controlled, and cohort matched studies thus not permitting cause and effect interpretations. Great variability in patient demographics, surgical procedures performed, drugs and interventions used, often absent control or measurement of comorbidities, and methodological issues of all kinds threaten any reasonable generalizability. Likewise many studies failed to examine or control for issues such as vision or hearing impairment, psychological issues such as attention deficit or depression, any of which could create learning dysfunction or cognitive issues. This has created a need for prospective, carefully controlled studies.

Prospective Studies in Humans

Prospective studies are now under way to provide valid evidence regarding the impact of anesthetic management factors on the potential for neurotoxicity in the developing brain. The General Anesthesia Spinal (GAS) study is a multisite, randomized controlled trial comparing regional and general anesthesia for effects on neurodevelopmental outcome and apnea in infants. The GAS study aims to determine whether different types of anesthesia (regional versus general) given to 660 infants undergoing inguinal hernia repair result in equivalent neurodevelopmental outcomes. This multi-national study (Table 11.2) also aims to describe the incidence of apnea in the postoperative period after both regional and general anesthesia for inguinal hernia repair in infants. The general anesthesia group will receive sevoflurane plus bupivacaine (up to 2.5 mg/kg) administered via caudal route or an ilioinguinal nerve block. The regional anesthesia group will receive bupivacaine (up to 2.5 mg/kg) administered via caudal, subarachnoid, both caudal and subarachnoid, or subarachnoid and ilioinguinal block. Neurodevelopmental testing is designed

TABLE 11.2
Sites Participating in the GAS Study

GAS sites
Australia
Canada
Italy
United Kingdom
United States
The Netherlands
New Zealand

Note. GAS = General anesthesia spinal.

to take place at 2 years of age using the Bayley developmental scale and 5 years of age utilizing the Wechsler Preschool and Primary Scale of Intelligence-Third Edition full scale IQ score. Estimated completion date is January 2017.

The Mayo Anesthesia Safety in Kids study is a prospective, propensity matching, population-based study for children based in Olmsted County, Minnesota. Children exposed to no anesthesia, one anesthetic, or multiple anesthetics before the age of 3 years will be given the National Center for Toxicological Research Operant Test Battery between ages 8 and 12 or 15 and 19 during the 2012 to 2016 time period. This test battery has high reliability and validity and reveals cognitive deficits in nonhuman primates exposed to anesthesia. The results of the testing will be compared among children with different anesthetic exposures. Expected outcomes from this study will be a detailed phenotype of possible anesthetic-associated neurotoxicity in humans and the first opportunity to compare effects of anesthetic exposure on children and nonhuman primates performing the same test and tasks (Gleich et al., 2015).

The Pediatric Anesthesia and Neurodevelopment Assessment (PANDA) study is a multisite, sibling-matched cohort study that will enroll 500 subjects (Table 11.3). The anesthesia exposure will be limited to a single episode of general anesthesia for inguinal hernia repair in ASA I and II patients prior to 36 months of age. The study will perform extensive neuropsychological testing in children between 8 and 15 years of age. The results of this study will be applicable to healthy children undergoing elective procedures. This constitutes the vast majority of surgery done on children in the United States. The annual PANDA Symposium is a platform to review current preclinical and clinical data related to anesthetic neurotoxicity, to discuss relevant considerations in study design and

TABLE 11.3

Sites Participating in the PANDA Study

PANDA sites
Children's Hospital of Philadelphia
Boston Children's Hospital
Children's Hospital of New York (Columbia)
Cincinnati Children's Hospital
Vanderbilt University Children's Hospital
University of Michigan Children's Hospital
Pittsburgh Children's Hospital

Note. PANDA = Pediatric Anesthesia and Neurodevelopment Assessment.

approaches to future research among clinicians and researchers, and to engage key stakeholders in this controversial topic (Miller, Park, & Sun, 2014).

Sustaining the prospective work is a consortium, the Strategies for Mitigating Anesthesia Related neuroToxicity in Tots (SmartTots), a public–private partnership between the Food and Drug Administration (FDA) and the International Anesthesia Research Society (IARS). The mission of this partnership is to coordinate and fund research with the goal of ensuring safe surgery for the millions of infants and young children undergoing anesthesia and/or sedation each year. The FDA and IARS work together with multiple stakeholders to leverage their collective resources in an effort to address this important issue.

Major Limitations to Current Studies and Those Under Way

The complexity of performing studies involving humans is particularly noteworthy when children and CNS outcomes are involved. The rigor and limitations of such work are likely to generate critical commentary for years to come. Among the many limitations and obstacles that must be overcome in order to render valid conclusions are:

1. The consequences of anesthesia are difficult to separate from the consequences of surgery.
2. The impact of individual agents is challenging to identify when multiple anesthetic drugs are administered at the same time.
3. Children undergoing anesthesia and surgery may have a greater burden of illness (overt and covert) that may have effects on learning dysfunction with a subsequent decrement on exporting any conclusions to a broader population.

4. Many factors can influence learning dysfunction or cognitive capacity that may mirror any purported neurotoxic effect from drugs or procedures. Among the many are hearing impairment, visual impairment, and behavioral issues.
5. Is there good evidence that learning dysfunction, assessed as the outcome, is a good measure (mirror) of neurotoxicity?

CONCLUSIONS

The impact of early anesthetic exposure to children has captured the attention of anesthesia providers, researchers, governmental agencies, and parents. The multifactorial nature of cognitive, behavioral, and social development confounds the picture regarding the deleterious impact of anesthetic exposure. Fortunately, information from studies on animal models and retrospective human trials have set the stage for a new paradigm of clinical research. Current longitudinal and prospective studies focusing on the age at anesthetic exposure, number and duration of anesthetic exposure, type of surgery, and health status of the child will provide new insights into pediatric neurotoxicity.

NEUROTOXICITY IN THE OLDER PATIENT

Bedford (1955) was the first to formally recognize dysfunction of cognition following general anesthesia in aged adults, terming it "adverse cerebral effects of anaesthesia on old people." The relevance of that early report continues to gain traction as the number of older patients undergoing anesthesia for diagnostic and surgical procedures grows. One common manifestation of impairment in the aftermath of anesthetic drug exposure is termed postoperative cognitive dysfunction (POCD). We will use POCD as an indicator of neurotoxicity with the caveat that it occurs in the aftermath of anesthetic drug exposure.

The study of drug effects on the older brain, as with the younger brain, is complex and proves daunting for reasons related to ethical concerns, logistics, patient safety, and the many factors that independently, or in combination, serve to influence outcome. It is further complicated by the need to establish baseline function in order to systematically define POCD as a new cognitive impairment arising as a result of anesthetic exposure, and not simply a course of cognitive decline that was already in progress.

Based on the extant literature, age greater than 60 years defines the current review's threshold relevant to POCD. The epidemiology of POCD varies, in part because of the wide variety of methodological approaches used to identify it, the age of those studied, the need for an appropriate and well-matched control group, and the statistical control of confounding factors. While POCD can arise even in those younger, it occurs more often, lasts longer, and impacts quality of life greater in those over the age of 60 (Krenk, Ramussen, & Kehelt, 2010).

POCD Following Cardiac Surgery

The American College of Cardiology and the American Heart Association classify neurological complications after cardiac surgery into two domains. Type I refers to stroke, transient ischemic attacks, coma and fatal brain injury, while Type II refers to impairment of memory and concentration, and decrement in psychomotor speed (Eagle et al., 1999). Systematic review of high-quality studies reveals that at the time of hospital discharge the incidence of POCD is 30% to 65% and after several months it is in the range of 20% to 40% (Van Harten et al., 2012).

Hypotheses emerging over the decades tended to focus on perturbations in physiology from cardiopulmonary bypass. Recent, well-controlled trials reveal the incidence of POCD is similar whether the cardiac patient is "on-pump" or "off-pump," the latter referring to surgery on a beating heart without cardiopulmonary bypass (Sun et al., 2012; vanDijk et al., 2007; vanHarten, Scheeren, & Absalom, 2012). In fact, the incidence of POCD after cardiac surgery is similar to that seen in other types of major surgery when patient samples are otherwise well-matched. Current hypotheses regarding the etiology of POCD after cardiac surgery mirror those in major noncardiac surgery, focusing on three domains: (a) surgical insult, (b) drug exposure, and (c) patient-related factors (Figure 11.1). A growing body of work implicates inflammation as the key factor, and one that may be initiated or exacerbated by each of the domains (Figure 11.1).

The advent of off-pump cardiac surgery was likely precipitated by the attempt to deal with a perceived public health crisis (cognitive insult attributed to on-pump surgery) that lacked strong evidence based rationale. It is now clear from a body of clinical research that there is no clinical or statistical difference in cognitive outcomes related to the use or nonuse of cardiopulmonary bypass for cardiac surgery.

POCD Following Noncardiac Surgery

Postoperative delirium (PD) is an acute manifestation of some type of neurotoxic event and must be differentiated from POCD. As with POCD, there are patient-specific, procedure-specific, and drug-specific factors that can overlap and intersect complexly. PD can be thought of as "acute brain failure" that is well known to be associated with significant poor outcome unless remedied. PD is defined as altered and fluctuating mentation occurring acutely with the hallmarks of inattention and altered level of consciousness. Delirium may manifest

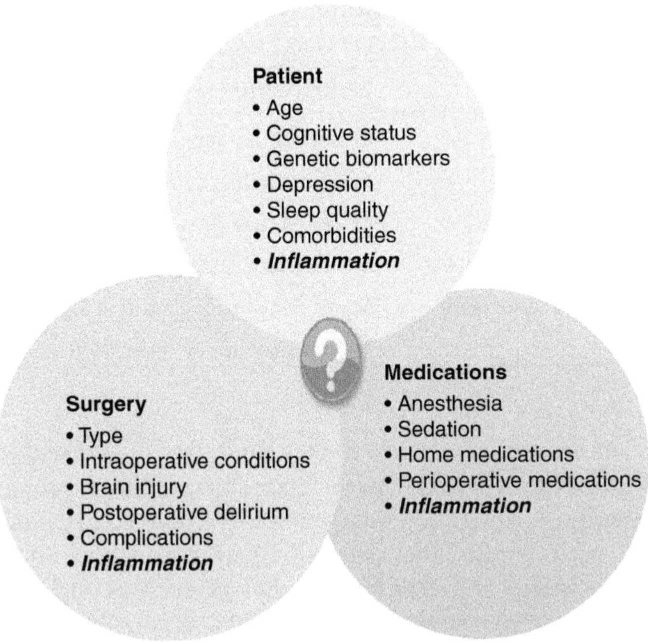

FIGURE 11.1 Multiple theories may help explain POCD. It is likely the intersection or overlap of many different factors predisposes to its occurrence.
Note. POCD = postoperative cognitive dysfunction.

as hyperactivity (restlessness, irritability, combativeness) or hypoactivity (lethargy, unawareness of the environment), with a highly variable incidence of 9% to 87% (Demeure & Fain, 2006). Table 11.4 provides some differential attributes of PD and POCD.

There is great variation, thus confounding its reported incidence, depending on the cohort of patients studied, the definition of POCD used, and the selection of the control group. Monk et al. (2008) observed POCD occurring at the time of hospital discharge in 36.6% of those aged 18 to 39, 30.4% in those aged 40 to 59, and 41.4% in those who are 60 years or older. Further confusing the domain is the observation that in carefully performed studies, regional anesthesia does not seem to reduce the incidence of POCD, demonstrating that any neurotoxic effects are likely due to a complex interaction of patient and care-provided factors (Rasmussen, 2006).

TABLE 11.4

Differentiating Postoperative Delirium From Postoperative Cognitive Dysfunction

Postoperative Delirium	Postoperative Cognitive Dysfunction
Acute onset	Onset subtle, weeks to months
Fluctuating course	Not fluctuating
Duration limited (days/weeks)	Duration may be weeks to months or beyond
Clouded consciousness	No clouding of consciousness
Inattentive/disorganized thought	Many domains of cognition affected
Usually reversible	May or may not be reversible

The literature and experience to date finds that the etiology, chronology, and ultimate outcome of POCD remains foggy, though there is strong association and overlap with risk factors and neuropathology observed in central degenerative processes such as Alzheimer's disease. Some suggest that anesthetics may exacerbate an existing, or occult neuropathology such as Alzheimer's disease (Planel et al., 2008; Planel et al., 2009). It should be noted that supporting evidence for this hypothesis is based on animal (murine) models although there are observational studies of older adults that show a strong association of sevoflurane use and POCD (Shoair et al., 2015).

Anesthesia exposure is not an isolated, independent event as it occurs when the need for a noxious intervention arises. Given the well appreciated inflammatory response associated with surgery, and severity and duration of the procedure as additional confounders, the role of neuroinflammation is gaining traction as a possible mechanism of POCD (Hovens et al., 2014). Ongoing work suggests that neuroinflammation impairs central neurotrophic factors, impairs neuronal plasticity, and weakens the blood–brain barrier, allowing pro-inflammatory molecules to enter the CNS and perturb neuronal function (Cibelli et al., 2010; Van Harten et al., 2012).

What We Know, and Don't Know, About the Major Anesthetic Drugs

Intravenous Agents

Research with respect to ketamine and propofol is particularly extensive. Ketamine is an NMDA antagonist that induces neuronal apoptosis in animal models. A proposed hypothesis suggests upregulation of NMDA receptors sensitizes the response to endogenous glutamate, leading to enhanced calcium influx and apoptosis (Wang et al., 2005). Likewise propofol, in various animal models, can induce neuroapoptosis via calcium dysregulation or tau protein hyperphosphorylation (Whittington et al., 2011).

Inhalational Agents

Sevoflurane and isoflurane are halogenated ethers that may induce apoptosis and elevate levels of beta-amyloid protein, activate caspase-3, increase the vulnerability in states of Alzheimer's disease like pathology, and impair neuronal signaling pathways (Zhang et al., 2013). It should be noted that these observations emerge from animal models.

Desflurane does not appear to cause caspase-3 activation or amyloid protein processing except under conditions of hypoxia in animal models (Zhang et al., 2008). That said, there are opposite observations that greatly complicate arriving at any consensus-based conclusions (Kodama et al., 2011).

Nitrous oxide is commonly used in conjunction with other agents due to its low solubility and ability to amplify the effect of other inhaled agents. As with other agents, human study is limited by technical and ethical issues and extant work is based on animal models performed under conditions of long duration and high concentrations. It may induce a neurotoxic reaction in the brain likely due to excitotoxicity and methionine synthetase inhibition (Jevtovic-Todorovic et al., 2003).

Further illustrating the daunting nature of unraveling the neurotoxic effects of anesthetic drugs is the observation that many of our anesthetic agents may promote hyperphosphorylation of the microtubule-associated protein tau when there is coexisting hypothermia (Planel et al., 2007). A follow-up study using a similar experimental model found that propofol during normothermia still increased tau phosphorylation (Whittington et al., 2011). The significance of these studies is grounded in the knowledge that hyperphosphorylated tau can self-assemble into neurofibrillary tangles that are microscopically observed in certain neurodegenerative diseases such as Parkinson's and Alzheimer's diseases.

Clinically the concerns of using these agents are primarily based on whether an older patient may have some existing level of neuropathology that may be exacerbated by the use of one or more of these agents. An inhaled agent may precipitate the onset of early onset POCD or it may promote other preexisting neurodegenerative disease progression, though studies, limited to controlled animal models and observational studies in humans, paint a complex and still ill-defined picture.

What can be concluded is that major surgery and general anesthesia do not cause persistent (beyond 6 months) POCD or dementia. Rather it appears that the preoperative condition of patients in terms of their cognitive trajectory and any concurrent disease that they experience are predictive of long-term POCD (Avidan & Evers, 2016).

Mechanisms and Risk Factors

There is an absence of fully clarified mechanisms that lead to or promote cognitive impairment. Animal experiments, where tight laboratory control and analysis are achievable, suggest a key role of the immune response in the genesis of cognitive insult that may be mediated by drugs, trauma, infectious processes, and even stress. Different mechanisms likely are relevant to different patients in their differing circumstances.

For example, it has long been appreciated by bedside nurses and clinicians in general that urinary tract infections are frequently attended by confusion or even delirium, especially in the older patient, strongly suggesting immune-mediated phenomena, with near 100% resolution once the infection resolves (Levkoff et al., 1988; Robinson & Eiseman, 2008). An immune-mediated response of inflammation is described in Figure 11.2.

Molecular Targets

A cholinergic deficiency or decrement in cholinergic neuronal function is likely implicated in many cases of anesthetic-related cognitive insult (Shoair et al., 2015). While pro-cholinergic drugs such as physostigmine can reverse anticholinergic poisoning, it is ineffective in remedying either PD or POCD (Beaver & Gavin, 1998). Additionally, the individual agents that are employed in achieving a state of general anesthesia each have unique and overlapping molecular targets of their own. These targets include ligand-gated ion inhibitory receptors (GABA and glycine), excitatory receptors (NMDA), as well as specific actions at channels that conduct sodium, potassium, and calcium. The complexities involved in neuronal activity provide many potential opportunities for drug effects to impair function.

In the aged patient, altered drug response, decrement in functional reserve, the cumulative effect of chronic disease, decreased neurogenesis and synaptogenesis, and the potential for by-products of neuronal degeneration to accumulate, may set the stage for adverse consequences of drugs that target the CNS, such as the general-anesthesia-inducing drugs. Thus the stage is set for anesthetic drugs exacting toxic effects on the brain and nervous system via a variety of putative pathways (Table 11.5).

To date we know little about possible molecular influences of drugs on the genesis of neurotoxicity in the aging brain. The complex intersection of the many known (and likely many to be discovered) factors that may influence neurotoxicity occurs in the presence of the unique genetics that each patient presents. The

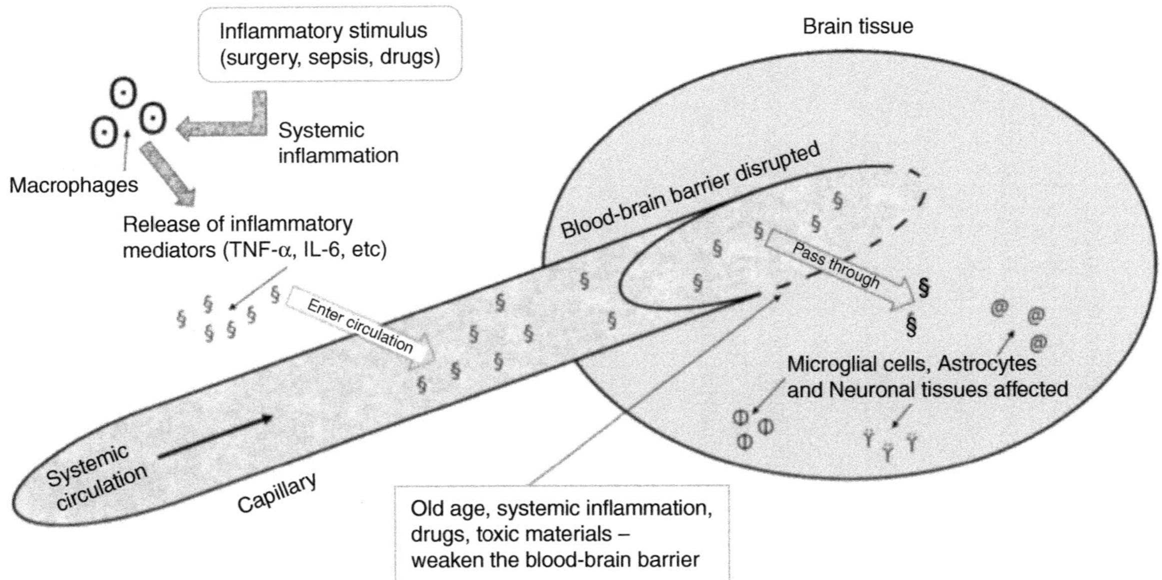

FIGURE 11.2 A theoretical model of cognitive impairment from inflammation starts with an insult (e.g., surgical trauma, drugs, infection, stress) provoking the release of inflammatory mediators from macrophages into the systemic circulation. Weakening of the blood–brain barrier allows these proinflammatory molecules to enter the brain and disrupt or impair neuronal function.

TABLE 11.5

Mechanism by Which Drugs May Impair Cognitive Function

Mechanism
Direct toxic effects/altered drug response
Altered calcium, potassium, and sodium homeostasis
Provoking systemic inflammatory effect that perturbs the CNS
Promote apoptosis and suppression of neuronal stem cell function
Acceleration of ongoing neurodegenerative processes
Accelerating acute and chronic disease that impairs neuronal performance
Impeding intracellular protein folding

future application of systematic principles of biology may elucidate pathogenic mechanisms that are currently unappreciated. Imaging technologies as well as living and computational experimental modeling may hold promise.

A Call for Action (At Last)?

That perioperative brain neurotoxicity or cognitive dysfunction is common in the early recovery phase has finally incited a call for action from the domestic and international anesthesiology communities. Recent work laments the absence of efforts to identify vulnerable patients and the need for assessing preoperative cognitive function (brain homeostasis) as aggressively as we currently interrogate the preoperative status of the heart, lungs, and kidneys (Hudson, 2011).

Neurotoxicity in the form of POCD or PD is associated with prolonged hospital stay, high cost, withdrawal from the workforce, decreased quality of life, and greater one-year mortality (Steinmetz et al., 2009). A strong case, therefore, can be made that the seriousness of neurotoxicity rivals or exceeds that of cardiopulmonary or other major system dysfunction.

Preoperative cognitive assessment permits the capture of a baseline metric, and if mild cognitive impairment is discovered then recognition of it, as with any systemic disease, might permit early diagnosis and intervention. How such information might influence perioperative management is not fully clear at this time, but it is difficult to argue that having such knowledge might prove clinically valuable.

In 2016 the time has come to recognize that the brain of the aged patient may be at risk in the same way that the heart, lungs, liver, or kidneys may be. Routine preanesthetic assessment that documents cognitive status, though long neglected, should become a standard part of the care provided to the aged patient. It is plausible that some older patients having surgery are already on a trajectory of cognitive decline or dementia that will be first detected in the aftermath of surgery and anesthesia. There is the tendency to seek temporal factors that may misleadingly point to the care that was received as part of their surgical intervention(s).

SUMMARY CONSIDERATIONS

A great deal of recent and ongoing work reveals concerns about the neurotoxicity of anesthetic drugs in the very young and older patient populations. A variety of agents, especially our inhalational anesthetics, may induce cellular apoptosis, dysregulate intra- and extracellular ions such as calcium, and cause protein malformation, maldistribution, and accumulation. These actions can be demonstrated very clearly in highly controlled cell cultures and subhuman animals. Likewise, neurotoxic effects in the older brain may accelerate, promote, or even initiate neurodegenerative processes, especially where plasticity or "cognitive reserve" may be limited or nonexistent.

There is current work in progress that is prospectively modeled to address many of the limitations of previous work. Additionally, out-of-the-box thinking has incited research models that are novel and hold great promise. One recent example is using the retina of the eye as a "window" or "lens" into the brain. Using a 7-day-old mouse model, researchers are revealing apoptotic changes in retinal tissue even after 1 hour of 2% isoflurane, suggesting that retinal tissue may mirror injury to brain neurons and offer real-time, early warning of adverse effects in humans (Cheng, He, Prasad, Wang, & Levy, 2015).

The cumulative effect of the ever-growing body of research is to reveal which anesthetics have the least theoretical impact on the developing or older brain. There will likely be continued efforts to develop drugs that have no lasting or toxic effect, as molecular mechanisms of neurotoxicity become illuminated. In the meantime we should tread cautiously and always be mindful of the potential downstream consequences of our interventions.

REFERENCES

Advidan, M. S., & Evers, A. S. (2016). The fallacy of persistent postoperative cognitive decline. *Anesthesiology, 124*(2), 255–258.

Aker, J., Block, R. I., & Biddle, C. (2015). Anesthesia and the developing brain. *American Association of Nurse Anesthetists Journal, 83*(2), 139–147.

Bedford, P. D. (1955). Adverse cerebral effects of anaesthesia on old people. *Lancet, 269*(6884), 259–263.

Beaver, K. M., & Gavin, T. J. (1998). Treatment of acute anticholinergic poisoning with physostigmine. *The American Journal Emergency Medicine*, *16*(5), 505–507.

Cheng, Y., He, L., Prasad, V., Wang, S., Levy, R. (2015). Anesthesia induced neuronal apoptosis in the developing retina. *Anesthesia and Analgesia*, *121*(5), 1325–1335.

Cibelli, M., Fidalgo, A., Terrando, N., Ma, D., Monaco, C., Feldmann, M., et al. (2010). Role of interleukin-1β in postoperative cognitive dysfunction. *Annals Neurology*, *68*(3), 360–368.

Creeley, C. E., Dikranian, K. T., Dissen, G. A., Back, S. A., Olney, J. W., & Brambink, A. M. (2014). Isoflurane-induced apoptosis of neurons and oligodendrocytes in the fetal rhesus macaque brain. *Anesthesiology*, *120*(3), 626–638.

Demeure, M. J., & Fain, M. J. (2006). The elderly surgical patient and postoperative delirium. *Journal of the American College of Surgeons*, *203*(5), 752–757.

Eagle, K. A., Guyton, R. A., Davidoff, R., Ewy, G. A., Fonger, J., Gardner, T. J., et al. (1999). ACC/AHA guidelines for coronary artery bypass graft surgery: Executive summary and recommendations: A report of the American College of Cardiology/American Heart Association Task Force on Practice Guidelines (Committee to revise the 1991 guidelines for coronary artery bypass graft surgery). *Circulation*, *100*, 1464–1480.

Gleich, S. F., Colligan, R., Katusic, S., Schroeder, D., Hanson, A., Buenvenida, S., et al. (2015). Neurodevelopment of children exposed to anesthesia: Design of the mayo anesthesia safety in kids (MASK) study. *Contemporary Clinical Trials*, *41*, 45–54.

Hovens, I. B., Schomaker, R. G., van der Zee, E. A., Absalom, A. R., Heineman, E., van Leeuwen, B. L., et al. (2014). Postoperative cognitive dysfunction: Involvement of neuroinflammation and neuronal functioning. *Brain, Behavior, Immunity*, *38*, 202–210.

Hudson, A. E., & Hemmings, H. C. (2011). Are anaesthetics toxic to the brain? *British Journal Anaesthesia*, *107*(1), 30–37.

Jevtovic-Todorovic, V. (2011). Anesthesia and the developing brain: Are we getting closer to understanding the truth? *Current Opinion in Anesthesiology*, *24*(4), 395–399.

Jevtovic-Todorovic, V., Beals, J., Benshoff, N., & Olney, J. W. (2003). Prolonged exposure to inhalational anesthetic nitrous oxide kills neurons in adult rat brain. *Neuroscience*, *122*(3), 609–616.

Kodama, M., Satoh, Y., Otsubo, Y., Araki, Y., Yonamine, R., Masui, K., et al. (2011). Neonatal desflurane exposure induces more robust neuroapoptosis than do isoflurane and sevoflurane and impairs working memory. *Anesthesiology*, *115*(5), 979–991.

Krenk, L., Rasmussen, L. S., & Kehlet, H. (2010). New insights into the pathophysiology of postoperative cognitive dysfunction. *Acta Anaesthiologica Scandinavica*, *54*(8), 951–956.

Levkoff, S. E., Safrean, C, Clearly, P. D., Gallop, J., & Phillips, R. S. (1988). Identification of factors associated with the diagnosis of delirium in elderly hospitalized patients. *Journal of the American Geriatrics Society*, *36*(12), 1099–1104.

Miller, T. L., Park, R., & Sun, L. S. (2014). Report of the Fourth PANDA Symposium on "Anesthesia and Neurodevelopment in Children." *Journal of Neurosurgical Anesthesiology*, *26*(4), 344–348.

Monk, T. G., Weldon, B. C., Garvan, C. W., Dede, D. E., van der Aa, M. T., Heilman, K. M., et al. (2008). Predictors of cognitive dysfunction after major noncardiac surgery. *Anesthesiology*, *108*(1), 18–30.

Paule, M. L., Liu, F., Zou, X., Hotchkiss, C., Hanig, J. P., Slikker Jr., W., et al. (2011). Ketamine anesthesia during first week of life can cause long-lasting cognitive deficits in rhesus monkeys. *Neurotoxicology Teratology*, *33*(2), 220–230.

Planel, E., Bretteville, A., Liu, L., Virag, L., Du, A. L., Yu, W. H., et al. (2009). Acceleration and persistence of neurofibrillary pathology in a mouse model of tauopathy following anesthesia. *FASEB Journal*, *23*(8), 2595–2604.

Planel, E., Krishnamurthy, P., Miyasaka, T., Liu, L., Herman, M., Kumar, A., et al. (2008). Anesthesia-induced hyperphosphorylation through inhibition of phosphatase detaches 3-repeat tau from microtubules without affecting their stability in vivo. *Journal of Neuroscience*, *28*(48), 12798–12807.

Planel, E., Richer, K. E., Nolan, C. E., Finley, J. E., Liu, L., Wen, Y., et al. (2007). Anesthesia leads to tau hyperphosphorylation through inhibition of phosphatase activity by hypothermia. *Journal Neuroscience*, *27*(12), 3090–3097.

Rasmussen, L. (2006). Postoperative cognitive dysfunction: Incidence and prevention. *Best Practice and Research Clinical Anaesthesiology*, *20*(2), 315–330.

Robinson, T. N., & Eiseman, B. (2008). Postoperative delirium in the elderly: Diagnosis and management. *Clinical Interventions in Aging*, *3*(2), 351–355.

Shen, X., Dong, Y., Xu, S., Wang, H., Maio, C., Soriano, S. G., et al. (2013). Selective anesthesia-induced neuroinflammation in developing mouse brain and cognitive impairment. *Anesthesiology, 118*(3), 502–515.

Shoair, O. A., Grasso, M. P., Lahaye, L. A., Daniel, R., Biddle, C. J., & Slattum, P. W. (2015). Incidence and risk factors for postoperative cognitive dysfunction in older adults undergoing major noncardiac surgery: A prospective study. *Journal Anaesthesiology Clinical Pharmacology*, *31*(1), 30–36.

Steinmetz, J., Christensen, K., Lund, T., Lohse, N., & Rasmussen, L. S. (2009). Long-term consequences of postoperative cognitive dysfunction. *Anesthesiology, 110*(3), 548–555.

Sun, J. H., Wu, X. Y., Wang, W. J., & Jin, L. L. (2012). Cognitive dysfunction after off-pump versus on-pump coronary artery bypass surgery: A meta-analysis. *Journal of International Medical Research, 40*(3), 852–858.

Sun, L. S. (2010). Early childhood general anesthesia exposure and neurocognitive development: What do we know? *British Journal of Anaesthesia, 105*(1), 61–68.

Van Dijk, D., Spoor, M., Hijman, R., Nathoe, H. M., Borst, C., Jansen, E. W., et al. (2007). Cognitive and cardiac outcomes five years after off-pump vs. on-pump coronary artery bypass graft surgery. *Journal of American Medical Association, 297*, 701–708.

Van Harten, A. E., Scheeren, T. W., & Absalom, A. R. (2012). A review of postoperative cognitive dysfunction and neuroinflammation associated with cardiac surgery and anaesthesia. *Anaesthesia*, *67*(3), 280–293.

Wang, C., Sadovova, N., Fu, X., Schmued, L., Scallet, A., Hanig, J., et al. (2005). The role of the NMDA receptor in ketamine induced apoptosis in rat forebrain culture. *Neuroscience*, *132*(4), 967–977.

Weiser, T. G., Regenbogen, S. E., Thompson, K. D., Haynes, K. B., Lipsitz, S. R., Berry, W. R., et al. (2008). An estimation of the global volume of surgery: A modelling strategy based on available data. *Lancet*, *372*(9633), 139–144.

Whittington, R. A., Virag, L., Marcouiller, F., Papon, M., Khoury, N. B., Julien, C., et al. (2011). Propofol directly increases tau phosphorylation. *PLoS One*, *6*, e16648.

Wise-Faberowski, L., Quinonez, Z. A., & Hammer, G. B. (2014). Anesthesia and the developing brain: Relevance to the pediatric cardiac surgery. *Brain Science, 4*(2), 295–310

Zhang, B., Dong, Y., Zheng, G., Moir, R. D., Xia, W., Yue, Y., et al. (2008). The inhalation anesthetic desflurane induces caspase activation and increases amyloid beta-protein levels under hypoxic conditions. *Journal of Biological Chemistry*, *283*(18), 11866–11875.

Zhang, Y., Dong, Y., Zheng, H., Shie, V., Wang, H., Busscher, Y., et al. (2013). Sevoflurane inhibits neurogenesis and the Wnt-catenin signaling pathway in mouse neural progenitor cells. *Current Molecular Medicine, 13*(9), 1446–1454.

Zou, X., Liu, F., Zhang, X., Patterson, T. A., Callicott, R., Liu, S., et al. (2011). Inhalation anesthetic-induced neuronal damage in the developing rhesus monkey. *Neurotoxicology and Teratology, 33*(5), 592–597.

CHAPTER 12

Wet or Dry?

A Review of Intravenous Fluid Administration in Anesthesia Practice

Matthew D'Angelo and R. Kyle Hodgen

ABSTRACT

Fluid therapy has dramatically changed since its early inception nearly 200 years ago. Administration of intravenous fluid (IVF) has evolved from a "drip" technique to the algorithmic approach of the anesthetic fluid plan, and is now moving toward Goal-Directed Fluid Therapy. As the science and culture of fluid management evolves, anesthetists must remain focused on "why" anesthetic fluid matters. The purpose of IVF administration is to support tissue perfusion and maintain euvolemia. As the evidence underlying perioperative practice matures and the science of anesthesia races to meet the evolving demands of surgery, anesthetists must align knowledge generation with the individualized needs of the patient. The future of perioperative IVF therapy will be patient centric. In the near future, anesthetists will know the patient's blood volume before, during, and after the surgery. They will no longer depend on inaccurate surrogates to estimate, but have the knowledge to titrate fluids to maintain a zero balance. Practice will move away from algorithms and toward individualized fluid administration based on reproducible end points. Decisions about fluid selection, timing, and volume will be driven by patient- and case-specific

http://dx.doi.org/10.1891/0739-6686.35.221

requirements as specific as when a patient is typed and crossed for blood transfusion. The greatest challenge for the anesthetist in perioperative fluid therapy is to move beyond the dogmatic practices of the past and toward fluid therapy guided by patient centric evidence.

CLINICAL VIGNETTE

A 38-year-old, male patient (172 kg, 71 inches) presented to the operating room for the repair of an abdominal wall defect (massive ventral hernia) that was due to a traumatic injury several months earlier. The abdominal wall hernia was a result of a liver injury repair status post damage control laparotomy technique. The surgical procedure included skin graph removal, the removal of bowel adhesions, and free flap harvest and graft placement over the defect.

The patient's previous medical history was significant for hypertension and morbid obesity. The patient had no significant surgical history prior to the traumatic event. The patient self-administered two oral bowel preparations as per the surgeon's request the evening before surgery. The patient's preoperative laboratory values were within normal limits: Hemoglobin (hgb) and hematocrit (HcT) were 12.1% and 38% respectively. The surgical team requested that anesthesia restrict fluid during the procedure, to mitigate tissue edema and the risks of abdominal compartment syndrome, as well as avoid vasopressors to facilitate free flap harvest and minimize graft failure.

The patient was brought to the operating room and placed on routine monitors. A lumbar epidural catheter was placed, but not dosed, for postoperative pain management. Induction of anesthesia was completed without incident, arterial access was quickly achieved, and two additional large bore intravenous (IV) catheters were placed in each upper extremity. The patient's vital signs were within 20% of his preoperative baseline, but remained toward the lower threshold of this range for the duration of surgery.

The procedure lasted approximately 10 hours and the patient incurred an estimated 450 milliliters (mL) of blood loss. Over the course of the procedure the patient's HcT fell from 38% to 29%. The patient received a total of 8.9 L of crystalloid and voided approximately 700 ml of urine (0.92 mL/kg/hour). At the conclusion of the case the patient's vital signs were "soft" (systolic blood pressure 90–100 mmHg), but still within 20% to 25% of preoperative baseline. The epidural catheter was retested (negative for cerebral spinal fluid) and dosed with 6 mL of 0.25% bupivacaine prior to the patient being moved to the hospital bed. The plan was to "slowly" emerge the patient and extubate the next morning.

Immediately following the administration of epidural bupivacaine the patient developed profound hypotension. The patient's systolic blood pressure decreased from the low 90s to 60s and the heart rate rose from 89 beats per minute (bpm) to greater than 120 bpm. The patient was immediately administered large volumes of IV crystalloid solutions, several units of packed red blood cells and vasopressors. Following vigorous fluid resuscitation in the recovery room the patient's HcT was measured and determined to be 19%. While the patient was successfully discharged from the hospital 22 days after surgery, he remained intubated in intensive care for several days and required additional surgeries for abdominal exploration. This case was examined shortly after patient discharge. While no "smoking gun" was identified, the general consensus among the review team was that the patient had received insufficient fluid resuscitation during the procedure. This vignette details many of the complexities that surround intravenous fluid (IVF) administration in the perioperative setting, and highlights the challenges that anesthetists face when administering IVFs.

Introduction

Each day, tens of thousands of liters of IVFs are administered in the United States and around the world. IVF administration is a mainstay of the practice of anesthesia. Ideally, IVFs are administered to replete fasting deficits, resuscitate fluid losses, and maintain normal intravascular volume to support and optimize tissue perfusion. Although commonplace, perioperative IVF administration remains controversial in clinical practice (Brandstrup, 2006; Corcoran, Rhodes, Clarke, Myles, & Ho, 2012; Joshi, 2005; Kampmeier, Rehberg, & Ertmer, 2014; Lobo, Macafee, & Allison, 2006). Anesthetists are left to decide the quantity (how much does the patient need?), quality (crystalloid, colloid or blood component therapy), and appropriate timing of IVF delivery with little guidance. This variance in anesthesia practice is due to limited availability of evidence about the influence of perioperative fluid therapy on patient outcomes (Hahn, Bahlmann, & Nilsson, 2014; Kampmeier et al., 2014; Lobo et al., 2006). Indeed, while the quality and quantity of IVF literature are growing there are few definitive answers for the perioperative setting (Kampmeier et al., 2014).

Translating available evidence into practice is further complicated by differing definitions within the literature, varying clinical research designs, inconsistent end points for analysis, and, maybe most importantly, limited evidence on euvolemia and normal blood volume (D'Angelo, Hodgen, Wofford, & Vacchiano, 2015; de Almeida et al., 2012; Doherty & Buggy, 2012; Lobo et al., 2006; Strunden, Heckel, Goetz, & Reuter, 2011; van Haren & Zacharowski, 2014; Veenstra, Ince, & Boerma, 2014). Therefore, the purpose of this chapter will be to (a) review the conventional methods for perioperative fluid administration and its underlying philosophy, (b) review the physiology of hypovolemia and hypervolemia, (c) review emerging technologies, (d) describe Goal-Directed Fluid Therapy (GDFT), and (e) provide a brief analysis and a look toward the future of perioperative IVF therapy.

The Anesthetic Fluid Plan

The use of IVFs has been standard anesthetic practice since the inception of IV anesthetics. Traditionally, the administration of perioperative IVF therapy is guided by the anesthetic fluid plan. The anesthetic fluid plan is the combination of an anesthetic fluid algorithm and the calculation of the allowable blood loss (ABL) as determined by the HcT. The anesthetic fluid algorithm consists of four major subcomponents: maintenance fluid, fasting deficits (nil per hour [NPO]), losses to the "third space" and/or evaporative losses, and estimated blood loss (Gallagher & Vacchiano, 2014).

Maintenance fluid was first described by Holliday and Segar in 1957, and has remained relatively unchanged and unchallenged for over 50 years (Bailey, McNaull, Jooste, & Tuchman, 2010). Holliday and Segar's original work addressed the perioperative IVF requirements for children (Holliday & Segar, 1957). Their work has commonly become known as the "4-2-1 Rule." The "4-2-1 Rule" is a fixed, weight-based method that is intended to compensate for patient sensible and insensible fluid losses. Sensible losses include measurable fluid deficits as a result of perspiration, feces, and urine. Insensible losses are evaporative fluid deficits from the skin and lungs and are estimated to be approximately 0.2 mL/kg/hr to 0.3 mL/kg/hr in the normothermic patient (Voldby & Brandstrup, 2016). In the years that followed, the "4-2-1 Rule" has become widely embraced by the anesthesia community and has become a pillar for standardized intraoperative IVF management for surgical patients of all ages (Arya, 2012; Bailey et al., 2010).

The second component of the fluid algorithm accounts for fasting deficits. The replacement of fasting deficits was recommended by Furman and colleagues in 1975 and based on the general belief that surgical patients are hypovolemic due to preoperative fluid restriction and fasting (Arya, 2012; Furman et al., 1975; Muller et al., 2014). Despite this common belief there is little evidence to support the notion of preoperative hypovolemia from NPO (Hahn et al., 2014; Muller et al., 2014). A growing body of research may actually refute this core belief; however, as fasting guidelines change and become less stringent this component may likely become less of a clinical issue (Arya, 2012; Voldby & Brandstrup, 2016).

The concept of "third space" losses was introduced by Shires and colleagues in 1961 (Shires, Williams, & Brown, 1961). According to Shires, the "third space" is a potential reservoir of nonfunctional fluid stores that is a result of capillary leak. Shires et al. postulated that there were decreases in extracellular fluid volume (ECFV) as a result of surgical trauma causing fluid to leak from the intravascular space into the "third space." Using an experimental design Shires measured ECFV before incision and at 2 hours following surgical procedures and determined a loss of intravascular fluid in the experimental (surgical) group (Bailey et al., 2010; Shires, 1968; Shires et al., 1961). Unfortunately, however, critics of Shires's work note flaws in design and question the true loss of ECFV as a result of surgical trauma (Bailey et al., 2010; Shires, 1968; Shires et al., 1961). Several studies refute the existence of the "third space" and Shires et al.'s postulated decreases in ECFV (Brandstrup et al., 2003). Without rigorous empirical support the concept of the "third space" should be abandoned.

Surgical wound evaporative loss was initially described by Lamke et al. (Lamke, Nilsson, & Reithner, 1977). Using a chamber above exposed viscera the researchers were able to demonstrate a great range of evaporative losses from tissue to the environment (Lamke et al., 1977). The authors found that the rate of evaporation correlated with surgical incision size. Through this work the anesthetic fluid algorithm was modified to accommodate the potential loss of fluids to the environment: Small incisions increased fluid administration by 2 g/hr and extensive, large incisions increased fluid administration by as much as 32 g/hr (Lamke et al., 1977; Voldby & Brandstrup, 2016).

In addition to the fluid plan, anesthetists routinely calculate the ABL. The ABL is used as a means to calculate the acceptable quantity of blood that can be shed before the anesthetist would consider transfusing blood products to the patient (Bourke & Smith, 1974). The ABL is calculated by calculating the patient's ideal blood volume (BVi) and multiplying the BVi by the change in HcT (HcT baseline – HcT target/Hct baseline; Gross, 1983). Like the anesthetic fluid plan, this practice is problematic as it assumes continuous maintenance of euvolemia with crystalloid/colloid during exsanguination. The HcT only defines the percentage of red cell mass as it relates to total blood volume (TBV). This number alone cannot be used to differentiate between anemia and hemodilution or between polycythemia and hemoconcentration (Jacob et al., 2012).

The historical foundation laid by the works of Holliday and Segar, Shires, and Furman has been passed from generation to generation of anesthetists. Multiple anesthesia texts have published the anesthetic fluid algorithm with very little variation for over half a century (Barash, Cullen, Stoelting, Cahalan, & Stock, 2009). For example, for the 38-year-old patient described in the vignette (ideal body weight 85 kg), the traditional IVF plan prescribes maintenance fluid of 125 mL/hour, fasting deficit replacement of 1.5 L (given over 2 hours), third space loss replacement of 680 mL/hr, and ongoing crystalloid replacement of blood loss of 1350 mL, for a total of 9.6 L of crystalloid given over the course of the case. The patient actually received 8.9 L of crystalloid, 93% of the volume prescribed by the algorithmic approach. However, the patient's instability at the conclusion of the case clearly demonstrates that he developed an intraoperative fluid volume deficit greater than the 700 mL difference between the volume prescribed by the algorithm and the volume actually administered. Given that the traditional proxy measures of fluid volume, including blood pressure, heart rate, and urine output, remained within normal limits during the case, this situation clearly demonstrates the inadequacy of the traditional fluid plan in meeting the individualized needs of this patient.

While the anesthetic fluid plan is commonly used to guide intraoperative IVF therapy, its implementation is provider-dependent (Lilot et al., 2015). Lilot et al. performed a retrospective data analysis of intraoperative fluid administration during open intra-abdominal procedures at two large medical centers in the United States. Variability of fluid administration between providers was expressed as the Corrected Coefficient of Variation (cCOV; Lilot et al., 2015). Mean fluid administration across centers was 7.1 (sd 4.9) mL/kg/h, and individual provider's administration ranged from 2.3 (sd 3.7) to 14 (sd 10) mL/kg/hr (Lilot et al., 2015; Minto & Mythen, 2015). Data from this study demonstrates that fluid administration is largely based on provider interpretation of clinical indicators and personal habits. One can only assume that this phenomenon is not unique to the context of this study and two medical centers. The results give rise to the question: Why is there so much variability in IVF administration practices between providers?

The answer to this question is largely speculative, but it likely stems from the discrepancy between the state of the science and the traditions of the anesthetic fluid plan. While the anesthetic fluid plan is commonly used to guide IVF therapy, it must be remembered that this fluid algorithm was intended for a euvolemic patient minus fasting deficits. The most practical use of the anesthetic fluid plan is for healthy patients. This assumption holds true for the ABL. In the absence of blood volume analysis the HcT (or hemoglobin) alone is relatively worthless. While the anesthetic fluid plan is oriented toward "optimized" patients in reality it is applied to patients undergoing complex, high-risk procedures. Thus, a substantial proportion of patients who present for surgery are not "normal" patients. Indeed, medications, diet, and physical health status can all alter normal blood volume (D'Angelo et al., 2015).

Therefore, the traditional anesthetic fluid plan is wrought with opportunities for error. Despite a growing body of contradictory research the anesthetic fluid plan continues to be utilized. While there are several limitations with the anesthetic fluid plan, none is greater than its inability to predict or compensate for deviations from euvolemia. Therefore, the anesthetist must rely on surrogate markers to detect, evaluate, and guide IVF administration. Unfortunately, the inability of clinicians to accurately identify blood volume abnormalities (Iregui et al., 2003) likely contributes to hypo- and hypervolemia.

The Physiology of Hypovolemia and Hypervolemia

The ultimate goal of perioperative IVF therapy is to optimize patient cardiovascular function and promote adequate tissue perfusion (Kampmeier et al., 2014). Assuming a nonseptic state, euvolemia represents an ideal relationship between blood volume, systemic vascular resistance (SVR), and cardiac output (CO). Through this relationship tissue receives adequate perfusion over a wide range of changes in metabolic demand. Euvolemia is most often cited as the desired "end state" for the administration of IVFs in the perioperative setting (Aditianingsih & George, 2014). Ideally, perioperative IVF therapy should be administered to maintain patient euvolemia and ultimately support adequate perfusion (Chappell, Jacob, Hofmann-Kiefer, Conzen, & Rehm, 2008). Generally speaking, too little IVF leads to hypovolemia and excessive fluid leads to hypervolemia (Chappell & Jacob, 2014).

Hypovolemia, or reduced circulating volume, is a serious concern in the perioperative arena (Navarro et al., 2015). Hypovolemia contributes to inadequate tissue perfusion and is associated with postoperative complications (Navarro et al., 2015). Dehydration and hemoconcentration are common events for patients who are malnourished, have not had oral fluids, have shed blood volume, or have had preoperative mechanical bowel preparations (Junghans et al., 2006; Lobo et al., 2006).

Although hypovolemia does not necessarily equate to shock it does share a common physiologic pathway. Hypovolemia has a very deliberate pathological progression that activates both a rapid and slow response. Decreased intravascular volume causes baroreceptors in the great vessels, heart, and carotid bodies to become activated (Frajewicki et al., 1997). This activation stimulates the afferent sympathetic nervous system (SNS) and the vasomotor center of the medulla (Guyton & Hall, 2006). Catecholamines released from efferent SNS neurons stimulate adrenergic receptors. These receptors trigger constriction of vascular smooth muscle and increasing SVR, cardiac inotropy and chronotropy with the goal of improving perfusion pressure (Guyton & Hall, 2006).

As hypovolemia progresses and glomerular filtration rate is reduced the juxtaglomerular cells of the afferent arterioles release renin (Guyton & Hall, 2006). Renin begins a negative feedback loop with the intent of reversing hypovolemia via the renin–angiotensinogen–aldosterone system (RAAS). The primary function of the RAAS is to produce angiotensin-II (A-II). A-II is a potent vasoconstrictor that acts directly on the vascular smooth muscle and indirectly by increasing the release and reducing the metabolism of SNS neurotransmitters yielding an increased SVR and improved perfusion pressure. Aldosterone, antidiuretic hormone and atrial natriuretic peptide are released to increase fluid reabsorption (Kampmeier et al., 2014). While the release of neuroendocrine hormone occurs with the sympathetic response, it is a time-dependent process, in many cases requiring more than 24 hours to increase plasma or intravascular volume (Mythen & Webb, 1994).

According to Starling's equation, intravascular hypovolemia will cause fluid from the extravascular compartment to mobilize and shift to the intravascular space. Increases in oncotic forces favor reabsorption of interstitial fluids while reductions in hydrostatic pressure reduce perfusion at the tissue (Guyton & Hall, 2006). Reabsorption of fluid from the interstitium to the vasculature may act as an "autotransfusion" temporarily masking the clinical indicators of hypovolemia.

The influence of hypovolemia at the level of tissue perfusion is variable based upon volume deficit, patient pathology, and metabolic demand of the tissue. In the early stages, decreased intravascular volume causes blood to shunt away from "ischemia tolerant" tissues (Dutton, 2002). While this can be tolerated in many patients for an extended period of time, if uncorrected, it can lead to anaerobic respiration and the accumulation of metabolic byproducts such as lactate (Dutton, 2001).

While fluid restriction and hypovolemia have been implicated with increased postoperative complications, excessive fluid administration and subsequent hypervolemia are also antithetical to euvolemia (Joshi, 2005; Voldby & Brandstrup, 2016). In the normal, well-functioning heart, hypervolemia exerts its most significant influence at the level of capillary. Using Starling's equation, increased intravascular volume will cause increases in hydrostatic pressure favoring filtration of intravascular fluid from the vasculature to the interstitium. Simultaneously, hypervolemia dilutes circulating plasma proteins and reduces overall oncotic pressure (Guyton & Hall, 2006). Increased filtration with reduced absorption will yield fluid accumulation in the interstitium and tissue edema.

Tissue edema is not benign nor without significant clinical impact for the patient. Edema has been shown to reduce tissue oxygenation, and obstruct and impair capillary blood flow (Larsen, Singh, Velocci, Nasser, & McCullough, 2016). Disruption to the capillary–tissue interface retards metabolite clearance and alters cellular interactions (Larsen et al., 2016). Fluid retention and weight gain as a result of excessive fluid administration is a common event following major surgery. On average, a patient's weight may increase 5 to 10 kg due to IVF administration (Holte, Sharrock, & Kehlet, 2002; Kudsk, 2003). Positive fluid balance has been shown as a predictor of hospital mortality and significantly impairs the pulmonary, cardiac, renal, and gastrointestinal systems (Larsen et al., 2016; Silva et al., 2013). In a retrospective evaluation of 48 patients admitted to the intensive care unit, Lowell, Schifferdecker, Driscoll, Benotti, and Bistrian (1990) observed that patients whose weight increased greater than 10% of their baseline demonstrated 32% greater incidence of mortality when compared to those who had a weight gain of less than 10% (Lowell et al., 1990).

Emerging Technologies

The relative failures of the anesthetic fluid plan and growing body of evidence for increased risk of morbidity and mortality associated with hypovolemia and hypervolemia have led to an increased effort to develop and refine methods to assess tissue perfusion. Clinically, perfusion is routinely evaluated by blood pressure, guided by the belief that tissue oxygenation is dependent on adequate perfusion. Unfortunately, normal blood pressure does not necessarily equate to adequate perfusion (Menon et al., 2000). Assuming normal cardiac function, blood pressure can be viewed as a dynamic continuum between intravascular volume and SVR. In a nonseptic state, this relationship is inversely proportional. As intravascular volume decreases (i.e., dehydration and hemorrhage) vascular tone increases (vasoconstriction) to support and maintain perfusion. While this relationship maintains homeostasis, it can mislead the anesthetist.

Clinical investigation has demonstrated that a healthy patient can tolerate in excess of 20% blood volume deficit with little to no change in vital signs (Dutton, 2001). During this period, the pathologic effects of hypovolemia and hypoperfusion can occur. Current methods of assessing intravascular volume, including blood pressure, heart rate, central venous pressure, and pulmonary artery pressure, have demonstrated mixed results at accurately predicting blood volume abnormalities (Birkhahn, Gaeta, Terry, Bove, & Tloczkowski, 2005; Sinert & Spektor, 2005).

The late 1990s brought a dramatic change to the way anesthetists and surgeons viewed IVF therapy (Thiele, Bartels, & Gan, 2015). The dawn of the 21st century introduced the perioperative community to innovative practices like Enhanced Recovery After Surgery (ERAS) and brought older concepts like GDFT to the forefront of the IVF therapy discussion (Thiele et al., 2015). ERAS protocols and GDFT typically involve algorithmic-like processes that are targeted to guide IVF administration with the intent to maximize perfusion during complex surgical procedures (Thiele et al., 2015; Van der Linden, Dierick, Wilmin, Bellens, & Hert, 2010). While ERAS and GDFT will be discussed in detail later in this chapter, the implementation of these strategies has created a technological wave to meet the growing, and evolving, demands of clinicians who manage intraoperative IVF therapy. Indeed, CO monitoring during high-risk abdominal surgery has been shown to reduce cost, postoperative complications, and mortality (Legrand, Ruscio, Benhamou, & Pelletier-Fleury, 2015).

Goal-Directed Fluid Therapy is a general term used to describe the use of CO, or some other similar physiologic parameter, to guide IVF administration and titrate inotropic agents. Many of the evolving technologies have focused on providing measurements of CO or, more recently, indices of patient fluid responsiveness from a fluid bolus (Thiele et al., 2015). Existing technologies described in the literature include the pulmonary artery catheter (PAC), photoplethysmography (PPG), bioimpedance, bioreactance, esophageal Doppler (ED), and arterial waveform analysis (AWA); see Thiele et al. (2015). Although each of these technologies will be described, the greatest emphasis and discussion of this section will focus on ED and AWA. While all technologies have limitations, the current data strongly supports the use or implementation of ED and AWA (SITE; Thiele et al., 2015) when euvolemia is critical to ensuring patient survival (or well-being, or whatever).

Pulmonary Artery Catheter

The PAC was introduced into practice in the 1970s and has long been considered the "gold standard" to measure CO (Chatterjee, 2009). A PAC is a flexible, flow-directed, balloon-tipped catheter that is directed into a branch of the pulmonary artery through access from the right side of the heart. Cardiac output is determined by the injection of cool fluids (typically room temperature) that are diluted in the right atrium and measured by a thermistor further down the PAC (Dulak, 2003). Although PACs have been evaluated for use in GDFT trials (Gurgel & do Nascimento, 2011), their efficacy and safety in "routine" practice, along with the development of less invasive CO monitors, makes the PAC a less attractive option (Thiele et al., 2015).

Photoplethysmography

PPG is the use of a red or near-infrared light (pulse oximeter) to illuminate the skin and measure changes in light absorption (Nilsson, 2013). Partridge (1987) identified PPG as a potential tool for the noninvasive evaluation of fluid responsiveness (Partridge, 1987). PPG works by leveraging absorption of light by hemoglobin and the pressure change exerted on the vasculature by respiration. The change in light absorption from pulsatile blood flow, along with the oscillation from breathing, creates a large and a small oximeter pulse pressure (Partridge, 1987; Thiele et al., 2015). The change in pulse pressures is used to calculate the Pleth Variability Index (PVI).

PPG and PVI technology is packed in a variety of devices by developers. Its use and value to guide IVF therapy is in its infancy. Forget et al. employed PVI technology in a randomized study of general surgery patients (Forget, Lois, & de Kock, 2010). The PVI group demonstrated lower levels of lactate development despite receiving lower quantities of IVFs (Forget et al., 2010). While data appears promising, it is too early to determine what value PPG will have to effectively guide intraoperative IVF therapy.

Bioimpedance and Bioreactance

Bioimpedance technologies are noninvasive monitors that have the potential to measure body water volumes (Earthman, Traughber, Dobratz, & Howell, 2007). Bioimpedance monitors are based on Ohm's law and apply a small amount of electrical current over the thorax and measure the resistance of electrical current that flows through biological material (Thiele et al., 2015). In the ideal situation, bioimpedance monitors continuously measure the changes in intrathoracic blood volume and the change of impedance as a result of pulsatile flow (Thiele et al., 2015). Despite the relative ease of use, bioimpedance is susceptible to inaccurate measurement due to a variety of factors to include electrical noise and pulmonary edema (Thiele et al., 2015). One clinical study demonstrated agreement between ED and bioimpedance for the decision to administer IVFs despite variation in estimated stroke volume (SV; Waldron et al., 2014). This may suggest reliability between methods (Thiele et al., 2015; Waldron et al., 2014).

Because of the limitations of bioimpedance, bioreactance is an emerging technology that was developed by Cheetah Medical to measure CO. Bioreactance is based on the principle of thoracic phase shifts. Phase shifts are a result of alternating current in the thoracic cavity that results from a time delay between the current and the electrical voltage (Keren, Burkhoff, & Squara, 2007). Several authors have evaluated the efficacy of bioreactance when compared to other methods and support both the accuracy of the technology and its utility in fluid administration. Benomar et al. demonstrated that bioreactance could accurately predict fluid responsiveness and CO during passive leg raises (Benomar, Ouattara, Estagnasie, Brusset, & Squara, 2010). Waldron and colleagues compared ED with bioreactance for patients undergoing major colorectal surgery (Waldron et al., 2014). Early research has demonstrated a close correlation between ED and bioreactance and no difference in patient outcome when comparing methods.

Esophageal Doppler

ED is a minimally invasive hemodynamic monitor that can evaluate CO and volume status. ED assesses CO and volume status by calculating the heart rate and estimating the SV (Atlas, Brealey, Dhar, Dikta, & Singer, 2012). This technology is based upon the Doppler principle where the sound wave of a moving object is reflected back toward a probe. ED monitors measures blood flow velocity in the descending thoracic aorta (Thiele et al., 2015). CO and SV are estimated using nomograms that incorporate age, height, and weight that calibrates the monitor to the patient.

ED has the greatest and most compelling body of literature to support its use to guide the perioperative administration of IVFs, and has a demonstrated validity in estimating CO. Dark and Singer (2004) determined the validity of the ED in measuring CO in the critically ill when compared with the PAC thermodilution (PAC-TD) technique. The analysis incorporated a total of 11 validation papers that included 314 patients (Dark & Singer, 2004). The pooled median bias for PAC-TD versus ED was 0.19 L/min (range of –0.69–2.00 L/min) for CO (16 studies) and 0.6% (range of 0–2.3%) for changes in CO (5 studies). The pooled median percentage of clinical agreement (PCA) for PAC-TD versus ED was 52% (interquartile range [IQR] of 42%–69%) for CO and 86% (IQR of 55%–93%) for changes in CO. These differences in PCA were significant ($p = .03$ Mann–Whitney) for bolus PAC-TD as the clinical "gold standard." They concluded that the ED has high validity (no bias and high clinical agreement with PAC-TD) for monitoring changes in CO (Dark & Singer, 2004).

GDFT guided by ED has been demonstrated to positively impact clinical outcomes, such as length of postoperative hospital stay. In a study by Gan et al. (2002), a total of 100 subjects scheduled for major elective general, urologic, or gynecologic surgery with an anticipated blood loss greater than 500 mL were randomly assigned to a control group ($n = 50$) that received standard intraoperative care or to a protocol group ($n = 50$) that received intraoperative plasma volume expansion guided by the ED monitor (Gan et al., 2002). The protocol group demonstrated a significantly higher SV and CO at the end of surgery when compared with the control group. Patients in the protocol group received more fluid, had a reduced length of stay (LOS; $p = .03$), and had a faster return of bowel function ($p = .01$) when compared with the control group. The authors concluded that ED goal-directed intraoperative fluid administration contributed to the return of bowel function, lower incidence of postoperative nausea and vomiting, and decrease in LOS (Gan et al., 2002).

More recently, Chattopadhyay et al. (2013) examined the effect of fluid optimization using ED compared to standard fluid management on postoperative morbidity in women who underwent major gynecological cancer surgery (Chattopadhyay et al., 2013). Cases were sampled from two surgeons. A total of 198 subjects were enrolled; 79 were in the experimental group (ED) and 119 in the control, or standard anesthetic care group. The use of ED was associated with earlier postoperative recovery (adjusted *OR*, 2.83; 95% CIs [1.20, 6.68]; $p = .02$), fitness for discharge (adjusted *OR*, 2.81; 95% CIs [1.01, 7.78]; $p = .05$), and oral diet resumption than women in the "control group" group (median, 1 day versus 2 days; $p = .02$). The authors concluded that intraoperative fluid optimization with ED may be associated with improved postoperative recovery and early fitness for discharge (Chattopadhyay et al., 2013).

The most compelling evidence to date that supports the use of ED is a collection of seven prospective, randomized trials that included a total of 694 patients (Chytra et al., 2007; Gan et al., 2002; Noblett, Snowden, Shenton, & Horgan, 2006; Pillai et al., 2011; Sinclair, James, & Singer, 1997; Thiele et al., 2015; Venn et al., 2002; Wakeling et al., 2005). Using ED, these seven articles demonstrated a weighted average reduction in hospital LOS of 3.7 days (Thiele et al., 2015). These results were corroborated by a United Kingdom National Health Service study. In this study, ED was used to guide fluid therapy in 649 patients (in comparison with 658 who received standard treatment). The study demonstrated a 3.6-day reduction in stay for the ED group as compared with standard treatment for major abdominal, urologic, and gynecologic surgeries (Thiele et al., 2015).

Arterial Waveform Analysis

The bedside measurement of arterial waveforms has been used for over 50 years (Esper & Pinsky, 2014). AWA measures stroke volume variation (SVV). SVV can indicate a patient's volume status based upon the Frank–Starling curve (Esper & Pinsky, 2014; Thiele et al., 2015). AWA has been evaluated as a means to administer fluid in several GDFT settings. Like ED, most studies have shown that AWA demonstrates a reduction in hospital LOS (Thiele et al., 2015). Five articles demonstrated that the use of AWA for fluid management had a mean weighted average reduction in hospital LOS by 2.2 days in comparison to standard treatment (Buettner et al., 2008; Thiele et al., 2015). Despite these positive findings, the total number of studies to date does not have statistically meaningful comparisons between AWA and improved outcomes.

Although the methods to administer IVF therapy are not without limitations, the great majority of the literature supports the use of ED and AWA. The results of work by Pestaña and colleagues support the notion that perioperative hemodynamic protocol guided by invasive CO monitoring is superior to noninvasive or standard methods (Pestana et al., 2014). As technology emerges and practices evolve, standard practice will progress to therapy that is individualized to the patient and targeted toward a fluid therapy goal.

Goal-Directed Fluid Therapy

Aside from PPG, bioreactance, and ED, few methods of guiding fluid therapy have been correlated to improved patient outcomes. To address this limitation, GDFT has been proposed as an alternative fluid management technique to the traditional anesthetic fluid plan. GDFT emerged in anesthetic practice from the critical care community near the turn of the millennium and has increasingly gained acceptance as evidence mounts to support its use (Mayer, Boldt, Mengistu, Röhm, & Suttner, 2010). As previously noted, GDFT employs a variety of monitoring techniques that are intended to drive or orient the patient's IVF therapy toward a predetermined goal; most often to optimized cardiac performance by SV or CO.

GDFT has been shown to reduce hospital LOS. Lopes et al. (2007) demonstrated reductions in patient LOS as a result of GDFT using AWA (Lopes et al., 2007). This study design included 33 randomly assigned subjects to GDFT or standard care. Subjects assigned to the GDFT protocol had a shorter LOS, fewer complications, and shorter duration of mechanical ventilation (Lopes et al., 2007). In another study by Gan et al., patients receiving GDFT were shown to reduce LOS compared to standard operative care (5,420 mL vs. 4,775 mL; Gan et al., 2002; Voldby & Brandstrup, 2016).

Several meta-analyses have been conducted that have evaluated and summarized the overall effects of GDFT. Benes, Giglio, Brienza, and Michard (2014) included 14 studies (961 participants) in their analysis (Benes et al., 2014). Authors of this study noted a reduction in postoperative morbidity with GDFT (OR = 0.51; CI 0.34 to 0.75; $p < .001$; Benes et al., 2014). It is believed that the reduction in morbidity was due to a significant reduction in infectious (OR = 0.45; CI 0.27 to 0.74; $p = .002$), cardiovascular (OR = 0.55; CI 0.36 to 0.82; $p = .004$), and abdominal (OR = 0.56; CI 0.37 to 0.86; $p = .008$) complications. Additionally, GDFT was associated with a significant decrease in intensive care LOS (Weighted Mean Difference [WMD] −0.75 days; CI −1.37 to −0.12; $p = .02$).

A meta-analysis by Ripolles-Melchor et al. (2016) included five randomized controlled trials that used supraphysiologic hemodynamic targets. This meta-analysis demonstrated that there was a significant reduction in mortality for patients who received GDFT versus standard therapy (risk ratio, 0.63; 95% CIs [0.42, 0.94]; $p = .02$; Ripolles-Melchor et al., 2016). Although GDFT demonstrated some significant benefits for the reduction in mortality, Ripolles-Melchor and colleagues were unable to show that GDFT reduced patient complications (risk ratio, 0.75; 95% CIs [0.50, 1.17]; $p = .21$; Ripolles-Melchor et al., 2016).

In another meta-analysis, Rollins and Lobo (2016) evaluated 23 studies that included 2,099 patients (1,040 GDFT and 1,059 conventional fluid therapy). GDFT demonstrated many positive findings to include: a reduction in morbidity (risk ratio 0.76, 95% CIs [0.66, 0.89], $p = .0007$), reduced hospital LOS (mean difference 1.55 days, 95% CIs [2.73, 0.36], $p = .01$), reduced intensive care LOS (mean difference 0.63 days, 95% CIs [1.18, 0.09], $p = .02$), and reduced time to passage of feces (mean difference 0.90 days, 95% CIs [1.48, 0.32], $p = .002$; Rollins & Lobo, 2016).

CONCLUSIONS

While GDFT has generated significant support it continues to require scrutiny. Research has shown that not all GDFT protocols reduce morbidity and mortality when compared with traditional methods (Buettner et al., 2008). Additionally, there is no consensus as to which technologies to guide GDFT are most efficacious. Indeed, while GDFT has challenged the traditional paradigm it may be too early to declare victory for GDFT or defeat for traditional methods.

REFERENCES

Aditianingsih, D., & George, Y. W. (2014). Guiding principles of fluid and volume therapy. *Best Practice & Research Clinical Anaesthesiology, 28*(3), 249–260. http://dx.doi.org/10.1016/j.bpa.2014.07.002

Arya, V. K. (2012). Basics of fluid and blood transfusion therapy in paediatric surgical patients. *Indian Journal of Anaesthesia, 56*(5), 454–462. http://dx.doi.org/10.4103/0019-5049.103960

Atlas, G., Brealey, D., Dhar, S., Dikta, G., & Singer, M. (2012). Additional hemodynamic measurements with an esophageal Doppler monitor: A preliminary report of compliance, force, kinetic energy, and afterload in the clinical setting. *Journal of Clinical Monitoring and Computing, 26*(6), 473–482. http://dx.doi.org/10.1007/s10877-012-9386-5

Bailey, A. G., McNaull, P. P., Jooste, E., & Tuchman, J. B. (2010). Perioperative crystalloid and colloid fluid management in children: Where are we and how did we get here? *Anesthesia and Analgesia, 110*(2), 375–390.

Barash, P. G., Cullen, B. F., Stoelting, R. K., Cahalan, M. K., & Stock, M. C. (2009). *Clinical anesthesia* (6th ed.). Philadeplhia, PA: Wolters, Kluwer, Lippincott, Williams & Wilkins.

Benes, J., Giglio, M., Brienza, N., & Michard, F. (2014). The effects of goal-directed fluid therapy based on dynamic parameters on post-surgical outcome: A meta-analysis of randomized controlled trials. *Critical Care, 18*(5), 584. http://dx.doi.org/10.1186/s13054-014-0584-z

Benomar, B., Ouattara, A., Estagnasie, P., Brusset, A., & Squara, P. (2010). Fluid responsiveness predicted by noninvasive bioreactance-based passive leg raise test. *Intensive Care Medicine, 36*(11), 1875–1881. http://dx.doi.org/10.1007/s00134-010-1990-6

Birkhahn, R. H., Gaeta, T. J., Terry, D., Bove, J. J., & Tloczkowski, J. (2005). Shock index in diagnosing early acute hypovolemia. *The American Journal of Emergency Medicine, 23*(3), 323–326.

Bourke, D. L., & Smith, T. C. (1974). Estimating allowable hemodilution. *Anesthesiology, 41*(6), 609–612.

Brandstrup, B. (2006). Fluid therapy for the surgical patient. *Best Practice & Research Clinical Anaesthesiology, 20*(2), 265–283.

Brandstrup, B., Tønnesen, H., Beier-Holgersen, R., Hjortsø, E., Ørding, H., & Lindorff-Larsen, K. (2003). Effects of intravenous fluid restriction on postoperative complications: Comparison of two perioperative fluid regimens: A randomized assessor-blinded multicenter trial. *Annals of Surgery, 238*(5), 641–648.

Buettner, M., Schummer, W., Huettemann, E., Schenke, S., van Hout, N., & Sakka, S. G. (2008). Influence of systolic-pressure-variation-guided intraoperative fluid management on organ function and oxygen transport. *British Journal of Anaesthesia, 101*(2), 194–199. http://dx.doi.org/10.1093/bja/aen126

Chappell, D., & Jacob, M. (2014). Role of the glycocalyx in fluid management: Small things matter. *Best Practice & Research Clinical Anaesthesiology, 28*(3), 227–234. http://dx.doi.org/10.1016/j.bpa.2014.06.003

Chappell, D., Jacob, M., Hofmann-Kiefer, K., Conzen, P., & Rehm, M. (2008). A rational approach to perioperative fluid management. *Anesthesiology, 109*(4), 723–740. http://dx.doi.org/10.1097/aln.0b013e3181863117

Chatterjee, K. (2009). The Swan-Ganz catheters: Past, present, and future. A viewpoint. *Circulation, 119*(1), 147–152. http://dx.doi.org/10.1161/circulationaha.108.811141

Chattopadhyay, S., Mittal, S., Christian, S., Terblanche, A. L., Patel, A., Biliatis, I., et al. (2013). The role of intraoperative fluid optimization using the esophageal Doppler in advanced gynecological cancer: Early postoperative recovery and fitness for discharge. *International Journal of Gynecological Cancer, 23*(1), 199–207. http://dx.doi.org/10.1097/igc.0b013e3182752372

Chytra, I., Pradl, R., Bosman, R., Pelnar, P., Kasal, E., & Zidkova, A. (2007). Esophageal Doppler-guided fluid management decreases blood lactate levels in multiple-trauma patients: A randomized controlled trial. *Critical Care, 11*(1), R24. http://dx.doi.org/10.1186/cc5703

Corcoran, T., Rhodes, J. E. J., Clarke, S., Myles, P. S., & Ho, K. M. (2012). Perioperative fluid management strategies in major surgery: A stratified meta-analysis. *Anesthesia & Analgesia, 114*(3), 640–641.

D'Angelo, M., Hodgen, R. K., Wofford, K., & Vacchiano, C. (2015). A theoretical mathematical model to estimate blood volume in clinical practice. *Biological Research For Nursing, 17*(5), 478–486. http://dx.doi.org/10.1177/1099800414555410

Dark, P. M., & Singer, M. (2004). The validity of trans-esophageal Doppler ultrasonography as a measure of cardiac output in critically ill adults. *Intensive Care Medicine, 30*(11), 2060–2066. http://dx.doi.org/10.1007/s00134-004-2430-2

de Almeida, J. P., Palomba, H., Galas, F. R., Fukushima, J. T., Duarte, F. A., Nagaoka, D.,et al. (2012). Positive fluid balance is associated with reduced survival in critically ill patients with cancer. *Acta Anaesthesiologica Scandinavica, 56*(6), 712–717. http://dx.doi.org/10.1111/j.1399-6576.2012.02717.x

Doherty, M., & Buggy, D. J. (2012). Intraoperative fluids: How much is too much? *British Journal of Anaesthesia, 109*(1), 69–79. http://dx.doi.org/10.1093/bja/aes171

Dulak, S. B. (2003). A PA catheter refresher course. *Resonance, 66*(4), 28–34; quiz 35.

Dutton, R. P. (2001). Resuscitation from traumatic shock. *Current opinion in anaesthesiology, 14*(2), 217–220.

Dutton, R. P. (2002). Low-pressure resuscitation from hemorrhagic shock. *International anesthesiology clinics, 40*(3), 19–30.

Earthman, C., Traughber, D., Dobratz, J., & Howell, W. (2007). Bioimpedance spectroscopy for clinical assessment of fluid distribution and body cell mass. *Nutrition in Clinical Practice, 22*(4), 389–405.

Esper, S. A., & Pinsky, M. R. (2014). Arterial waveform analysis. *Best Practice & Research Clinical Anaesthesiology, 28*(4), 363–380. http://dx.doi.org/10.1016/j.bpa.2014.08.002

Forget, P., Lois, F., & de Kock, M. (2010). Goal-directed fluid management based on the pulse oximeter-derived pleth variability index reduces lactate levels and improves fluid management. *Anesthesia & Analgesia, 111*(4), 910–914. http://dx.doi.org/10.1213/ane.0b013e3181eb624f

Frajewicki, V., Kahana, L., Yechieli, H., Brod, V., Kohan, R., & Bitterman, H. (1997). Effects of severe hemorrhage on plasma ANP and glomerular ANP receptors. *The American Journal of Physiology, 273*(5 Pt 2), R1623–R1630.

Furman, E. B., Roman, D. G., Lemmer, L. A., Hairabet, J., Jasinska, M., & Laver, M. B. (1975). Specific therapy in water, electrolyte and blood-volume replacement during pediatric surgery. *Anesthesiology, 42*(2), 187–193.

Gallagher, K., & Vacchiano, C. (2014). Reexamining traditional intraoperative fluid administration: Evolving views in the age of goal-directed therapy. *American Association of Nurse Anesthetists Journal, 82*(3), 235–242.

Gan, T. J., Soppitt, A., Maroof, M., Moalem, H., Robertson, K. M., & Moretti, E. (2002). Goal-directed intraoperative fluid administration reduces length of hospital stay after major surgery. *Anesthesiology, 97*(4), 820–826.

Gross, J. B. (1983). Estimating allowable blood loss: Corrected for dilution. *Anesthesiology, 58*(3), 277–280.

Gurgel, S. T., & do Nascimento, P., Jr. (2011). Maintaining tissue perfusion in high-risk surgical patients: A systematic review of randomized clinical trials. *Anesthesia & Analgesia, 112*(6), 1384–1391. http://dx.doi.org/10.1213/ane.0b013e3182055384

Guyton, A., & Hall, J. (2006). *Textbook of medical physiology* (11th ed.). Philadelphia, PA: W.B. Saunders.

Hahn, R. G., Bahlmann, H., & Nilsson, L. (2014). Dehydration and fluid volume kinetics before major open abdominal surgery. *Acta Anaesthesiologica Scandinavica, 58*(10), 1258–1266.

Holliday, M., & Segar, W. E. (1957). The maintenance need for water in parenteral fluid therapy. *Pediatrics, 19*(5), 823–832.

Holte, K., Sharrock, N. E., & Kehlet, H. (2002). Pathophysiology and clinical implications of perioperative fluid excess. *British Journal of Anaesthesia, 89*(4), 622–632.

Iregui, M. G., Prentice, D., Sherman, G., Schallom, L., Sona, C., & Kollef, M. H. (2003). Physician's estimates of cardiac index and intravascular volume based on clinical assessment versus transesophageal Doppler measurements obtained by critical care nurses. *American Journal of Critical Care, 12*(4), 336–342.

Jacob, M., Annaheim, S., Boutellier, U., Hinske, C., Rehm, M., Breymann, C., et al. (2012). Haematocrit is invalid for estimating red cell volume: A prospective study in male volunteers. *Blood Transfus, 10*(4), 471–479. http://dx.doi.org/10.2450/2012.0111-11

Joshi, G. P. (2005). Intraoperative fluid restriction improves outcome after major elective gastrointestinal surgery. *Anesthesia & Analgesia, 101*(2), 601–605. http://dx.doi.org/10.1213/01.ane.0000159171.26521.31

Junghans, T., Neuss, H., Strohauer, M., Raue, W., Haase, O., Schink, T., et al. (2006). Hypovolemia after traditional preoperative care in patients undergoing colonic surgery is underrepresented in conventional hemodynamic monitoring. *International Journal of Colorectal Disease, 21*(7), 693–697.

Kampmeier, T., Rehberg, S., & Ertmer, C. (2014). Evolution of fluid therapy. *Best Practice & Research Clinical Anaesthesiology, 28*(3), 207–216.

Keren, H., Burkhoff, D., & Squara, P. (2007). Evaluation of a noninvasive continuous cardiac output monitoring system based on thoracic bioreactance. *Heart and Circulatory Physiology, 293*(1), H583–H589. http://dx.doi.org/10.1152/ajpheart.00195.2007

Kudsk, K. A. (2003). Evidence for conservative fluid administration following elective surgery. *Annals of Surgery, 238*(5), 649–650. http://dx.doi.org/10.1097/01.sla.0000094389.57819.82

Lamke, L. O., Nilsson, G. E., & Reithner, H. L. (1977). Water loss by evaporation from the abdominal cavity during surgery. *Acta Chirurgica Scandinavica, 143*, 279–284.

Larsen, T. R., Singh, G., Velocci, V., Nasser, M., & McCullough, P. A. (2016). Frequency of fluid overload and usefulness of bioimpedance in patients requiring intensive care for sepsis syndromes. *Proceedings (Baylor University. Medical Center), 29*(1), 12–15.

Legrand, G., Ruscio, L., Benhamou, D., & Pelletier-Fleury, N. (2015). Goal-directed fluid therapy guided by cardiac monitoring during high-risk abdominal surgery in adult patients: Cost-effectiveness analysis of esophageal doppler and arterial pulse pressure waveform analysis. *Value Health, 18*(5), 605–613. http://dx.doi.org/10.1016/j.jval.2015.04.005

Lilot, M., Ehrenfeld, J. M., Lee, C., Harrington, B., Cannesson, M., & Rinehart, J. (2015). Variability in practice and factors predictive of total crystalloid administration during abdominal surgery: Retrospective two-centre analysis. *British Journal of Anaesthesia, 114*(5), 767–776. http://dx.doi.org/10.1093/bja/aeu452

Lobo, D. N., Macafee, D. A., & Allison, S. P. (2006). How perioperative fluid balance influences postoperative outcomes. *Best Practice & Research. Clinical Anaesthesiology, 20*(3), 439–455.

Lopes, M. R., Oliveira, M. A., Pereira, V. O. S., Lemos, I. P. B., Auler, J. O. C., & Michard, F. (2007). Goal-directed fluid management based on pulse pressure variation monitoring during high-risk surgery: A pilot randomized controlled trial. *Critical Care Medicine, 11*(5), R100.

Lowell, J. A., Schifferdecker, C., Driscoll, D. F., Benotti, P. N., & Bistrian, B. R. (1990). Postoperative fluid overload: Not a benign problem. *Critical Care Medicine, 18*(7), 728–733.

Mayer, J., Boldt, J., Mengistu, A. M., Röhm, K. D., & Suttner, S. (2010). Goal-directed intraoperative therapy based on autocalibrated arterial pressure waveform analysis reduces hospital stay in high-risk surgical patients: A randomized, controlled trial. *Critical Care, 14*(1), R18.

Menon, V., Slater, J. N., White, H. D., Sleeper, L. A., Cocke, T., & Hochman, J. S. (2000). Acute myocardial infarction complicated by systemic hypoperfusion without hypotension: Report of the SHOCK trial registry. *The American Journal of Medicine, 108*(5), 374–380.

Minto, G., & Mythen, M. G. (2015). Perioperative fluid management: Science, art or random chaos? *British Journal of Anaesthesia, 114*(5), 717–721. http://dx.doi.org/10.1093/bja/aev067

Muller, L., Briere, M., Bastide, S., Roger, C., Zoric, L., Seni, G., et al. (2014). Preoperative fasting does not affect haemodynamic status: A prospective, non-inferiority, echocardiography study. *British Journal of Anaesthesia, 112*(5), 835–841.

Mythen, M. G., & Webb, A. R. (1994). The role of gut mucosal hypoperfusion in the pathogenesis of post-operative organ dysfunction. *Intensive care medicine, 20*(3), 203–209.

Navarro, L. H. C., Bloomstone, J. A., Auler, J. O. C., Cannesson, M., Rocca, G. D., Gan, T. J., et al. (2015). Perioperative fluid therapy: A statement from the international Fluid Optimization Group. *Perioperative Medicine, 4*(1), 1–20. http://dx.doi.org/10.1186/s13741-015-0014-z

Nilsson, L. M. (2013). Respiration signals from photoplethysmography. *Anesthesia & Analgesia, 117*(4), 859–865. http://dx.doi.org/10.1213/ane.0b013e31828098b2

Noblett, S. E., Snowden, C. P., Shenton, B. K., & Horgan, A. F. (2006). Randomized clinical trial assessing the effect of Doppler-optimized fluid management on outcome after elective colorectal resection. *British Journal of Surgery, 93*(9), 1069–1076.

Partridge, B. L. (1987). Use of pulse oximetry as a noninvasive indicator of intravascular volume status. *Journal of Clinical Monitoring, 3*(4), 263–268.

Pestana, D., Espinosa, E., Eden, A., Najera, D., Collar, L., Aldecoa, C., et al. (2014). Perioperative goal-directed hemodynamic optimization using noninvasive cardiac output monitoring in major abdominal surgery: A prospective, randomized, multicenter, pragmatic trial: POEMAS Study (PeriOperative goal-directed thErapy in Major Abdominal Surgery). *Anesthesia & Analgesia, 119*(3), 579–587. http://dx.doi.org/10.1213/ane.0000000000000295

Pillai, P., McEleavy, I., Gaughan, M., Snowden, C., Nesbitt, I., Durkan, G., et al. (2011). A double-blind randomized controlled clinical trial to assess the effect of Doppler optimized intraoperative fluid management on outcome following radical cystectomy. *The Journal of Urology, 186*(6), 2201–2206. http://dx.doi.org/10.1016/j.juro.2011.07.093

Ripolles-Melchor, J., Espinosa, A., Martinez-Hurtado, E., Abad-Gurumeta, A., Casans-Frances, R., Fernandez-Perez, C., et al. (2016). Perioperative goal-directed hemodynamic therapy in noncardiac surgery: A systematic review and meta-analysis. *Journal of Clinical Anesthesia, 28*, 105–115. http://dx.doi.org/10.1016/j.jclinane.2015.08.004

Rollins, K. E., & Lobo, D. N. (2016). Intraoperative goal-directed fluid therapy in elective major abdominal surgery: A meta-analysis of randomized controlled trials. *Annals of Surgery, 263*(3), 465–476. http://dx.doi.org/10.1097/sla.0000000000001366

Shires, G. T. (1968). Fluid and electrolyte needs at operation. *South African Medical Journal, 42*(33), 867–872.

Shires, T., Williams, J., & Brown, F. (1961). Acute change in extracellular fluids associated with major surgical procedures. *Annals of Surgery, 154*, 803–810.

Silva, J. M, Jr., de Oliveira, A. M., Nogueira, F. A., Vianna, P. M., Pereira Filho, M. C., Dias, L. F., et. al. (2013). The effect of excess fluid balance on the mortality rate of surgical patients: A multicenter prospective study. *Critical Care, 17*(6), R288. http://dx.doi.org/10.1186/cc13151

Sinclair, S., James, S., & Singer, M. (1997). Intraoperative intravascular volume optimization and length of hospital stay after repair of proximal femoral fracture: Randomized controlled trial. *British Medical Journal, 315*(7113), 909–912.

Sinert, R., & Spektor, M. (2005). Evidence-based emergency medicine/rational clinical examination abstract. Clinical assessment of hypovolemia. *Annals of Emergency Medicine, 45*(3), 327–329.

Strunden, M. S., Heckel, K., Goetz, A. E., & Reuter, D. A. (2011). Perioperative fluid and volume management: Physiological basis, tools and strategies. *Annals of Intensive Care, 1*(1), 2. http://dx.doi.org/10.1186/2110-5820-1-2

Thiele, R. H., Bartels, K., & Gan, T. J. (2015). Inter-device differences in monitoring for goal-directed fluid therapy. *Canadian Journal of Anesthesia, 62*(2), 169–181. http://dx.doi.org/10.1007/s12630-014-0265-z

Van der Linden, P. J., Dierick, A., Wilmin, S., Bellens, B., & Hert, S. G. (2010). A randomized controlled trial comparing an intraoperative goal-directed strategy with routine clinical practice in patients undergoing peripheral arterial surgery. *European Journal of Anaesthesiology, 27*(9), 788–793.

van Haren, F., & Zacharowski, K. (2014). What's new in volume therapy in the intensive care unit? *Best Practice & Research Clinical Anaesthesiology, 28*(3), 275–283. http://dx.doi.org/10.1016/j.bpa.2014.06.004

Veenstra, G., Ince, C., & Boerma, E. C. (2014). Direct markers of organ perfusion to guide fluid therapy: When to start, when to stop. *Best Practice & Research Clinical Anaesthesiology, 28*(3), 217–226. http://dx.doi.org/10.1016/j.bpa.2014.06.002

Venn, R., Steele, A., Richardson, P., Poloniecki, J., Grounds, M., & Newman, P. (2002). Randomized controlled trial to investigate influence of the fluid challenge on duration of hospital stay and perioperative morbidity in patients with hip fractures. *British Journal of Anaesthesia, 88*(1), 65–71.

Voldby, A. W., & Brandstrup, B. (2016). Fluid therapy in the perioperative setting—a clinical review. *Journal of Intensive Care, 4*(27). http://dx.doi.org/10.1186/s40560-016-0154-3

Wakeling, H. G., McFall, M. R., Jenkins, C. S., Woods, W. G., Miles, W. F., & Barclay, G. R. (2005). Intraoperative oesophageal Doppler guided fluid management shortens postoperative hospital stay after major bowel surgery. *British Journal of Anaesthesia, 95*(5), 634–642.

Waldron, N. H., Miller, T. E., Thacker, J. K., Manchester, A. K., White, W. D., Nardiello, J., et al. (2014). A prospective comparison of a noninvasive cardiac output monitor versus esophageal Doppler monitor for goal-directed fluid therapy in colorectal surgery patients. *Anesthesia & Analgesia, 118*(5), 966–975. http://dx.doi.org/10.1213/ane.0000000000000182

CHAPTER 13

The Role of Pharmacogenomics in Anesthesia Pharmacology

Brett Morgan, Edwin N. Aroke, and Jennifer Dungan

ABSTRACT

The field of pharmacogenomics seeks to identify the impact of genetic variants on drug dosing, response, metabolism, and safety outcomes. The narrow therapeutic indices for anesthesia drugs, variability of patient responses to anesthesia, and the risks associated with surgery make anesthetics and the perioperative period prime targets for pharmacogenetic research. Anesthesia providers strive to optimize anesthesia delivery and patient outcomes and to specifically reduce anesthesia-related risks and negative outcomes. Despite pharmacogenomics emerging from the field of anesthesia, the most significant advances to date in the understanding and application of genetics to pharmacology have occurred outside of anesthesiology. This chapter provides an overview of genetic concepts fundamental to understanding the pharmacogenetics of anesthesia practice and presents the current state of the science with respect to the genetic influence on the response to volatile and intravenous anesthetic agents and opioid receptor agonists commonly used in anesthesia practice. In addition, the chapter delineates U.S. Food and Drug Administration labeling tenets for pharmacogenetics, discusses clinical implications of pharmacogenomics for family members, and highlights the potential for future paradigm shifts in pharmacogenomics of anesthesia practice.

http://dx.doi.org/10.1891/0739-6686.35.241

INTRODUCTION

Ever since nurses began administering anesthesia, there has been significant interest in why patients respond so differently to drugs administered during the perioperative period. For many years, clinicians attributed differing responses to factors such as patient weight, co-morbidities, gender, and the type of surgical procedure being performed (Ama et al., 2010). While these factors do affect a patient's reaction to a drug, in recent years, significant work has been done to identify relationships between certain genetic variants and the way patients respond to various drugs. It is now well appreciated that genetic factors play a significant role in these differing responses (Chidambaran, Ngamprasertwong, Vinks, & Sadhasivam, 2012).

Anesthesia providers, such as nurse anesthetists, strive to deliver safe, high-quality care to patients undergoing surgical and diagnostic procedures. Within the specialty of anesthesiology, much attention has been focused on preventing adverse effects and optimizing therapeutic outcomes of pharmacologic interventions. In part, because anesthesia drugs have narrow therapeutic indices, and also because patients respond so differently to those drugs and surgery, the perioperative period carries an especially high risk for adverse reactions or subtherapeutic drug responses. By having a better understanding of the genetic influence on drug pharmacokinetic and dynamic variability, anesthesia providers would be better equipped to manage increasingly challenging patient populations. The field of pharmacogenomics seeks to identify the impact of genetic variation associated with variation in drug response and metabolism. The purpose of this chapter is to present pharmacogenomic principles and current evidence germane to contemporary issues in anesthesiology and perioperative nursing.

OVERVIEW OF GENETIC PRINCIPALS

Pharmacogenomics is the study of genomic variation that influences individual responses to drugs (American Medical Association, 2016). Three main clinical goals of pharmacogenomics are to maximize drug efficacy, select responsive patients, and avoid adverse drug reactions. Genetics may account for 20% to 95% of variability in drug disposition and effects, and for about 50% of adverse drug reactions (Chidambaran et al., 2012). Pharmacologic processes influenced by genetic factors involve: (a) interactions with drug targets to produce cellular effects and (b) drug disposition through effects on metabolizing enzymes, transporters, and receptors. Each of these processes can be affected by genetic variation.

DNA is housed within the nucleus of each cell and directs processes of homeostasis through its code. The code is made up of four types of nucleotides, also known as base pairs: adenine (A), cytosine (G), guanine (G), and thymine (T). The double-stranded DNA is bound together by phosphodiester bonds between adenine and thymine, as well as between cytosine and guanine. Segments of the nucleotide code constitute "genes" that encode for the production of specific proteins. Through a process called transcription, the double-stranded DNA divides into two single strands of messenger ribonucleic acid (mRNA) from which copies are made. The mRNA code is then "read" (or, transcribed) as triplet base pairs called codons, which code for individual amino acids that are strung together during the process of translation to form polypeptides, the building blocks of proteins. For example, the nucleotide codon "CGA" produces the single amino acid arginine, and additional amino acids are added based on the next series of codons, ending with a specific "stop codon" of either TAA, TAG, or TGA. Segments of nucleotides constitute genes and a series of genes are packaged together into a chromosome. Single chromosomes are inherited from each parent.

Variation in the genetic code is common, and can lead to disease or negative outcomes. Humans share about 99.5% similarity in their genetic code from one person to the next. The typical, more frequent version of genetic code is referred to as the "wild-type allele," while the less common version is the "variant allele." Among humans, roughly one nucleotide differs for every 1,000 bases (about 3 million differences among approximately 3 billion total nucleotides). Some of these differences are inherited, some are due to errors during meiosis and mitosis, and some occur when DNA is exposed to chemicals, radiation, or other teratogens. Genetic variations can be causative for disease (mutations) or can influence risk for disease (polymorphisms). While there are some exceptions, causative mutations almost always lead to significant protein alterations that result in disease or other negative outcomes. Polymorphisms can increase risk (sometimes through known protein alterations), but can also confer decreased risk or have no effect at all. Mutations tend to be rarer in the population (less than 1% frequency) and polymorphisms represent common variation.

The most notable genomic variation in pharmacogenomics is the single nucleotide polymorphism (SNP; pronounced "snip," and are cataloged by an "rs number"; e.g., rs123456) in the National Center for Biotechnology Information (NCBI) database of SNPs. SNPs are a single base pair change that occurs in the code, where the "wild-type" nucleotide is replaced by a less common nucleotide at that position. Building on our previous example, if the "G" nucleotide in codon "C**G**A" were replaced by an "A" at base pair position 224 in the code, the triplet codon would become "C**A**A," which would encode for glutamine instead of arginine at a certain amino acid position (such as position 60 in the amino acid strand). This SNP would be written as either C224A, 224C > A, or 224C/A, and the protein change would be written as Arg60Glx or R60Z, as arginine is represented by the letter R and glutamine by the letter Z in amino acid nomenclature. Because the "A" is present in about 10% of people in the population, this is known as a SNP (rather than a mutation), even though it results in a protein change. It may influence risk predisposition, but not always.

In pharmacogenomics, a different nomenclature is often used to denote SNPs. Often, an asterisk followed by a number is used to denote the genetic variant, with *1 representing the wild-type (common) variant for which other variants at that genetic location (*2,*3,*4, etc.) are compared. One reason for this naming convention is that it allows for a combination of different alleles within the same gene to be combined, so they can be examined at the same time in comparison to the wild-type allele. Aroke and Dungan provide a detailed example of this naming convention relevant to anesthetic agents:

> *CYP2B6*6* identifies the allelic variant due to *785A>G (rs2279343)* and *516G>T (rs3745274)* SNPs in the cytochrome P450, 2B6 subtype (*CYP 2B6*) gene. Given the importance of the cytochrome P450 enzymes (CYP) in drug metabolism, their nomenclature warrants close attention (Dungan & Aroke, 2016). As shown in represented in Figure 13.1, the nomenclature for the CYP super family of enzymes is broken down into indicates family, subfamily, isoenzyme, and allelic variants.

In short, variations in the genome can lead to variation in pharmacokinetics and pharmacodynamics of drugs, which may have consequences for drug efficacy, dosing, and likelihood of adverse effects. A review of gene associations with contemporary anesthetic agents (volatile and intravenous anesthetics and opioid receptor agonists) is summarized in what follows.

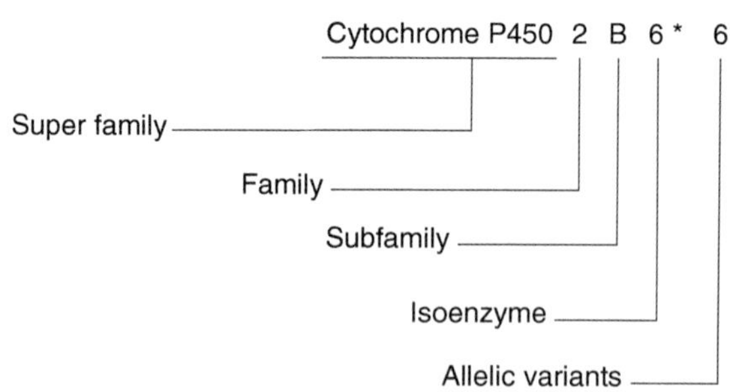

FIGURE 13.1 Nomenclature of the cytochrome P450.
Source: Bukaveckas, Valdes, and Linder (2004). Reprinted with permission.

VOLATILE ANESTHETIC AGENTS

Volatile anesthetics such as isoflurane, sevoflurane, and desflurane are delivered via inhalation to the lungs, subsequently taken up in the bloodstream and delivered to the central nervous system (CNS). It is in the CNS that they exert their effects either by suppressing excitatory neurotransmitters such as acetylcholine or by potentiating inhibitory neurotransmitters such as gamma-amino butyric acid (GABA) at GABA receptors. Thus, genes encoding for neurotransmitters may be potential "candidate genes" (a priori identified genes of interest) for pharmacogenomic investigation of volatile anesthetics. While about 95% of volatile anesthetics are excreted unchanged in the lungs, possible candidate genes of interest are those encoding cytochrome P450 enzymes. One strong candidate gene is *CYP 2E1*, which encodes for the primary isoenzyme (one of a number of specific forms of enzyme with variation in structure and properties), which metabolizes the remaining 5% of these agents (Kharasch et al., 1995; Kharasch, Hankins, Jubert, Thummel, & Taraday, 1999).

Genetic association studies of volatile anesthetics are limited to the past two decades, and while much attention has been paid to *CYP 2E1*, no significant genetic associations have been reported with polymorphisms of this gene and volatile agents. Others have looked at variation in the gene encoding human endogenous glutathione S-transferases (GSTs) that are responsible for phase II metabolism of many drugs. The link between genetic variation in glutathione S-transferase pi (*GSTP1*) gene polymorphism and increases in serum gamma glutamyl transferase (gamma-GST) enzyme protein level with exposure to sevoflurane has been established (Kaymak, Karahalil, Ozcan, & Oztuna, 2008). Genetic variability in the GST enzyme has been associated with alteration in hepatocyte integrity. Therefore, one group of investigators examined the relationship between *GSTP1* polymorphisms and hepatocellular integrity, as measured by alpha-GST in sevoflurane-exposed patients. Heterozygous carriers of the *GSTP1* Ile105Val polymorphism had greater hepatocellular injury (via increased alpha-GST) compared to homozygous wild-type carriers, just 24 hours after exposure to the anesthetic (Kaymak et al., 2008). Another pharmacogenetic study of sevoflurane administration reported lack of association between GABAAγ2 protein receptor polymorphism (known to affect receptor function) and the incidence and severity of emergence agitation in 5,000 Korean children (Park, Park, Kim, Kang, & Lee, 2008). A small study comparing 10 women with red hair to 10 women with black or brown hair revealed that an increased minimum alveolar concentration of desflurane was required to prevent response to noxious electrical stimuli in females with red hair who harbored certain polymorphisms of the melanocortin 1 receptor (*MC1R*) gene that encodes for red hair color (Liem et al., 2004).

INTRAVENOUS ANESTHETIC AGENTS

The cytochrome P450 (CYP P45) enzymes are responsible for the extensive metabolism of intravenous anesthetics, which include: propofol, ketamine, etomidate, thiopental, and methohexital. The metabolites of these agents are then excreted by the kidneys. Two main candidate genes persist in the pharmacogenomics study of intravenous anesthetics: *CYP 2B6* and uridine diphosphate glucuronosyltransferase (*UGT*) gene *UGT 1A9*. A majority of studies evaluate exposure to propofol and ketamine. While *CYP 2C9* and *CYP 3A4* are biologically plausible candidate genes, limited evidence exists for their association with intravenous anesthetics.

CYP 2B6 variants have been associated with variation in metabolism of both propofol and ketamine. This is no surprise, as the CYP 2B6 enzyme is the primary isoenzyme responsible for the hydroxylation of propofol and N-demethylation of ketamine; thus, enzymes coded by the *CYP2B6* gene catalyze the oxidation (phase I metabolism) of propofol and ketamine (Aroke & Dungan, 2016). In particular, *CYP 2B6* genetic variation is responsible for the interindividual variability in propofol metabolism (Court, Duan, Hesse, Venkatakrishnan, & Greenblatt, 2001; Iohom et al., 2007; Takahashi et al., 2008) even though the drug is primarily metabolized via glucuronidation by *UGT1A9,* which is discussed later in the chapter. Genes that code for the CYP 2B6 enzyme are highly polymorphic, meaning a great deal of genetic variation exists within the gene, and among populations. The *CYP2B6*4* allele is associated with increased expression and enzyme activity, while the *CYP2B6*6* allele is associated with loss of function and lower expression of functional mRNA.

Individuals with the *CYP 2B6**6 variant (correlating to coding SNP, c.516G > T) had high plasma concentrations of propofol and experienced delayed (increased) wakening time and risk of adverse reactions compared to those without the *6 gene variant (Kansaku et al., 2011). The same investigation found no association with propofol concentrations and outcomes and genetic variation in *CYP2B6* SNP, *c.G516T,* or *UGT1A9* SNP, 1366C > T (Kansaku et al., 2011). Sex differences in propofol response have prompted pharmacogenomic research. Given that women typically require higher doses of propofol for induction and recover more quickly than men (Choong et al., 2013; Loryan et al., 2012), a group of researchers explored association of CYP 2B6 SNPs and propofol concentration in women. They revealed that women with the T allele of *CYP 2B6* c.516G>T had greater plasma concentrations of propofol compared to G carriers ($p = .027$), utilizing a highly sensitive measure of propofol concentration to strengthen the internal validity of the study (Mastrogianni et al., 2014). This study was preliminary in nature and the finding inconsistent with other studies (Mastrogianni et al., 2014); however, future research may lead to better understanding of whether there may be a relationship between the *CYP2B6* c.516T allele and speculatively greater propofol protein binding or more rapid distribution in women.

CYP 2B6 is equally important in ketamine metabolism, as it is primarily responsible for N-demethylation into norketamine at clinically relevant plasma levels, with secondary involvement of CYP3A4 and CYP2C9 (Yanagihara et al., 2001). When ketamine achieves higher plasma concentrations, CYP3A4 takes over as the primary metabolic isoenzyme with some contribution from CYP2B6 and CYP2C9 (Hijazi & Boulieu, 2002). Such variability in this process has received interest with respect to pharmacokinetic associations with the corresponding genes CYP 2B6, CYP 3A4, and CYP 2C9. The *CYP2B6**6* allele significantly altered ketamine metabolism in a recent in vitro study (Li et al., 2013). The same investigators then performed an in vivo study that demonstrated a higher median steady state plasma level and lower plasma clearance of ketamine and norketamine in CYP2B6*6/*6 (those having two copies of the *6 allele) compared to those with only one *6 allele or *1 wild-type carriers (Li et al., 2015). In addition, investigators reported that decreased plasma clearance of ketamine was associated with an increase in drowsiness, thereby implying a relationship between *6/*6 genotype, ketamine metabolism, and ketamine-related drowsiness (Li et al., 2015).

As previously noted, enzymes coded by the *UGT* gene are responsible for glucuronidation (phase II metabolism) of propofol. Variations in the *UGT1A9* gene that encodes for the enzyme catalyst, UDP-glucuronosyltransferase, have been shown to significantly affect propofol metabolism (Takahashi et al., 2008). The *UGT1A9* 726G/G variant was associated with a loss of UGT 1A9 activity (Saeki et al., 2003), which could theoretically affect metabolism. Another SNP in UGT1A, D256N decreased propofol glucuronidation (Takahashi et al., 2008). A pilot study found no association between observed sex differences in propofol glucuronidation and *UGT1A9* gene expression (Loryan et al., 2012), with negative association confirmed in a later replication by the same group (Choong et al., 2013). Significantly higher induction doses were required of patients who were homozygous with the *UGT1A9*-188T/G variant, and higher propofol clearance was observed in those heterozygous for *UGT1A9*-188T/C compared to other genetic variants in *UGT 1A9*, *CYP 2B6*, or *GABRE* (Khan et al., 2014). A haplotype investigation (study evaluating the combined effect of specific combinations of genetic alleles) of *GABRE* that encodes the GABA receptor examined combinations of alleles inherited together among four different *GABRE* variants (mRNA358G/T, 20118C/T, 20502A/T, and 20326C/T) and found no significant associations between the haplotypes and induction time with propofol among 150 White patients (Iohom et al., 2007).

OPIOID RECEPTOR AGONISTS

Opioid administration remains a mainstay treatment for acute perioperative pain; however, there is significant interindividual variability that exists in patient sensitivity to both the analgesic effects of the medications and adverse effects such a nausea, vomiting, and respiratory depression. Polymorphisms that affect opioid therapy include those found in metabolizing enzymes, opioid receptors, transporters, and structures that impact perception and processing of afferent nociception (Stoelting & Hillier, 2006). For the purposes of this review, genetic influences on receptor efficacy, metabolism, and dosing will be described as they relate to the most common genes affecting anesthesia practice and perioperative nursing.

Mu-Opioid Receptor Gene

Morphine is the prototype in the class of drugs known as opioids. The clinical effects of morphine are predominately caused by interactions that occur at the mu-opioid receptor, and polymorphisms that occur in the mu-opioid receptor gene (*OPRM1*) are associated with a change in efficacy of the receptor. Studies have identified that the haplotype of *OPRM1* includes greater than 100 polymorphisms. Of those 100, only 6 are clinically relevant to the analgesic effect of the receptor (Gong et al., 2013). The most commonly studied SNP is 118A > G (aka, A118G), which leads to a substitution of asparagine for aspartate at position 40 on *OPRM1* (Skorpen et al., 2016). Ren and colleagues conducted a meta-analysis of 13 studies to investigate the relationship between A118G and opioid consumption following surgery (Ren et al., 2015). They found that during the first 24 hours following surgery, 118G allele carriers required more opioids to control their pain compared to AA homozygotes, indicating a greater consumption of opioid pain medications. In addition to typical A118G mutations, case reports have identified instances of complete knockout of the mu-opioid receptor, rendering patients completely or significantly nonresponsive to opioid therapy (Skorpen et al., 2016). In addition to surgical pain, A118G is associated with an increased requirement for opioids in treating other types of pain. Gong and colleagues implicated A118G in influencing opioid requirement variability in patients experiencing cancer-related pain, citing it as a key variable in interindividual variability in pain control (Gong et al., 2013).

Cytochrome P450 2D6 Gene

In addition to changes in receptor efficacy, some genetic variants affect drug metabolism, which in turn has implications for dosing and side effects. The cytochrome P450 (CYP) 2D6 produces the hepatic drug-metabolizing enzyme CYP2D6. There is great variability in expression of the *CYP2D6* gene, with some patients having more than one copy of functional *CYP2D6* alleles and some having two nonfunctional alleles. Based on the functionality of their alleles, patients can be characterized as ultra-metabolizers, extensive metabolizers, intermediate metabolizers, or poor metabolizers. Codeine is metabolized by *CYP2D6* to morphine, which ultimately interacts with MORs to produce analgesia (Kelly et al., 2012). Pharmacokinetic studies have shown that patients identified as *CYP2D6* poor metabolizers have decreased morphine levels and higher pain scores compared to patients following the administration of codeine, as compared to patients who are nonpoor metabolizers. The opposite is true for ultra-metabolizers, who show increased conversion of codeine to morphine, ultimately leading to toxicity (Crews et al., 2012). In 2013, three children died after receiving "normal" doses of codeine following routine tonsillectomy surgeries (Kelly, 2013). These deaths were attributed to respiratory depression associated with toxic levels of morphine resulting from ultra-metabolism of codeine. As a result, the Clinical Pharmacogenetics Implementation Consortium (CPIC) Guidelines for *CYP P450 D6* Genotype and Codeine Therapy were developed (Crews et al., 2012; U.S. Food and Drug Administration [FDA], 2016) and updated (Crews et al., 2014; Table 13.1). In addition to codeine, genetic polymorphisms affecting CYP2D6 activity have been investigated for methadone (Kharasch, Regina, Blood, & Friedel, 2015), oxycodone, tramadol, and hydrocodone (Lotsch & Geisslinger, 2006). For each of these drugs, altered function of CYP2D6 affected postadministration plasma concentrations similar to that of codeine.

P-glycoprotein Transporter ABCB1

P-glycoprotein ABCB1 (ABCB1) is a transporter protein located at the blood–brain barrier that is responsible for morphine transport into the brain, and polymorphisms of *ABCB1* have been associated with varying CNS levels of morphine (Kesimci, Engin, Kanbak, & Karahalil, 2012). In a study investigating the effect of polymorphism of *ABCB1* in children undergoing tonsillectomy surgery, children with GG and GA genotypes of SNP rs9282564 demonstrated a higher risk of developing respiratory depression following surgery (Sadhasivam et al., 2015). Adding one copy of the minor allele (G) led to a 4.7-fold increase in the incidence of prolonged hospital stay due to postoperative respiratory depression (Sadhasivam et al., 2015). A study conducted on adults also noted that *ABCB1* mutations were associated with increased respiratory depression after receiving fentanyl for postoperative pain (Oertel & Lotsch, 2008). Interestingly, a meta-analysis of a total of 11 studies failed to demonstrate significant differences in opioid consumption for analgesia between patients with wild-type *ABCB1* and mutation carriers (Ren et al., 2015).

TABLE 13.1

Drug Metabolism Categories With Codeine Example

Category	Pharmacokinetic Response	Genotypes	Examples of *CYP2D6* Diplotypes	Implications for Codeine Metabolism	Recommendations for Codeine Therapy
Ultra-rapid metabolizer (UM)	Enzymes process the drug in a highly efficient manner	An individual carrying more than two copies of functional alleles	*1/*1xN *1/*2xN	Increased formation of morphine following codeine administration, leading to higher risk of toxicity	Avoid codeine use due to potential for toxicity
Extensive metabolizers (EM)	Normal/typical rate of enzyme activity to process the drug	An individual carrying two alleles encoding full or reduced function or one full function allele together with either one nonfunctional or one reduced-function allele	*1/*1, *1/*2, *2/*2, *1/*41, *1/*4, *2/*5, *10/*10	Normal morphine formation	Use label recommended age- or weight-specific dosing

Intermediate metabolizers (IM)	Decreased (but not poor) enzyme activity for processing the drug	An individual carrying one reduced and one nonfunctional allele	*4/*10, *5/*41	Reduced morphine formation	Use label recommended age- or weight-specific dosing. If no response, consider alternative analgesics such as morphine or a nonopioid
Poor metabolizers (PM)	Enzymes processes the drug poorly, at a very slow rate	An individual carrying no functional alleles	*4/*4, *4/*5, *5/*5, *4/*6	Greatly reduced morphine formation following codeine administration, leading to insufficient pain relief	Avoid codeine use due to lack of efficacy

Adapted and used with permission from PharmGKB (2016b) and Crews et al. (2014).

CLINICAL IMPLICATIONS OF PHARMACOGENETIC FDA LABELS

Health care providers need to be up to date on the FDA-approved labels for drugs with pharmacogenetic associations (FDA, 2015) and the implications for clinical practice. Where pharmacogenetic associations are established in the research literature, the FDA has a role in the evaluation of evidence and oversight of clinical application regarding pharmacologic prescribing. Currently there are no volatile or intravenous anesthetic agents with FDA-approved pharmacogenetic labels; however, it is important for anesthesia providers to understand the four FDA-approved drug labels relevant to pharmacogenomics for two reasons: (a) non-anesthetic drugs that are used within anesthesia practice (such as codeine) have pharmacogenomic FDA-approved labels and (b) future scientific evidence could result in anesthetics achieving such labels.

The first is an FDA-approved "Genetic Testing Required" label, which indicates that genetic testing is required prior to initiation of pharmacologic therapy to determine whether the drug is appropriate (efficacious) for the patient (PharmGKB, 2016a). The "Recommended" FDA-approved label indicates that genetic testing is recommended prior to initiation of therapy (PharmGKB, 2016a), and sometimes in the context of only a certain subset of patients for whom the evidence is applicable (such as among population ethnicities). An "Actionable PGx" (pharmacogenomics) label indicates changes in efficacy, dosage, or toxicity due to certain genetic variants among subgroups of patients in the population, but does not require or recommend genetic testing for the recommended prescribing or doses (PharmGKB, 2016a). The last FDA-approved label is deemed "Informative PGx," and is used to indicate that genetic variation is associated with the drug's metabolism or pharmacodynamics but does not result in different patient responses (PharmGKB, 2016a). The FDA publishes a curated table of Pharmacogenomic Biomarkers in Drug Labeling online (FDA, 2015).

CLINICAL IMPLICATIONS OF PHARMACOGENOMICS IN ANESTHESIA: FAMILY MEMBERS

Where genetic risk is of concern, potential impact of genetic risk for relatives of the person being tested (proband) is often of greatest concern. The decisions around screening and notification of family members for potential genetic risk are less complicated when a clear inheritance pattern is established for a genetic variant (e.g., autosomal dominant and recessive transmission from generation to generation). Such inheritance patterns have not been clearly established for pharmacogenetic variants. This is because the numbers of related family members (twins, sibling, or multiple generations) having *well-defined* drug responses are often inadequate for conclusive heritability analyses (Roden, Wilke, Kroemer, & Stein, 2011). Despite the lack of clear heritability information for drug response, certain clinical contexts necessitate implications for family members.

A caveat to pharmacogenomics is that the relevance of genetic risk to families is specific to the context of whether family members are likely to receive the same drug in question. It is assumed that shared genetic and shared environmental factors may increase the likelihood that similar disease processes and the need for similar pharmaceutical management may occur (Mills, Voora, Peyser, & Haga, 2013). While the need for surgery and anesthesia may be much more limited in terms of shared variance among families, significant (and especially serious) anesthetic drug reactions should be documented and the proband should be prompted to consider sharing this information with first-degree family members (parents, siblings). Two specific and rare situations in anesthesia practice impacting family members involve *RYR1* mutations in malignant hyperthermia and *MTHFR* mutations in nitrous oxide toxicity, wherein nitrous oxide should not be delivered to family members of probands with known mutations in these genes (Searle & Hopkins, 2009).

CONCLUSION

As anesthesia providers become more aware of the pharmacogenomic implications to their practice, there could be a movement toward tailoring anesthetic plans toward specific genetic profiles. This type of genetic-guided drug therapy is becoming more sought after as patients have begun to show increasing interest in their genetic profile (Chang, Weitzel, & Schmidt, 2015). Selecting the correct drug, correct dose, and the timing of administration could all be guided by matching a patient's genetic profile to a database of genetic variants known to contribute to drug efficacy, response, and safety. This could potentially lead to better patient outcomes and improved anesthesia safety (Ama et al., 2010). However, there are acknowledged barriers for clinical application of pharmacogenomics in anesthesia practice, namely cost and logistics of receipt of genetic testing results in a timely enough way to be clinically useful in the perioperative setting. Recent trends in preemptive pharmacogenomic testing could cause a paradigm shift in future demand and uptake for personalized anesthesia approaches (Aroke & Dungan, 2016; Dunnenberger et al., 2015). Nurses and nursing educators will need to pay close attention to this emerging field as it will likely have significant implications on future practice.

REFERENCES

Ama, T., Bounmythavong, S., Blaze, J., Weismann, M., Marienau, M. S., & Nicholson, W. T. (2010). Implications of pharmacogenomics for anesthesia providers. *American Association of Nurse Anesthetists Journal, 78*(5), 393–399.

American Medical Association. (2016). *Pharmacogenomics*. Retrieved from http://www.ama-assn.org/ama/pub/physician-resources/medical-science/genetics-molecular-medicine/current-topics/pharmacogenomics.page?

Aroke, E., & Dungan, J. R. (2016). Pharmacogenetics of anesthesia: An integrative review. *Nursing Research, 65*(4), 318–330.

Bukaveckas, B. L., Valdes, R, Jr., & Linder, M. W. (2004). Pharmacogenetics as related to the practice of cardiothoracic and vascular anesthesia. *Journal of Cardiothoracic Vascular Anesthesia, 18*(3), 353–365.

Chang, K. L., Weitzel, K., & Schmidt, S. (2015). Pharmacogenetics: Using genetic information to guide drug therapy. *American Family Physician, 92*(7), 588–594.

Chidambaran, V., Ngamprasertwong, P., Vinks, A. A., & Sadhasivam, S. (2012). Pharmacogenetics and anesthetic drugs. *Current Clinical Pharmacology, 7*(2), 78–101.

Choong, E., Loryan, I., Lindqvist, M., Nordling, A., el Bouazzaoui, S., van Schaik, R. H., et al. (2013). Sex difference in formation of propofol metabolites: A replication study. *Basic and Clinical Pharmacology Toxicology, 113*(2), 126–131. http://dx.doi.org/10.1111/bcpt.12070

Court, M. H., Duan, S. X., Hesse, L. M., Venkatakrishnan, K., & Greenblatt, D. J. (2001). Cytochrome P-450 2B6 is responsible for interindividual variability of propofol hydroxylation by human liver microsomes. *Anesthesiology, 94*(1), 110–119.

Crews, K. R., Gaedigk, A., Dunnenberger, H. M., Klein, T. E., Shen, D. D., Callaghan, J. T., et al. (2012). Clinical pharmacogenetics implementation consortium (CPIC) guidelines for codeine therapy in the context of cytochrome P450 2D6 (CYP2D6) genotype. *Clinical Pharmacology and Therapeutics, 91*(2), 321–326. http://dx.doi.org/10.1038/clpt.2011.287

Crews, K. R., Gaedigk, A., Dunnenberger, H. M., Leeder, J. S., Klein, T. E., Caudle, K. E., et al. (2014). Clinical Pharmacogenetics Implementation consortium guidelines for cytochrome P450 2D6 genotype and codeine therapy: 2014 update. *Clinical Pharmacology and Therapeutics, 95*(4), 376–382. http://dx.doi.org/10.1038/clpt.2013.254

Dunnenberger, H. M., Crews, K. R., Hoffman, J. M., Caudle, K. E., Broeckel, U., Howard, S. C., et al. (2015). Preemptive clinical pharmacogenetics implementation: Current programs in five US medical centers. *Annual Review of Pharmacology Toxicology, 55*, 89–106. http://dx.doi.org/10.1146/annurev-pharmtox-010814-124835

Gong, X. D., Wang, J. Y., Liu, F., Yuan, H. H., Zhang, W. Y., Guo, Y. H., et al. (2013). Gene polymorphisms of OPRM1 A118G and ABCB1 C3435T may influence opioid requirements in Chinese patients with cancer pain. *Asian Pacific Journal Cancer Prevention, 14*(5), 2937–2943.

Hijazi, Y., & Boulieu, R. (2002). Contribution of CYP3A4, CYP2B6, and CYP2C9 isoforms to N-demethylation of ketamine in human liver microsomes. *Drug Metabolism Disposition, 30*(7), 853–858.

Iohom, G., Ni Chonghaile, M., O'Brien, J. K., Cunningham, A. J., Fitzgerald, D. F., & Shields, D. C. (2007). An investigation of potential genetic determinants of propofol requirements and recovery from anaesthesia. *European Journal Anaesthesiology, 24*(11), 912–919. http://dx.doi.org/10.1017/s0265021507000476

Kansaku, F., Kumai, T., Sasaki, K., Yokozuka, M., Shimizu, M., Tateda, T., et al. (2011). Individual differences in pharmacokinetics and pharmacodynamics of anesthetic agent propofol with regard to CYP2B6 and UGT1A9 genotype and patient age. *Drug Metabolism Pharmacokinetics, 26*(5), 532–537.

Kaymak, C., Karahalil, B., Ozcan, N. N., & Oztuna, D. (2008). Association between GSTP1 gene polymorphism and serum alpha-GST concentrations undergoing sevoflurane anaesthesia. *European Journal Anaesthesiology, 25*(3), 193–199. http://dx.doi.org/10.1017/s0265021507002724

Kelly, L. E., Rieder, M., van den Anker, J., Malkin, B., Ross, C., Neely, M. N., et al. (2012). More codeine fatalities after tonsillectomy in North American children. *Pediatrics, 129*(5), e1343–e1347. http://dx.doi.org/10.1542/peds.2011-2538

Kelly, P. A. (2013). Pharmacogenomics: why standard codeine doses can have serious toxicities or no therapeutic effect. *Oncology Nursing Forum, 40*(4), 322–324. http://dx.doi.org/10.1188/13.onf.322-324

Kesimci, E., Engin, A. B., Kanbak, O., & Karahalil, B. (2012). Association between ABCB1 gene polymorphisms and fentanyl's adverse effects in Turkish patients undergoing spinal anesthesia. *Gene, 493*(2), 273–277. http://dx.doi.org/10.1016/j.gene.2011.11.040

Khan, M. S., Zetterlund, E. L., Green, H., Oscarsson, A., Zackrisson, A. L., Svanborg, E., et al. (2014). Pharmacogenetics, plasma concentrations, clinical signs and EEG during propofol treatment. *Basic and Clinical Pharmacology Toxicology, 115*(6), 565–570. http://dx.doi.org/10.1111/bcpt.12277

Kharasch, E. D., Armstrong, A. S., Gunn, K., Artru, A., Cox, K., & Karol, M. D. (1995). Clinical sevoflurane metabolism and disposition. II. The role of cytochrome P450 2E1 in fluoride and hexafluoroisopropanol formation. *Anesthesiology, 82*(6), 1379–1388.

Kharasch, E. D., Hankins, D. C., Jubert, C., Thummel, K. E., & Taraday, J. K. (1999). Lack of single-dose disulfiram effects on cytochrome P-450 2C9, 2C19, 2D6, and 3A4 activities: Evidence for specificity toward P-450 2E1. *Drug Metabolism Disposition, 27*(6), 717–723.

Kharasch, E. D., Regina, K. J., Blood, J., & Friedel, C. (2015). Methadone pharmacogenetics: CYP2B6 Polymorphisms determine plasma concentrations, clearance, and metabolism. *Anesthesiology, 123*(5), 1142–1153. http://dx.doi.org/10.1097/aln.0000000000000867

Li, Y., Coller, J. K., Hutchinson, M. R., Klein, K., Zanger, U. M., Stanley, N. J., et al. (2013). The CYP2B6*6 allele significantly alters the N-demethylation of ketamine enantiomers in vitro. *Drug Metabolism and Disposition, 41*(6), 1264–1272. http://dx.doi.org/10.1124/dmd.113.051631

Li, Y., Jackson, K. A., Slon, B., Hardy, J. R., Franco, M., William, L., et al. (2015). CYP2B6*6 allele and age substantially reduce steady-state ketamine clearance in chronic pain patients: impact on adverse effects. *British Journal Clinical Pharmacology, 80*(2), 276–284. http://dx.doi.org/10.1111/bcp.12614

Liem, E. B., Lin, C. M., Suleman, M. I., Doufas, A. G., Gregg, R. G., Veauthier, J. M., et al. (2004). Anesthetic requirement is increased in redheads. *Anesthesiology, 101*(2), 279–283.

Loryan, I., Lindqvist, M., Johansson, I., Hiratsuka, M., van der Heiden, I., van Schaik, R. H., et al. (2012). Influence of sex on propofol metabolism, a pilot study: Implications for propofol anesthesia. *European Journal of Clinical Pharmacology, 68*(4), 397–406. http://dx.doi.org/10.1007/s00228-011-1132-2

Lotsch, J., & Geisslinger, G. (2006). Current evidence for a genetic modulation of the response to analgesics. *Pain, 121*(1–2), 1–5. http://dx.doi.org/10.1016/j.pain.2006.01.010

Mastrogianni, O., Gbandi, E., Orphanidis, A., Raikos, N., Goutziomitrou, E., Kolibianakis, E. M., et al. (2014). Association of the CYP2B6 c.516G>T polymorphism with high blood propofol concentrations in women from northern Greece. *Drug Metabolism Pharmacokinetics, 29*(2), 215–218.

Mills, R., Voora, D., Peyser, B., & Haga, S. B. (2013). Delivering pharmacogenetic testing in a primary care setting. *Pharmacogenomics and Personalized Medicine, 6*, 105–112. http://dx.doi.org/10.2147/pgpm.s50598

Oertel, B., & Lotsch, J. (2008). Genetic mutations that prevent pain: Implications for future pain medication. *Pharmacogenomics, 9*(2), 179–194. http://dx.doi.org/10.2217/14622416.9.2.179

Park, C. S., Park, H. J., Kim, K. N., Kang, H. S., & Lee, S. K. (2008). The influence of GABAAγ2 genetic polymorphism on the emergence agitation induced by sevoflurane. *Korean Journal of Anesthesiology, 55*, 139–144. http://dx.doi.org/10.4097/kjae.2008.55.2.139

PharmGKB. (2016a). Drug Label Information and Legend. Retrieved from https://www.pharmgkb.org/page/drugLabelLegend

PharmGKB. (2016b). *Clinical pharmacogenetics implementation consortium (CPIC) guideline information for codeine and CYP2D6 website*. Retrieved June 10, 2016 from https://www.pharmgkb.org/guideline/PA166104996

Ren, Z. Y., Xu, X. Q., Bao, Y. P., He, J., Shi, L., Deng, J. H., et al. (2015). The impact of genetic variation on sensitivity to opioid analgesics in patients with postoperative pain: A systematic review and meta-analysis. *Pain Physician, 18*(2), 131–152.

Roden, D. M., Wilke, R. A., Kroemer, H. K., & Stein, C. M. (2011). Pharmacogenomics: The genetics of variable drug responses. *Circulation, 123*(15), 1661–1670. http://dx.doi.org/10.1161/circulationaha.109.914820

Sadhasivam, S., Chidambaran, V., Zhang, X., Meller, J., Esslinger, H., Zhang, K., et al. (2015). Opioid-induced respiratory depression: ABCB1 transporter pharmacogenetics. *The Pharmacogenomics Journal, 15*(2), 119–126. http://dx.doi.org/10.1038/tpj.2014.56

Saeki, M., Saito, Y., Jinno, H., Sai, K., Komamura, K., Ueno, K., et al. (2003). Three novel single nucleotide polymorphisms in UGT1A9. *Drug Metabolism Pharmacokinetics, 18*(2), 146–149.

Searle, R, & Hopkins, P. M. (2009). Pharmacogenomic variability and anaesthesia. *British Journal of Anesthesia, 103*(1), 14–25. http://dx.doi.org/10.1093/bja/aep130

Skorpen, F., von Hofacker, S., Bjorngaard, M., Skogholt, A. H., Dale, O., Kaasa, S., et al. (2016). The rare Arg181Cys mutation in the mu opioid receptor can abolish opioid responses. *Acta Anaesthesiologica Scandinavica, 60*(8), 1084–1091. http://dx.doi.org/10.1111/aas.12739

Stoelting, R. K, & Hillier, S. C. (2006). *Pharmacology and physiology in anesthetic practice*. Philadelphia, PA: Lippincott Williams & Wilkins.

Takahashi, H., Maruo, Y., Mori, A., Iwai, M., Sato, H., & Takeuchi, Y. (2008). Effect of D256N and Y483D on propofol glucuronidation by human uridine 5'-diphosphate glucuronosyltransferase (UGT1A9). *Basic and Clinical Pharmacology and Toxicology, 103*(2), 131–136. http://dx.doi.org/10.1111/j.1742-7843.2008.00247.x

Yanagihara, Y., Kariya, S., Ohtani, M., Uchino, K., Aoyama, T., Yamamura, Y., et al. (2001). Involvement of CYP2B6 in n-demethylation of ketamine in human liver microsomes. *Drug Metabolism Dispositon, 29*(6), 887–890.

U.S. Food and Drug Administration. (2015). *Pharmacogenomic biomarkers in drug labeling*. Silver Spring, MD: Author. Retrieved from http://www.fda.gov/Drugs/ScienceResearch/ResearchAreas/Pharmacogenetics/ucm083378.htm

U.S. Food and Drug Administration. (2016). *FDA drug safety communication: Safety review update of codeine use in children; New boxed warning and contraindication on use after tonsillectomy and/oradenoidectomy.* Silver Spring, MD: Author. Retrieved from http://www.fda.gov/Drugs/DrugSafety/ucm339112.htm

Index

NOTE: Page references followed by *f* and *t* denote figures and tables, respectively.

www.ingramcontent.com/pod-product-compliance
Ingram Content Group UK Ltd.
Pitfield, Milton Keynes, MK11 3LW, UK
UKHW021845100926
8556IPUK00019B/1056

9 780826 142849